THE COMPLETE HOMEOPATHY HANDBOOK

Miranda Castro was born in London and grew up in a family converted to the benefits of alternative medicine. She trained in iridology, psychotherapy and acupuncture before specialising in homeopathy, and in 1989 she developed her individual practice from a small base to the multi-practitioner Spectrum Clinic in Finsbury Park, London.

She is not married, does not live in Surrey, does not have a degree, does not have two children, and does not work out in her spare time. She lives happily in North London with her son Daniel and their dog Rosie.

THE COMPLETE HOMEOPATHY HANDBOOK

A Guide to Everyday Health Care

Miranda Castro *F.S.Hom.*

PAPERMAC

First published 1990 by
Macmillan London Limited

First published in paperback 1991 by
PAPERMAC
a division of Pan Macmillan Publishers Limited
Cavaye Place London SW10 9PG
and Basingstoke

Associated companies in Auckland, Budapest, Dublin,
Gaborone, Harare, Hong Kong, Kampala, Kuala Lumpur,
Lagos, Madras, Manzini, Melbourne, Mexico City, Nairobi,
New York, Singapore, Sydney, Tokyo and Windhoek

Reprinted 1991, 1992

ISBN 0-333-55581-3

A CIP catalogue record for this book is available from
the British Library.

Illustrations by Liz Pepperell

Typeset by Rowland Phototypesetting Limited
Bury St Edmunds, Suffolk
Printed in Hong Kong

For my son Daniel

CONTENTS

Acknowledgements   ix
Introduction   xi
How To Use This Book   xiii

PART I: History, Principles and Prescribing

1 The History of Homeopathy   *3*
2 Principles and Concepts   *11*
3 Myths and Misapprehensions   *17*
4 Taking the Case   *20*
5 Prescribing   *24*

PART II: The Materia Medicas and Repertories

External Materia Medica and Repertory   *31*
Internal Materia Medica   *38*
Internal Repertory   *165*

PART III: Prescribing Guidelines and Follow-through

Stress as a Cause of Disease   *201*
Diseases You Can Treat Using This Book   *203*
Case-taking Questionnaire and Symptom Checklists   *227*
Repertorising Chart   *230*
Sample Cases   *231*

PART IV: The Appendices

List of Remedies   *246*
Glossary   *247*
First-Aid Kits, Pharmacies and Courses   *249*
Homeopaths and Homeopathic Organisations   *251*
Useful Reading and Bookshops   *252*

Index   254
Last Word   258

ACKNOWLEDGEMENTS

I wish to thank first my author friends who helped me organise the chaos – Robin Shohet and Jane Howard for enabling me actually to sit down and write, and Maggi Sikking and Silvie Turner for their constant support and encouragement.

Sincere thanks to all who helped with this project over the past four years, especially Andree Ryan, Erica Day, Francis Treuherz, Jane Harter, Jenny Haxworth, John Tomlinson, Lynda Ballinger, Mahavir Ball, Mike Strange, Rachel Packer, and Roz Fishel. Also thanks to Liz Pepperell for her delightful drawings.

Special thanks to the team at Macmillan who supported me unstintingly in my struggles as a first-time author . . . especially to Katrina Whone whose patience and sense of humour kept me going when all else failed.

I would like also to express much love for, and appreciation of, my teachers; my parents who sowed the seeds of who and what I am today; J. R. Worsley who helped me dig those seeds into the earth; Terry Cooper and Jenner Roth who helped me find those seeds again and rediscover their worth; all the great homeopathic teachers, both dead and alive, who, both in word and spirit, watered regularly the growing plant; my friends and family who have supported me in all weathers; and my patients who taught me so much and who finally made it possible for this tree of mine to bear fruit. Thank you.

INTRODUCTION

The practice of homeopathy, whether in the consulting room or in the home, is a delight and a challenge. Used carefully and wisely, it is highly effective in curing a wide range of illnesses, from minor health problems to very serious conditions. This book focuses on everyday complaints that you can treat yourself.

I am concerned that people who are using homeopathic medicines should know their potential and use them with respect, especially since they are now sold over the counter in most chemists and health-food shops, with very few guidelines.

In this climate of greater life expectancy and yet increasing ill-health and disillusionment with modern wonder drugs, people are questioning the quality of their health care and looking for safe and effective ways to treat illness as well as to improve their health. Homeopathy offers a safe alternative as it seeks to improve the general level of health of the whole person, emotionally as well as physically, and as such is playing an important role in the movement back to a more holistic approach to health.

I believe that conventional medicines should be used sparingly and that their indiscriminate use for minor ailments is inappropriate. I do not intend to make comparisons between orthodox and alternative medicine in this book; nor do I wish to belittle the work and intentions of orthodox doctors. Nonetheless, many people are undermining their general health by abusing (over-using) antibiotics and other strong medications for trivial complaints. This extended use can lead eventually to resistance to the drugs themselves; to allergies; and, of course, to an eventual breakdown of the immune system. Homeopathy carries none of these risks and in fact boosts the body's vitality.

I anticipate that many users of this book will already have had some experience of homeopathy and the use of homeopathic medicines in the home, and will be familiar with the approach of some of the first-aid guides already obtainable. Many books currently available on first-aid homeopathy oversimplify the 'art' of homeopathic prescribing and have given the false impression that prescribing a homeopathic remedy is simply a matter of looking up, say, 'boils', and giving the one remedy that is listed. This will always be a hit-or-miss affair, with the remedy working for only a percentage of those people who take it.

Homeopathic prescribing is not that simple. This book mimics the way a professional homeopath works. As a homeopath, my tools for prescribing are the Materia Medica and the Repertory. The Materia Medica is simply a full account of the homeopathic remedies and the Repertory is a cross-referenced index of the information presented in the Materia Medica. What I present here is a simplified form of these books where they apply to first-aid prescribing, translated where possible into lay-person's terms.

Within the limitations imposed by the size of this book, the information here will help you to make remedy selection more accurate. This book *also* looks at the principles underlying the theory of homeopathy, as well as at how to prescribe – how to spot the symptoms or signs of disease and how to classify them so that they can be used to find the best remedy. My aim is to help the serious first-aider to use these principles to prescribe successfully, as I introduce you to a whole new way of defining and treating illness.

Miranda Castro
London, 1990

HOW TO USE THIS BOOK

The goal of this book is to enable you to use homeopathic medicines safely and effectively at home in a variety of first-aid situations, from accidents and injuries to backache, coughs, colds, childhood illnesses, earaches, flu, food-poisoning, sore throats, teething and many other common complaints.

Most of the homeopathic first-aid books currently available have attempted to simplify the process of finding a remedy (as homeopathic medicines are called) in order to make homeopathy more accessible. This has resulted in some disappointment, as many people have found their attempts to use 'natural' medicine to be a hit-or-miss affair. This book aims to right this error by mimicking the method that a professional homeopath uses. To this end there are three main sections:

Part I: History, Principles and Prescribing

This section (Chapters 1–5) introduces the history and theory of homeopathy, including its guiding principles; it defines those complaints you can safely treat yourself and guides you through taking a case and prescribing.

Part II: The Materia Medicas and Repertories

This is the main part of the book and is divided into two sections: external remedies (drops, lotions, creams and ointments) and internal remedies (tablets taken internally). Each has a Materia Medica – an alphabetically arranged list of detailed descriptions of the remedies; and a Repertory – an index of symptoms or complaints to guide you to the correct remedy in the Materia Medica.

Part III: Prescribing Guidelines and Follow-through

This part includes clear guidelines on which complaints you can treat using this book. It also gives practical measures that may be helpful or important in each complaint. *It is essential to read this in conjunction with the remedy pictures in Part II.* Following this are questionnaires and charts to assist you in 'taking your case' and prescribing. Finally, there are ten sample cases illustrating the application of the principles of homeopathy, which you can use as examples or to test yourself to see how well you have understood the homeopathic processes outlined in this book.

Part IV: The Appendices

These include a glossary providing brief definitions of any unusual terms used in the book; a section on how to stock up a first-aid kit; a bibliography of further reading and information about pharmacies stocking homeopathic remedies and bookshops stocking useful books.

PART I
HISTORY, PRINCIPLES AND PRESCRIBING

·1·
THE HISTORY
OF
HOMEOPATHY

ORIGINS OF HOMEOPATHIC THOUGHT

In the fifth century BC Hippocrates (c.470–400 BC), the 'father of medicine', wrote that there were two methods of healing: by 'contraries' and by 'similars'. His writings show his insistence on a high ethical standard, on accuracy of observation and clarity of recording cases rather than on theory and symptomatology. He refuted the common idea that illness was punishment from the gods: 'Every disease has its own nature and arises from external causes, from cold, from the sun, from changing winds.' He advised against meddlesome interference, saying, 'Our natures are the physicians of our diseases.'

His observations on cure by 'similars' were not followed by the medical profession and over the next thousand years they seemed to lie dormant – except, of course, that country people throughout the world have used this principle successfully in their own folk-medicines for many hundreds of years.

Paracelsus (1493–1541), a German doctor born Philippus Aureolus Theophrastus Bombastus von Hohenheim, was unconventional even by the standards of his time. He was one of the natural philosophers who sought to overthrow what he called the 'logico-mathematical' theorising of the time. He saw the earth as a great chemical laboratory and recognised the value of chemical experiments in medicine, both as the basis for understanding physiological processes and as a source of medicinal preparations. He is called the 'father of chemistry', for he updated alchemy by moving it away from its search for the elixir of life towards treating illness and practical pharmaceutical studies; he based it firmly on the observation of plants, animals and minerals, and stressed the importance of direct, practical experience and experimentation. He railed against those who believed that contraries cure.

Paracelsus believed in the harmony of the whole universe. He turned to German folk-medicine, which believed in 'like curing like', or that the poison that causes a disease should become its cure. As a result he was accused of advocating the internal use of lethal poisons, but in fact he gave careful attention to dosage and noted that a very small dose could overcome a great disease. He also used only one medicine at a time. He saw nature in each and every person as a vital spirit, and predicted the germ theory of disease by stating that the causes of disease were external, seed-like factors introduced into the body through air, food and drink; these then became localised, growing in specific organs as the seeds of disease which combated the local vital spirit of the organ and the body. He also believed in the natural recuperative power of the human body. Again, his observations on the law of similars were not taken up for over two hundred years.

THE FOUNDER OF HOMEOPATHY: SAMUEL HAHNEMANN (1755–1843)

Samuel Hahnemann was born in Meissen in Saxony (now in East Germany) on 10 April 1755 into an era of enormous change and political upheaval. During his lifetime the Seven Years' War, the French Revolution and the Napoleonic Wars threw Europe into turmoil. The Industrial Revolution brought social change and great advances in technology, and there were developments in science. Hahnemann was born one year before Mozart, and the writers Goethe and Schiller were his contemporaries.

This period also saw a revolution in thought. Eighteenth-century Germany was the birthplace of the political, spiritual and intellectual movement now known as the Enlightenment; the freedom of thought and opinion it encouraged was important for the birth and development of homeopathy.

Hahnemann was the third of five children born into a poor but upright and devoutly Protestant family. He was educated initially by his parents. His father, a man of high principles and deep religious belief, taught him never to learn or listen passively but to question everything. Legend tells us that before his father went to work he would lock the boy in his room with a 'problem' to think through, releasing him on his return only if he had the correct answer. The young Samuel appears to have taken learning very seriously; he certainly had an inordinate thirst for knowledge and is reported to have been a gifted and clever child, though often ailing from over-studying and his family's economic circumstances. At school, his teachers recognised his unusual intelligence and he was not charged the usual fees. His greatest talents were for languages, mathematics, geometry and botany.

By teaching and translating, Hahnemann paid his way through the University of Leipzig, where he studied medicine and chemistry. He qualified as a doctor in 1791 and practised medicine for about nine years, during which time he married. Increasingly, however, he became disillusioned by the cruel and ineffective treatments of his time (blood-letting, purgings, poisonous drugs with horrendous side effects) and took the courageous decision to give up his practice, concentrating instead on study, research, writing and translation:

I cannot reckon on much income from practice . . . I am too conscientious to prolong illness or make it appear more dangerous than it really is. . . . It was agony for me to walk always in darkness, when I had to heal the sick, and to prescribe, according to such or such an hypothesis concerning diseases, substances which owed their place in the Materia Medica to an arbitrary decision. . . . Soon after my marriage, I renounced the practice of medicine, that I might no longer incur the risk of doing injury, and I engaged exclusively in chemistry and in literary occupations.

This meant that for many years his family was extremely poor, with Hahnemann, his wife and a growing number of children living at times in only one room and with little more than bread and fresh air as sustenance.

The first proving

One of the major works Hahnemann translated was Dr William Cullen's *A Treatise on Materia Medica*. Cullen (1710–90) was an Edinburgh teacher, physician and chemist, and his book included an essay on Peruvian bark or Cinchona (which homeopaths call *China*), from which quinine, the treatment for malaria, is derived. Cullen attributed Cinchona's ability to cure malaria, with its symptoms of periodic fever, sweating and palpitations, to its bitterness. Hahnemann, sceptical of this explanation, tested small doses on himself and wrote in a letter:

I took by way of experiment, twice a day, four drachms of good China. My feet, finger ends, etc., at first became quite cold; I grew languid and drowsy; then my heart began to palpitate, and my pulse grew hard and small; intolerable anxiety, trembling, prostration throughout all my limbs; then pulsation, in the head, redness of my cheeks, thirst, and, in short, all these symptoms which are ordinarily characteristic of intermittent fever, made their appearance, one after the other, yet without the peculiar chilly, shivering rigor. Briefly, even those symptoms which are of regular occurrence and especially characteristic – as the stupidity of mind, the kind of rigidity in all the limbs, but above all the numb, disagreeable sensation, which seems to have its seat in the periosteum, over every bone in the whole body – all these made their appearance. This paroxysm lasted two or three hours each time, and recurred, if I repeated this dose, not otherwise; I discontinued it and was in good health.

In other words, Hahnemann observed that Cinchona produced in a healthy person the symptoms of malaria, the very disease that it was known to cure.

This discovery was to be of great importance in the development of homeopathic theory and practice. By observing the symptoms any substance produced when given to a healthy person, Hahnemann could discover the healing properties of that substance. Physicians had long grappled with this problem and the Doctrine of Signatures, which states that a plant will act on that part of the body which it most resembles in appearance, was an attempt to understand the healing powers of natural remedies. Hahnemann had discovered an experimental basis that would systematically yield vastly more accurate and specific information about the individual substances tested. The procedure was called 'proving' (i.e. testing) a remedy.

Like cures like: the first law of homeopathy discovered

The standard medical assumption had always been that if the body produced a symptom the appropriate treatment would be an antidote, an opposite or 'contrary' medicine to that symptom. For example, constipation would be treated with laxatives, which produce diarrhoea. Hahnemann's experience with

Cinchona indicated that a different principle of treatment might apply. Hahnemann would have been familiar with Hippocrates' writings on curing with 'similars', and so it must have been with great excitement that he embarked on further experiments that confirmed this principle.

He called this *similia similibus curentur*, or 'let likes be cured with like', and this principle of curing with similars became the first law of a system of healing he called 'homeopathy', from the Greek *homoios* (similar) and *pathos* (suffering or disease), in order to differentiate it from orthodox medicine, which he called 'allopathy', meaning 'opposite suffering'.

> *If I mistake not, practical medicine has devised three ways of applying remedies for the relief of disorders of the human body. The first method, that of removing or destroying the causes of the malady, that is preventive treatment. . . . The second and most common,* contraria contraris, *that is healing by opposites, such as the palliative treatment of constipation by laxatives . . . the third . . .* similia similibus, *that is, in order to cure disease, we must seek medicines that can excite similar symptoms in the healthy body.*

Hahnemann wrote this in 1796. During the next six years he conducted many provings on his family and friends, and also studied accounts of the symptoms shown by victims of accidental poisonings.

Finally he set up in medical practice again, but with a different basis for his prescriptions. He used the material he had gathered from the provings and in his patients looked for the *similimum* – the remedy whose 'symptom picture' (based on the provings) most matched that of his patient. His methods were met with disbelief and he was ridiculed by colleagues, but the patients flowed in and the astonishing results Hahnemann achieved verified his theory.

He also differed from conventional practitioners in giving only one remedy at a time, which was unheard of in an age when apothecaries made fortunes by mixing numerous substances, many of which were highly noxious. This earned him enemies among the pharmacists.

The minimum dose

Hahnemann did not stop there. Dissatisfied with the side effects of his diluted medicines, he experimented with smaller and smaller doses of these single remedies in order to minimise the side effects. He found, however, that when he diluted a medicine sufficiently to eradicate the side effects, it no longer effected a cure. He therefore developed a new method of dilution: instead of simply stirring the substance after each dilution he shook it vigorously. This shaking he called

'succussion' and the resultant remedy a 'potentised remedy'.

He found that not only did he now obtain a remedy that had no side effects but that the more he diluted using succussion, the more effectively his remedy cured. He believed that the shaking released the strength or energy of the substance (involving some sort of imprinting on the water/alcohol solvent), with none of its toxic effects remaining.

Hahnemann numbered the potentised remedies according to the number of times they had been diluted: a remedy diluted six times (taking out one-hundredth of the liquid each time and adding $^{99}/_{100}$ alcohol) was called a 6C (see page 13). Initially he prescribed remedies that had been diluted up to the sixth potency; then he experimented with the higher dilutions, finding them more effective still. In his lifetime he prescribed up to the thirtieth potency. His followers took dilution even further.

This process of dilution incurred yet more wrath and derision from the medical establishment, who could not explain, and therefore could not accept, how anything so dilute could have any effect. Yet despite opposition, homeopathy survived and spread remarkably quickly – because it was remarkably effective.

The Organon and other publications

Hahnemann's literary output during his life was prodigious. He proved about one hundred remedies, wrote over seventy original works and translated about twenty-four English, French, Italian and Latin texts on a wide range of subjects. He also corresponded with homeopaths, colleagues and friends throughout the world, all in addition to his vast daily practice.

In 1810 Hahnemann published the first edition of *The Organon of Rational Medicine* (later *The Organon of the Healing Art*), which ran to six editions, each one modified and expanded. In it he set out clearly the homeopathic philosophy or system of belief. In the same year, when Leipzig was attacked in the Napoleonic campaigns and 80,000 men were slaughtered, Hahnemann's treatments of the survivors and also of victims of the great typhus epidemic that followed the siege were highly successful and further increased his reputation.

He lectured at Leipzig University, where his theoretical lectures, which often deteriorated into violent tirades against the medical practices of doctors and apothecaries, earned him the nickname 'Raging Hurricane'. However, a few medical practitioners were prepared to go against the mainstream of opinion and a number trained under him and took his teachings out into the world. By the early 1820s he had also built up a thriving practice.

Between 1811 and 1821 Hahnemann published his *Materia Medica Pura* in six volumes; this represented the results of the provings so far undertaken – thousands of symptoms for sixty-six remedies. The provings were meticulous and painstaking, but it is worth remembering that in Hahnemann's experiments nothing was done to eliminate the power of suggestion: provers knew what substance they were taking. Remedies were given in weak dilutions and not in potentised doses. Coffee, tea, wine, brandy and spicy or salty food were all banned from the provers' diets, although a little beer was allowed. Games and work activity were restricted, but moderate exercise was encouraged.

In 1828 Hahnemann's *Chronic Diseases and Their Homeopathic Cure* appeared (it eventually ran to five volumes). In it he elaborated on the philosophy of *The Organon*, adding more remedies as a result of his experiences in successfully treating chronic patients. He discussed the use of higher potencies – up to the 30th potency – and introduced the concept of 'miasms' to account for the failure of some patients to respond to treatment with remedies which clearly matched their symptoms. Among such people he found a history of certain diseases and discovered that he was able to link the tendency to particular types of condition to a legacy in the patient's inherited health. He developed a way of treating these blocks to health homeopathically.

Success with cholera

In 1831 cholera swept through Central Europe. Hahnemann published papers on the homeopathic treatment of the disease, advocating the administration of the remedy *Camphor* in the early stages and *Cuprum metallicum*, *Veratrum album*, *Bryonia alba* and *Rhus toxicodendron* in the later stages. He also stressed that clothing and bedding should be heated to destroy 'all known infectious matters' and advised cleanliness, ventilation and disinfection of the rooms, and quarantine. In such respects his ideas were far ahead of his time: the work of Pasteur on the germ theory of disease and that of Lister on disinfection were still to come. In Raab in Hungary, only six out of 154 homeopathically treated patients died, compared with almost 59 per cent of those treated conventionally. Elsewhere throughout Europe, cholera was more successfully treated with homeopathy than with orthodox medicine; mortality rates varied between 2.4 and 21.1 per cent compared with 50 per cent or more in conventional treatment.

In 1833 the Leipzig Homeopathic Hospital was opened, but in-fighting between homeopaths, the autocratic controlling influence of Hahnemann and the extreme polarisation that homeopathy caused within the medical profession created tensions that finally led to its dissolution in 1842.

Hahnemann's final years

In 1834 a certain Mademoiselle Marie Melanie d'Hervilly travelled from Paris to consult Hahnemann (now aged seventy-nine and a widower) in Kothen, where he was established. She was an attractive, intelligent society lady of about thirty, and a self-styled artist who had caused a minor scandal by dressing as a man.

After reading *The Organon* she came to study with Hahnemann, claiming that she had a vocation for medicine. Within six months of her arrival in Kothen they were married, much to the horror of Hahnemann's remaining family. They moved to Paris and set up house in the fashionable rue de Milan, where Hahnemann established a prosperous practice, continuing to work long days with his patients, rich and poor alike, maintaining his 'no cure, no fee' system. Melanie helped her husband by taking notes and began to treat patients under his supervision.

On 2 July 1843, at the age of eighty-eight, Hahnemann died in Paris after a few months of bronchial catarrh. Melanie refused to allow friends and family to visit the body; there were no invitations to the funeral and Hahnemann was buried in a public grave in the cemetery at Montmartre. Fifty-five years later his body was exhumed and reburied in the famous Père Lachaise cemetery along with poets, musicians and field marshals.

Melanie Hahnemann continued to practise after his death; as she had had no formal medical training, she was the first woman lay homeopath. Presumably wealthy after Hahnemann's death, she refused to help her German relations, and withheld various of her husband's notes and writings, including the sixth edition of *The Organon*, against repeated requests from homeopaths. She held out for enormous sums, gaining a reputation for being shrewd and calculating. Unpopular and isolated, she died at the age of seventy-eight.

Samuel Hahnemann lived before the germ theory of disease had been proposed, before thermometers, the X-ray and antibiotics made medicine appear increasingly 'scientific'. Yet, as we have seen, in his ideas and in his approach, he was certainly a man of science and an innovator. He was a man of sufficient intellect and culture to combine science and metaphysics. Consciously or unconsciously, he drew on the traditions of German folk-medicine, alchemy and magic, as well as the developments in chemistry, pathology, pharmaceutics and medicine which in the late eighteenth and early nineteenth centuries were beginning to make medical diagnosis and treatment both more accurate and more humane. Although brought up in a Protestant household, in later life he became a religious free-thinker, believing that God permeated every living thing. He also seems to have believed that he was divinely chosen and guided in his work. His development of a safe and effective system of medicine has given the world a priceless gift.

HAHNEMANN'S FOLLOWERS

Hahnemann was apparently an irritable (and irritating) man with a penchant for antagonism which seems to have lived on in many of his followers. They were mostly doctors who became 'converted' to homeopathy. Two such converts were Constantine Hering and James Tyler Kent.

Constantine Hering (1800–80)

Hering studied medicine at Leipzig University, where, after publication of *The Organon*, his professor asked him to write a paper disproving Hahnemann's theories. Far from being able to discredit Hahnemann, he found himself greatly interested and abandoned the paper. He was also successfully treated for an inflammation of the hand that threatened amputation after a wound became infected while he was dissecting, and this convinced him further. He became involved in the homeopathic world and joined the Provers' Union, which meant he had to move to another university in order to complete his medical training because of the hostility at Leipzig towards homeopathy.

In 1827 Hering travelled to South America on a voyage of botanical exploration (financed by the King of Saxony) and sent details of his researches back to Germany – including the provings of *Lachesis* the bushmaster snake (see page 105), which he personally undertook, asking his wife to record everything that he said and did while he was delirious from the venom.

On his way back to Europe he stopped off in Philadelphia and was persuaded to stay to become one of the founding fathers of homeopathy in the USA. He set up the first training academy (which closed down after the funds were embezzled by a dishonest secretary), then opened the Hahnemann Medical College, which flourished and grew almost to university status. It had 70 professors and lecturers, and 300 students training at any one time, treating 50,000 patients and 6000 out-patient cases a year in a general hospital with 200 beds as well as a special wing for midwifery. In all, 3500 homeopaths were trained by the college.

Hering continued to prove remedies throughout his life and wrote extensively. He is best remembered today for his Laws of Cure (see page 15). He also took Hahnemann's miasm theories a stage further, developing the idea that any disease could leave a 'taint' or miasm. He developed potentised disease products with which he experimented by giving them to people who had never been well since suffering from a particular disease. For example, he potentised the sputum of a person suffering from tuberculosis and gave it to patients who had never been really well since suffering from tuberculosis themselves. This method of treatment cleared the miasm, and enabled the indicated remedies to work. This was not 'classical' homeopathy as Hahnemann had developed it, and has since been called 'isopathy' – that is, treating with the *same* thing rather than with a *similar* thing.

James Tyler Kent (1849–1916)

After qualifying as a physician in his native America, Kent practised orthodox medicine until his first wife became ill and demanded homeopathic treatment. The success of this treatment converted Kent and he devoted his remarkable energy to homeopathy. A man with a high moral sense and an equally strong belief in his own rightness and authority, Kent's writings are dogmatic, much like Hahnemann's later works.

He advocated the use of very high potencies – up to CM and MM (see page 13) and mainly prescribed above the 30th potency. (Machinery had by then been invented to succuss the remedies and facilitate the making of higher dilutions.) The practice of high-potency prescribing led to a split among American homeopaths and to much in-fighting between 'high' (30 and above) and 'low' (up to 30) prescribers.

Kent's major published works are his *Repertory*, his *Philosophy* and his *Materia Medica*. The Repertory, which is more systematic and readable – and therefore more accessible – than earlier ones, is the one still most in use today. His Materia Medica was – and is – also the most accessible to date. He developed 'pictures' of the remedies – 'constitutional types', as they became known – from the patients' emotional symptoms, identifying, for example, 'Sulphur patients', who were scruffy and lazy ('ragged philosophers', as he termed them). This approach moved away from the purely scientific and pathological understanding of the remedies. Those who adopted Kent's new methods, along with high-potency prescribing, became known as Kentians. His influence increased after his death, both in the USA and abroad.

THE NINETEENTH CENTURY

Homeopathy in the USA

In the 1820s, when homeopathy arrived in the USA, the state of orthodox medicine was, if anything, worse than it was in Europe. The practice of almost completely draining the body of blood (four-fifths were let) was advocated, even for children. A drug known as 'Calomel' (*Mercurius chloride*), which had been introduced originally to cure syphilis, was used as a standard 'purgative'; its side effects were loss of teeth and seizure of the jaws necessitating major surgery, and/or death from mercury poisoning.

As many ordinary people consulted herbalists and bone-setters, homeopathy was easily accepted and quickly flourished. Homeopaths were seen to be well-educated and hard-working people, and the 'metaphysical' background appealed to many church people. It was adopted in particular by followers of Swedenborg (1689–1772), a visionary who 'received' information about the spirit world and the cosmos and believed that he was a vehicle for a new religious revelation. His writings appealed to people who were studying the new sciences, such as Darwinism, and who were concerned about the conflict between science and orthodox religion. For many homeopaths this blend of reason and mysticism was ideal. Kent, like Hering and many other American homeopaths, was a Swedenborgian.

In 1846 the American Medical Association was founded. It adopted a code of ethics which forbade its members from consulting homeopaths, and local and state medical societies were told to purge themselves of homeopaths and their sympathisers. Nonetheless, homeopathy had made a positive mark on orthodox medicine – blood-letting abated, medical training improved and several homeopathic remedies found their way into allopathic prescribing. Public demand for homeopathic treatment continued.

The 1860s through to the 1880s saw the heyday of American homeopathy. Practitioners proved every conceivable remedy, often at great cost to their own health; some even involved their children in the provings. Hospitals and training programmes were established and, at its peak, there were fifty-six homeopathic hospitals, thirteen mental asylums, nine homeopathic children's hospitals and fifteen sanatoriums, with thousands of trained homeopaths throughout the country. The homeopathic training colleges excluded neither women nor black people, as was the case with their allopathic counterparts.

As homeopathy appeared to become more settled in the USA both financially and politically, intense battles developed between high- and low-potency prescribers. The purists became high-potency prescribers, centred around Kent's teachings; the revisionists became low-potency prescribers who moved towards pathological diagnosis, giving, for example, a homeopathic prescription for an ulcer rather than treating the patient's constitution (i.e. taking into account the whole person and the 'total symptom picture'). British homeopaths maintained a more balanced practice than in the USA, using both high and low potencies for prescribing.

Homeopathy in Britain

In 1826 a young doctor called Frederick Hervey Foster Quin visited Hahnemann in Germany and spent some time studying with the Leipzig homeopaths; later he studied for a year with Hahnemann in Paris. He was a very well connected young man with a flourishing practice and a social network to match. He had been appointed physician to Napoleon in exile on St Helena, but Napoleon had died before he could take up the post. In 1831 Quin caught cholera while visiting Europe to study homeopathic treatments for the epidemic and was cured with Hahnemann's prescription of *Camphor*.

In 1832 Quin set up a homeopathic practice in London, where he treated many famous people, including Dickens and Thackeray, and in 1844 he established the British Homœopathic Society (later the Faculty of Homœopathy). He founded the London Homœopathic Hospital in 1849.

It is interesting to note that during the cholera outbreak of 1854 in London, the Board of Health suppressed the fact that deaths at the Homœopathic Hospital were a mere 16.4 per cent, compared with the 50 per cent average for other hospitals. When challenged, the Board explained: 'The figures would give sanction to a practice opposed to the maintenance of truth and the progress of science.'*

After the Crimean War (1853–6), which led to the formation of a proper nursing service under Florence Nightingale, a medical bill was introduced to Parliament which would have made homeopathy illegal, but Quin's friends in the House of Lords secured a saving amendment.

If Quin was the practical and fashionable force behind the establishment of homeopathy in England, the two most influential writers and teachers were Robert Dudgeon, who translated Hahnemann's texts into English, and Richard Hughes, a mild man with a conciliatory attitude towards the orthodox medical establishment as well as a rigorous and scientific attitude towards homeopathy. Hughes rejected the vital-

*Pinchuck and Clark, *Medicine for Beginners*, Writers and Readers, London, 1984.

force theories of Hahnemann and took a stricter attitude towards provings and Materia Medica than Hahnemann had done in his later years. He distrusted high-potency prescribing and ridiculed the American high-potency machines. Hughes looked to a world 'where the rivalry between homeopathic and allopathic practitioners would no longer embitter doctors and perplex patients', which would have meant the assimilation of homeopathy into allopathy. He was dubbed a 'half-homeopath' and his influence faded after his death.

Queen Adelaide, wife of King William IV, brought homeopathy from her native Saxony to the English royal family. Albert, Queen Victoria's consort, was the son of Duke Ernst of Saxe-Coburg who had employed Hahnemann in 1792 to run a humane lunatic asylum in Germany. The English royal family maintains an active involvement in homeopathy to this day. The Queen has her own consultant homeopath and carries her 'black box' of homeopathic remedies with her on all her travels.

THE TWENTIETH CENTURY

By the time of Hahnemann's death in 1843, homeopathy was established throughout the world, although the mutual antagonism and distrust between homeopaths and allopaths continued to hinder its progress.

Developments in medicine around the close of the nineteenth century strengthened the orthodox camp: science had proved the existence of microbes, the old practices Hahnemann had condemned were diminishing, and powerful new drugs were being developed. The rise of medicine became synonymous with the rise of the pharmaceutical industry – an effective and wealthy lobbying force behind allopathic medicine. As the position of allopathy became stronger, the homeopathic establishment was weakened by internal division. The confused general public was drawn to the side that could put its case most clearly and strongly.

Medicine became increasingly involved with economic and political factors far removed from the health of the patient, but advertising became a powerful force and the public – and many of the homeopaths – were swept up by the tide. In 1911 the American Medical Association moved to close many homeopathic teaching institutions because they were considered to provide a poor standard of education. The AMA also mounted a huge anti-homeopathy propaganda campaign. Consequently, by 1918 the number of homeopathic hospitals in the USA had dwindled to

seven. Great optimism accompanied the introduction of penicillin: doctors thought that a sort of medical Nirvana had arrived. The time involved in the taking of a homeopathic case was regarded as a thing of the past. The five-minute prescription and a cure for every ill had arrived. Little did they realise that it was the dawn of a medical nemesis.

Homeopathy around the world today

Homeopathy is popular over much of Asia from Pakistan, Bangladesh and Nepal to Sri Lanka. In India homeopathy is now officially recognised as a separate branch of medicine and flourishes there, fully supported by the government. It has the largest number of homeopathic hospitals in the world, 300,000 full-time homeopaths (70,000 registered with state boards), forty homeopathic medical schools with four- to six-year training programmes, and a thriving publishing outlet.

Homeopathy has spread throughout Europe, although it is poorly represented in some countries, like Spain, Iceland and Denmark. In others – France for example – there is a larger and fast-growing interest. Homeopathic medicines are readily available in most pharmacies and there are homeopathic consultants at some hospitals. In France the Napoleonic Laws banned the use of all potencies above 30C and this has led to a complicated use of the lower potencies, with, for example, 3C, 4C and 5C all in the same remedy being used for different complaints. France also subscribes to combination remedies, moving away from the holistic or classical approach. The country boasts several fine laboratories producing remedies to a very high standard.

In West Germany, the birthplace of homeopathy, it is extremely popular with several thousand practitioners, but, as in France, German homeopaths are extremely fond of combinations, using mixtures of up to twenty remedies.

In Eastern Europe homeopathy is poorly represented, although there is some interest in Poland. The exact extent of homeopathy in the USSR is not known, although it is certainly available in the main cities. In 1935 an official decree allowed doctors to prescribe orthodox or homeopathic medicines according to their choice.

Homeopathy is highly respected in many South American countries, with Mexico, Argentina and Brazil at the forefront, each with many thousands of homeopaths. The standard of practice is high.

In Australia and New Zealand homeopathy is spreading rapidly, with both doctors and professional homeopaths taking part.

A small but dedicated number of homeopaths were

practising in South Africa when in 1974 an Act of Parliament closed down the homeopathic colleges (in a move identical to that in the USA in the early 1900s). It is not officially accepted, but a few practitioners continue to work.

Homeopathy is non-existent in the Arab states. It is gaining in popularity in Israel.

In Greece George Vithoulkas, author of *The Science of Homeopathy*, is a professional practitioner who has set up a clinic and training school in Athens. His clinic has treated hundreds of thousands of patients over the twenty years since its foundation and has developed a remarkable reputation. Vithoulkas is as concerned with the importance of *how* homeopathy works as he is with the more metaphysical aspects. He follows Hahnemann and Kent in his purely classical approach, and has drawn together much material from observation. He has updated Kent's repertory in terms of language and accessibility, but also with respect to the mental and emotional states. These he has re-interpreted in the light of modern psychology and by so doing has made an invaluable contribution to homeopathy. He has called his remedy pictures 'essences', and the publication of his Materia Medica is eagerly awaited.

Homeopathy in Britain today

Throughout the late nineteenth century and early twentieth century, homeopathic hospitals were opened in Bristol, Liverpool, Glasgow and Tunbridge Wells, as well as in London, and in 1946, when the National Health Service was established, homeopathy was included as an officially approved method of treatment. As we have seen, it did not grow to become a real rival to orthodox medicine, but in Britain today its popularity is increasing rapidly. It is still practised under the National Health in these five hospitals and by GPs, although the limit of time on consultations often means that antibiotics are handed out with the homeopathic medicines just in case the latter do not work.

Professional homeopaths run private practices and many participate in almost-free clinics for the needy. The Society of Homœopaths, the organisation which represents the professional homeopath in this country, promotes the practice of homeopathy to a high standard. From small beginnings in 1974, the number of registered members (who use the initials RSHom. after their names) increases annually and there are now at least six colleges training several hundred professional homeopaths each year.

·2·
PRINCIPLES AND CONCEPTS

'The highest ideal of therapy is to restore health rapidly, gently, permanently; to remove and destroy the whole disease in the shortest, surest, least harmful way, according to clearly comprehensible principles.'

So it was that Samuel Hahnemann, in *The Organon*, defined his goals for a new system of medicine. It is hard to imagine a description that could express more concisely the needs of both practitioner and patient.

Homeopathy strengthens the body's vitality and its ability to respond to stress without recourse to other medicines. The principles of homeopathy as a whole represent a complete view of the processes of health and disease. Since 1810, when *The Organon* was first published, they have proved very resistant to major re-interpretation. Homeopathy, as a system of medicine, is practised within the framework of these principles and, because they are crucial to successful prescribing, I hope they will become as familiar to you as old friends.

THE SIMILIMUM OR LAW OF SIMILARS

This basic law of homeopathy is *similia similibus curentur*: 'let likes be cured with like'. Based on this premise, the first homeopathic principle states that any substance that can make you ill can also cure you – anything that is capable of producing symptoms of disease in a healthy person can cure those symptoms in a sick person.

By 'symptom' the homeopath means those changes that are felt by the patient (subjective) or observed (objective), which may be associated with a particular disease, or state of dis-ease, and which are the outward expression of that state.

PROVINGS

'Proving' is the name given to the homeopathic method of testing substances in order to establish their 'symptom pictures'. Since Hahnemann's first proving in 1790 (see page 4), hundreds of provings have been carried out and their results collated in the great Materia Medicas. In the 1940s the Americans organised a programme of re-proving remedies, but it was abandoned when identical symptoms were elicited all over again.

Today, healthy volunteer provers of new, potentially medicinal substances are divided into two groups, according to double-blind trial rules, with one group being given the unnamed substance and the other a placebo. Neither the provers nor the conductor of the proving knows at the time who is taking what. The remedies are sometimes tested in their diluted – potentised – form or, if they are not poisonous, in crude doses (in the 'mother tincture'). Once the proving is complete and the individuals who have produced a symptom picture have returned to a state of health, the results are collated. Not everybody who proves a substance will provide symptoms: only a proportion of people are susceptible to any one substance, as is the case with diseases. All symptoms – physical, emotional and mental – are noted in painstaking detail, then gathered in a schematic way and common themes noted.

Apart from the symptoms that have been deliberately proved by homeopaths over the years, two other types of symptom are taken into account:

Accidental provings have provided a rich source of valuable information that might not otherwise be available to us. Substances such as deadly nightshade, snake venoms, hemlock and many others are of great value: because they can *cause* extremely serious conditions, they also have the ability to cure them.

Understandably, not all the volunteers who willingly proved remedies were as keen as Constantine Hering (see page 7) to risk their health by testing highly poisonous substances. However, homeopaths have been able to add symptom pictures of substances such as deadly nightshade, the remedy *Belladonna*, or snake venoms such as *Lachesis* to the Materia Medica by drawing on detailed accounts of accidental poisonings. Deliberate poisonings, such as the death of Socrates by hemlock (the remedy *Conium*), have also provided homeopaths with much useful information.

Cured symptoms. After a remedy has been successfully prescribed, symptoms cured by it which did not emerge either in the provings or in the accidental provings are noted. If the remedy consistently cures these symptoms in many people, then they are added to the picture.

THE MATERIA MEDICA

The Materia Medica (Latin for 'Medical Matter' or 'Material') lists the symptom pictures of each remedy, as discovered in the provings. The many hundreds of remedies are arranged alphabetically and the symptoms of those remedies are arranged according to body area. New remedies are constantly being discovered and added.

The professional homeopath works with a number of Materia Medicas compiled by different homeopaths, each reflecting personal experience over their careers. They all have the same basic information, as they are based on the original provings; it is how the individual homeopath presents the material and interprets the information that is interesting.

Within this vast amount of information certain patterns emerge and it is these patterns with which the homeopath becomes familiar. He or she will memorise the strong symptoms or keynotes of a remedy, but the small or the obscure symptoms will need looking up in the Materia Medica. For example, if a person is suffering from a cold after being caught out in the rain, a number of remedies come to mind, but it is the particular symptoms of the patient's cold that may then need to be looked up in order to decide between the different remedies.

THE REPERTORY

The Repertory is an index of symptoms from the Materia Medica listed in alphabetical order and there-by providing a valuable cross-referencing system. A good Repertory is essential as it is impossible to memorise the vast number of symptoms in the Materia Medica.

THE SINGLE REMEDY

The classical homeopath gives one remedy at a time in order to gauge its effect more precisely than would be possible if two or more remedies were given together. Indeed, the remedies were all originally proved separately and it is consequently not known how they inter-react if mixed; it would make sense to use combined remedies only if they have been proved in combination.

However, this most difficult aspect of homeopathic prescribing deters many people. Finding a single remedy to match the patient's symptoms is a constant challenge and can involve an enormous amount of hard work. The lazy, busy or misguided homeopath may mix several remedies together in the hope that one will work. This hit-or-miss approach is not true classical homeopathy as Hahnemann defined it and shows a lack of understanding of the fundamental principles.

THE MINIMUM DOSE

The more a remedy is diluted and succussed (vigorously shaken), the stronger it becomes as a cure (see page 13). This idea – the infinitesimal dose, as it is called – is one of the great stumbling blocks for a conventionally trained scientific mind. I always tell cynics that they must see homeopathy work in order to believe it because no amount of theory is acceptable without some sort of tangible proof. People who find this concept baffling are known to laugh like drains at the thought that a very dilute solution of sea salt – beyond the point where there is any salt left in the solution – is capable of curing a wide range of complaints, from cold sores, hayfever and headaches to depression (see *Natrum muriaticum*, page 117). Logically, it does seem unlikely that a substance that can cause high blood pressure in its crude form could become a strong and effective agent for healing when it is so dilute.

There is a pharmacological law that states that although a large dose of a poison can destroy life, a moderate dose will only paralyse and a very small dose will actually stimulate those same life processes.

New discoveries in physics are beginning to explain this phenomenon. One theory is that the succussion creates an electrochemical pattern which is stored in the dilutant and which then spreads like liquid crystal through the body's own water. Another hypothesis suggests that the dilution process triggers an electromagnetic imprinting which directly affects the electromagnetic field of the body.

Potencies

There are two scales for diluting substances – the decimal and the centesimal. In all cases the starting remedy is made from a mixture of the substance itself which has been steeped in alcohol for a period of time and then strained. This starting liquid is called a 'tincture' or 'mother tincture'.

For the decimal scale, one-tenth of the tincture is added to nine-tenths of alcohol and shaken vigorously; this first dilution is called a 1X. The number of a homeopathic remedy reflects the number of times it has been diluted and succussed: for example, *Sulphur 6X* has been diluted and succussed six times.

The centesimal scale is diluted using one part tincture in a hundred (as opposed to ten) and the letter C is added after the number (although in practice homeopaths have omitted the C and just use the numbers for the centesimal scale).

Paradoxically, a 6X is called a low potency and 200 (C) a high potency – the greater the dilution, the greater the potency.

The most commonly used potency in the decimal scale is the 6X, although the 9X, 12X, 24X and 30X are used by some. In the centesimal scale those low potencies most commonly used are the 6, 12 and 30. The higher potencies – 200, 1M (diluted one thousand times), 10M (ten thousand times) and CM (one hundred thousand times) – are highly respected by homeopaths and should not be used by the home prescriber.

'Inert' substances are ground for many hours with a pestle and mortar until they become soluble, a process called 'trituration' which is used for metals as well as other substances that do not dissolve easily.

THE WHOLE PERSON

The concept of treating the 'whole person' is an essential element of classical homeopathy. The basis of this belief is that symptoms, diseases or pains do not exist in isolation, but are a reflection of how the person as a whole is coping with stress. It is the whole person that counts – not just the physical body but also the mental and/or emotional 'bodies'. The homeopath looks beyond the 'presenting complaint', beyond the label of the disease (for example 'tonsillitis' or 'migraines' or

'food poisoning') to the 'totality of symptoms' a person experiences.

I always ask myself, 'How is this person different from another with this particular complaint?' The homeopath individualises the prescription to fit the patient – rather like a tailored suit. Imagine that the whole person is like a jigsaw. Prescribing on one symptom alone is like seeing only a small part of the jigsaw; it does not give you enough information to work out what the whole picture is.

As far as first-aid prescribing is concerned, it *is* possible to prescribe on a single symptom – like, for example, chilblains or mouth ulcers. But it is always preferable to find a remedy that matches the totality of symptoms, taking into account as many pieces of the jigsaw as possible. If you are able to locate at least most of the pieces and fit them together (see 'The Symptom Picture' and 'Working Out the Remedy', pages 20 and 22), then you will be able to make sense of the whole picture *and* match it to a single remedy.

CONSTITUTION AND SUSCEPTIBILITY

I often hear people say enviously about a friend, 'He smokes like a chimney, drinks like a fish, works like a maniac and has never had a day's illness in his life. It's not fair. I struggle constantly to stay healthy and need nine hours' sleep a night, otherwise I get sick. Why?'

Well, the answer lies in the constitution. The person who works all hours and smokes and drinks as if there were no tomorrow has a strong constitution – and may well be wasting his 'inheritance', because there *will* come a time when it will run out, when even *he* will get sick.

George Vithoulkas, in *The Science of Homeopathy*, defines the constitution as 'the genetic inheritance tempered or modified by our environment', that is, a person's fundamental structure – their state of health *and* their temperament. Basically, a strong constitution is one that can withstand considerable pressure without falling ill. A weak constitution is one that has an increased susceptibility to illness.

Susceptibility is simply the degree to which a person is vulnerable to an outside influence. In an epidemic not everyone will be affected (the germ theory of disease fails to take this into account). We call those who are affected 'susceptible'. Their predisposition is due to an underlying constitutional weakness that is either inherited or due to past and/or current stress (mental, emotional or physical), and which makes the person open to certain disease conditions.

If your grandparents all died of old age and your parents have been basically healthy all their lives; if your birth was planned and your mother was healthy throughout her pregnancy (didn't smoke, drink, etc.); if your parents' marriage is happy and your birth was uneventful, then your constitution should be of the strongest variety.

If, on the other hand, all your grandparents died at early ages of cancer or heart disease and one of your parents had tuberculosis as a child and the other suffered from asthma and eczema, then your chances of inheriting a weak constitution are greater. You can still escape the worst of a poor inheritance if your parents' marriage is a happy one and they have taken good care of their own health.

It may help you to think of your constitution as a huge energy bank. At birth some people have vast reserves, both on deposit and in their current account. Others have only a nominal amount in the current account and need to be paying into that account constantly throughout their lives in order to 'stay in the black' – in order to stay healthy.

And that is where alternative medicine comes in. Many people come to a homeopath for 'constitutional treatment' – in other words to improve their general health rather than wait until they fall ill. The value of constitutional treatment is that it boosts the weak constitution and decreases its susceptibility to disease.

VITAL FORCE

Homeopaths believe there is a balancing mechanism that keeps us in health, provided that the stresses on our constitutions are neither too prolonged nor too great. This balancing mechanism Hahnemann called the 'vital force' and he believed it to be that energetic substance, independent of physical and chemical forces, that literally gives us life and is absent at our death.

The human organism, indeed any living thing, has a unique relationship with its environment. Biologists call it 'homeostasis', by which they mean that a healthy living being is self-regulating, with an innate (protective) tendency to maintain equilibrium and compensate for disruptive changes. Homeopaths believe that the vital force produces symptoms to counteract the various stresses we experience, and that it makes adjustments moment by moment throughout our lives to keep us healthy and balanced. These symptoms, then, are simply the body's way of telling us how it is coping with stress. Obvious examples are shivering when cold, perspiring when overheated and eating or drinking when hungry or thirsty. All these reactions help to ensure the regulation of a constant, life-preserving environment within the body.

Familiar expressions such as 'defence mechanism', and 'immune system' are another way of referring to the vital force. Homeopaths believe that disease 'attacks' only when this vital force is weakened.

Homeopathic medicines act as a catalyst, the energy of the remedy stimulating the body's own vital force (its immune system or defence mechanism) to heal itself. They do not weaken the defence mechanism by suppressing it as do many orthodox medicines. The correct homeopathic treatment not only alleviates the symptoms but enables the patient to feel that life is once again flowing harmoniously. Patients often remark that they haven't felt so well in a long time.

ACUTE AND CHRONIC DISEASES

Acute disease is self-limiting; in other words, it is not deep-seated and, given time, will usually clear of its own accord. Some acute illnesses, such as pneumonia, meningitis or nephritis for example, are extremely serious and can, rarely, be fatal. These are not within the scope of the home prescriber and always need expert advice.

An acute disease has three definite stages: *the incubation period*, when there may be no symptoms of disease: *the acute phase*, when the recognisable symptoms surface; *the convalescent stage*, when a person usually improves.

Coughs, colds, flus, food poisoning and children's illnesses such as chicken pox are all examples of acute illnesses. Well-chosen homeopathic remedies will speed up recovery, alleviate pain and ensure that there are no complications.

See pages 203–26 for the acute illnesses you can and cannot treat using this book.

Chronic disease is more deep-seated than acute disease. It develops slowly, continues for a long time and is often accompanied by a general deterioration in health. The development of the disease does not take a predictable course; neither is it possible to say for how long it will last. (An acute illness that is followed by complications can develop into a chronic, long-term illness.)

Arthritis, heart disease, cancer and mental illness are all examples of chronic illness. Homeopaths believe that the increase in incidence of these conditions we are now seeing is in part due to the chemical stresses the individual has to put up with, including the over-use of orthodox medicines and environmental pollution.

MIASMS

In the early years of his practice Hahnemann was puzzled to find that some patients failed to respond to their constitutional remedies and some patients who did improve relapsed after only a short time. He collected these 'difficult' cases together and after much painstaking study found a common factor in the presence of certain diseases in the personal or family history of such patients. He realised these diseases must constitute blocks to health which stopped the indicated constitutional remedy from working. He called these blocks 'miasms' and developed a comprehensive and complex theory around them. His insights have enabled the professional homeopath to assess through the history of a patient (both personal and inherited) their likely constitutional strength and, in many cases, to predict the sort of blocks that he or she might encounter during the course of constitutional treatment.

Hahnemann defined three basic miasms which he believed to be the underlying causes of chronic disease, each of which predisposes a person to a particular range of health problems which he also defined at length. The three miasms were: *Psora*, which he associated with suppressed skin diseases and with leprosy; *Sycosis*, associated with suppressed gonorrhoea; and *Syphilis*, associated with suppressed syphilis.

Homeopaths have since added many more and believe that cancer is a 'marriage' of the miasms – it is present in people whose inherited picture includes all three miasms and more.

When the homeopath encounters a 'miasmatic block' in a patient, and the indicated remedy does not act, the block must be cleared. There are various methods for doing this, but it is a matter for the professional homeopath, not for self-treatment.

THE LAWS OF CURE

The Laws of Cure were formulated by Constantine Hering (see page 7), who based them on a lifetime's observation of the processes involved when sick patients became cured. Throughout his years of practice he was able to draw the following conclusions:

- As someone is cured, symptoms move from the innermost organs of the body (those most vital to life) to the outer organs. In other words, cure moves from within to without. For example, someone with heart disease (serious, life threatening) may experience stomach or bowel problems during the process of cure.
- Cure also takes place from above to below, so that symptoms usually 'drip off' the body, starting from the head and clearing downwards, with the hands and the feet (sometimes simultaneously) being the last to be affected (with, say, a skin eruption).

- Symptoms that have been suppressed in the past often resurface during the process of cure and usually do so in the reverse order from their original sequence. For example, if a patient with heart disease had been successfully treated with orthodox medicines for a stomach ulcer before the heart condition, then the appearance of stomach symptoms (less severe than in the original complaint) would be welcomed as a sign that the old suppressed symptoms were being cleared out. These laws apply to the treatment of chronic complaints but occasionally also to acute prescribing – so if an old symptom surfaces after a good prescription, wait to see if it will clear of its own accord. If it does, the remedy is still working . . . carry on waiting.

The suppression of a disease usually leads to a more deep-seated illness surfacing. For example, many children whose eczema has been 'successfully' treated with steroids may suffer from asthma at a later date. These two events are seen by the orthodox medical profession as having only a casual connection, whereas the homeopath believes that the suppression of the eczema has caused the asthma. Successful homeopathic treatment involves the eczema reappearing at some point.

It is also possible to suppress with homeopathic medicines by treating a single symptom and not therefore taking the whole person into account.

Homeopaths use these Laws of Cure to monitor treatment, to check whether the cure is going in the 'right' direction. As far as acute treatment or home prescribing is concerned, occasionally a very well-selected constitutional remedy will push to the surface old symptoms that may have been forgotten. These will clear of their own accord. It is important not to prescribe another remedy and by so doing encourage the chronic condition to go back 'in' again.

HEALTH

Health is more than simply the absence of disease. Being healthy gives us a sense of well-being, of being balanced, of personal freedom. It is above all the ability to withstand stress.

When we are physically healthy we have strength and flexibility, and a reservoir of energy to draw on should we need it. Being emotionally healthy means we can acknowledge and express our feelings and by so doing maintain rewarding relationships. Being mentally healthy enables us to think clearly, to formulate ideas, solve problems and make decisions easily.

Disease limits that personal freedom; a broken leg, for example, limits a person's physical freedom by making it difficult to walk, to be physical. A depression can limit a person's emotional freedom because of his or her difficulty in interacting with other people, and so on. Mental exhaustion after, say, a taxing exam makes it difficult to concentrate and to make decisions and therefore limits a person's mental freedom. If you do fall ill it is often useful to ask yourself how and why that illness is limiting you.

The orthodox medical view, or germ theory, of disease is that illness is a 'bad' thing. An alternative medical view is that disease is a 'good' thing, alerting the body to the necessity of taking some time and space to have a good clear-out. I think that disease is neither good nor bad. The disease we succumb to provides us with information about our personal weaknesses, about how we are living our lives and coping with stress. It alerts us to the fact that there are deficiencies or weaknesses that need attention.

Building health – preventative medicine

The desire to rid the body of disease is a healthy attitude, although any approach that involves building health and therefore preventing disease or ill-health will, of course, be of greater benefit in the long term than any temporary suppression of the symptoms alone. How we approach illness, as well as the treatment we choose, deserves some thought.

The presence of disease or pain often creates anxiety, which in turn can lead to fear and panic. In this situation most of us at one time or another have consulted an authoritative figure (a doctor) to allay our anxiety by putting a name to what is happening to our bodies, and to determine how it must be treated. The danger here is that, in looking outside ourselves for the answers and in asking too few questions, we experience a loss of personal control with consequent feelings of helplessness. We give up our responsibility

for our own health to the people 'in charge' and we become real patients, or, as I see it, victims.

In this situation we may find that we feel unable to confide misgivings, to express our instincts about our own health, or to explore other options. We become passive consumers of medical care. For example, women who are not well informed on the subject of contraception and who then begin to have trouble with the contraceptive pill, will, on voicing their worries and symptoms, be reassured that the Pill is perfectly safe, that there is nothing to worry about and that their problem is psychosomatic. This is usually not true and these women then suffer needlessly for months and sometimes years because they carry on taking a drug that doesn't suit them.

How do we, as patients, redress this balance? The first step is to become informed, by reading and talking to people who are sympathetic to our views (and doubts), and who may have had similar experiences. We also need to learn to ask for what we need, to make realistic demands of health-care professionals. We need to seek the help of doctors and specialists (both orthodox and alternative) who are willing to communicate with us, who are able to acknowledge that we, the patients, have a part to play in our own healing processes and are therefore able to give us the information we need (and deserve) about what they think is happening.

By taking responsibility for what happens to our bodies we can then start creating for ourselves the balance *we* want in our own lives, and we can start tuning into our own feelings, or inner sense, of what is wrong with us. By developing this positive approach towards creating a healthy life for ourselves we can move away from automatically taking a defensive position towards illness.

Ultimately, being involved in our own healing processes gives us self-confidence, increases our personal strength and gives us more choices.

·3·
MYTHS
AND
MISAPPREHENSIONS

Many homeopaths, believing that the explanation of how homeopathy works is secondary to its success with literally millions of patients, have traditionally refused to reveal the names of the medicines they give. This and the lack of information they have provided about their practice has led to an aura of secrecy in which myths abound. It is worth looking at a few of these misapprehensions.

Myth: 'Homeopathy is safe'

In the same way that homeopathy can cure – dramatically and permanently in many cases – it can also cause harm. Kent said that he would rather share a room with a nest of vipers than be subjected to the administrations of an inexperienced homeopath! Potential dangers are:

Unintentional provings

If you take too many homeopathic pills over a period of time it is possible to 'prove' the remedy – that is, to suffer from the symptoms that the remedy was supposed to cure. This can mean that although your own symptoms may improve initially, they may worsen again if you continue to take the pills. Worse still, if the remedy did not fit your picture – was not right for you – you may experience symptoms you never had before.

This is a danger with self-prescribing or over-the-counter prescribing, where there is no professional homeopath to monitor the symptoms. In my first year in practice a woman rang me one day in a frantic state, desperate for help. She told me the following story:

I asked for help at a homeopathic chemist for thrush, which I had suffered from for several months, and was prescribed Nux vomica 30 *over the counter and told to take it three times daily. After a few days I experienced a marked improvement in my condition, so I carried on taking it. After a week of no further changes my symptoms started to get worse so I carried on taking it. I finished the bottle of pills and went back to the pharmacy and told them my thrush was now as bad as when I had started taking the remedy. They gave me another bottle of* Nux vomica 30 *and told me to continue with the treatment. It is now two months since I started on this remedy and my thrush is unbearable. It is so bad I can't sleep at night and I am irritable all the time. Please help me.*

I advised this woman to stop taking the pills and to antidote the remedy with strong coffee and camphorated ointment (to counteract its effects) and within twenty-four hours she was back to her old self, having slept well for the first time in over a month. The thrush was back to where it had been before she took the *Nux vomica* – annoying but manageable.

A colleague of mine tells of a six-month-old baby who was treated at a local hospital as an emergency out-patient in a state of collapse. The nurse on duty was a student of my colleague's and discovered that the mother had been giving her baby *Chamomilla 6* several times a day for colic since soon after birth. As soon as the homeopathic remedy was discontinued for a period of time the muscle tone returned.

It is important to be on your guard against this over-use of homeopathic medicines. Read carefully Chapter 6 before you start prescribing.

Confusion of the symptom picture

If a remedy has not been prescribed on the whole person it will work in a limited way, curing a restricted number of symptoms. In these cases some complaints remain and it is possible to end up giving one remedy after another in order to try to 'get rid' of the remaining symptoms. In the end the whole picture becomes so changed that it is difficult to find the *similimum* (that single remedy that was needed at the very beginning).

The professional homeopath has different ways of dealing with this phenomenon in order to get back to the original symptom picture. If you find that you are prescribing one remedy after another with only limited effect, then do get professional help.

Suppression

A homeopathic remedy can cure a superficial symptom such as a skin eruption in the same way that, for example, the application of a Cortisone cream can. This will only be the case if the remedy has been prescribed on the skin complaint (single symptom) without taking into account the whole person and/or the cause. The effect is to push the disease further into the body (see Laws of Cure, page 15). Constitutional treatment will often commence with the original symptom resurfacing. Suppression is not common in homeopathy but *is* possible. In self-prescribing, if your complaint disappears but *you* feel much worse in yourself (i.e. your moods and your energy) then it is likely that you have made a poor choice of remedy – antidote it and get some professional advice.

Myth: 'Homeopathy is a form of herbalism'

In my experience, this is the commonest myth of all. While it is certainly true that a proportion of the remedies a homeopath uses are based on plants, and though, as in homeopathy, the herbalist prescribes on the individual, the principles that govern the two therapies are quite different.

Many plants have known healing properties; herbalism is concerned with the known sphere of action of a plant based on its chemical constituents as well as its known healing qualities. Herbalism has existed for thousands of years – for as long as we have records – in some form or another and has its roots in mother earth. It is the only form of medicine used by animals.

Homeopathy, on the other hand, is based on a very different set of principles (see Chapter 2). Homeopathic remedies are not used in the material dose; nor are they based solely on plants, using as they do poisons, metals and disease products. Homeopaths generally prescribe one remedy at a time rather than the mixtures of plant tinctures that herbalists employ. And, of course, homeopathy in its modern form is a mere 180 years old.

Myth: 'Homeopathy is a form of vaccination'

People often say that they understand homeopathy to be like a vaccination in that the patient is given a small quantity of the disease he already has in order to make him immune to it.

This is not true. Homeopathy and vaccination have *similar*, not the *same*, concepts and very different practices. Vaccines work on the physical body in a very specific way, in that they stimulate the immune system directly to produce specific antibodies *as if* that person had contracted that particular disease; in so doing they are, of course, stressing the immune system. Many vaccines have been known to produce permanent side effects. They must be tested on animals and then on humans to verify their safety, and even then children and adults are often damaged on a physical, emotional or mental level.

A homeopathic remedy works in a totally different way, as a reading of Chapter 2 will again bear out. Homeopathic remedies affect the energy patterns or the vital force of a person and by so doing stimulate the body to heal itself. They are administered orally in a diluted (and safe) dose as opposed to being introduced directly into the bloodstream, as is the case with vaccination, thereby bypassing the body's natural defence system and stressing it in a way that is not fully understood. Homeopathic medicines are not tested on innocent animals and do not have side effects.

Myth: 'Homeopathic remedies are placebos'

This myth can be rephrased to read 'You need to believe in it for it to work.' This is patently ridiculous to anyone who has experienced or prescribed a successful homeopathic cure for, say, a head injury or a middle-ear infection.

A placebo is an unmedicated pill which the patient believes contains something that will cure him or her. Double-blind trials always involve the inclusion of a control group taking a placebo instead of the medicine being tested in order to rule out the individual's 'suggestibility'.

It is because homeopathic remedies do not always work that they are sometimes believed to be ineffective, and, because routine prescriptions such as *Rhus toxicodendron* for rheumatism and *Chamomilla* for teething babies are freely available from high-street chemists, people are wrongly persuaded into thinking that they need not consult a homeopath (or an adequate first-aid book). If the remedies do not work it is assumed that homeopathy does not work; if they *do* work it is attributed to a placebo effect – some double blind!

Homeopathic medicines work effectively on babies and animals, neither of whom are open to being affected by placebos.

It is always essential to individualise the remedy to fit the patient and not the disease, to ensure that the underlying principles are observed so that the element of chance is decreased and homeopathy can be seen to work.

Of course, there are many people who will recognise the experience of consulting a practitioner who inspires belief and hope, who left them feeling buoyant and encouraged. But if this initial rapport is not backed up with good solid prescribing, then no amount of that positive 'transference' will cure the patient.

Myth: 'Homeopathy is mysterious and unscientific'

The fact that homeopathic medicines are prepared in a pharmacy or a laboratory and that their preparation involves a particular technique subject to precise and clearly stated controls (it does not involve mysterious and secret processes which put it into the realm of white magic or alchemy) is enough to convince many people of its validity.

Homeopaths have traditionally justified their practice by their results, without feeling a need to explain how their methods work. The homeopathic philosophy or doctrine is a set of rules for practice – one that hasn't changed since it was formulated 180 years ago. These rules and principles constitute a unified hypothesis whose validity is tested out empirically – with cured patients confirming the hypothesis.

Harris Coulter, in his book *Homœopathic Science and Modern Medicine (The Physics of Healing with Microdoses)*, discusses this issue at great length and also describes many of the trials that have been conducted over the past fifty years or so using plants, animals and humans as controls to prove the effectiveness of homeopathic medicines.

·4·
TAKING
THE
CASE

It is well worth the effort to approach first-aid prescribing seriously by teaching yourself how to take a case and how to work out the right remedy. That is the major concern of this book: to help you to prescribe in the same way that a professional homeopath would. There are many books on the market that take the 'symptomatic approach', directing you to a remedy on the strength of one symptom or complaint. In my opinion this is not thorough enough and the results cannot be guaranteed. In this book, therefore, I have taken a more classical approach, which involves looking at the whole person in a more detailed way.

Throughout the book I have assumed that you are prescribing for someone else. If you fall ill and wish to prescribe for yourself then the same principles apply, but it is important to remember that it is difficult to be objective about your own symptoms, and you may be fooled into prescribing the wrong remedy. For example, you may feel quite normal and calm in yourself while everyone around you has experienced a sharp increase in your levels of irritability and touchiness; and/or you may already have forgotten the drenching you got the day before you fell ill. It can be most useful to talk through your case before you self-prescribe. Some people are highly competent at knowing exactly what their 'symptom picture' is and are clear about the stresses that led up to their illness; others need more help. Do get that help if you need it.

Before you begin to take the case, check that the complaint is within the scope of this book. Don't attempt to prescribe for a chronic disease; these always need professional attention. See also pages 203–26 for diseases you can treat using this book.

THE SYMPTOM PICTURE

I have used the word **complaint** throughout the book to mean the disease itself, or rather its label; for example 'sore throat' or 'cough'. The **symptoms** are the visible signs of the complaint. Say your child is complaining of a barking cough that is worse at night and better for sitting up. The complaint is the cough, and the symptoms are barking, worse at night and better for sitting up. So the complaint expresses itself through the symptoms.

The **symptom picture** is a detailed account of what is wrong with you as a whole when you fall ill. Your symptoms – the signs or indications of your being ill – are a form of expression and a call for help from your body. A homeopathic prescriber is a symptom sleuth! In order for a remedy to work well you need to match, as accurately as possible, the patient's symptom picture with that of a **remedy picture** – the collection of symptoms produced by the remedy in its proving, as set out in the Materia Medica. It doesn't have to be identical, merely similar.

Your observations are therefore very important. You are not simply looking for aches and pains; you need to get a picture of the *differences* in the patient from her normal state of health. Gathering information is not always easy. Look for clear, strongly marked symptoms; vague, 'well . . . sometimes' symptoms don't count unless they present a 'changeable' symptom picture in themselves.

Certain symptoms are always present in any given disease and are indicated in its name. For example, pain during urination is usually called cystitis; certain types of skin rashes are called eczema; inflamed, bloodshot eyes are often called conjunctivitis. Homeopathy does not treat the labelled disease alone – the cystitis, the eczema, the conjunctivitis; it treats the individual who is sick. No two cases of cystitis are exactly the same. Every labelled disease (or complaint) is also accompanied by symptoms peculiar to the individual who has it, and differs from another case of the same 'disease'. It is these individual characteristics in the patient that guide us to the right homeopathic remedy.

Simply to write 'headache' or 'cough' is not enough. If you look either of these symptoms up in the Repertory you will find many remedies listed. It is the particular symptoms of the patient's headache or cough that enable you to begin to narrow down the choice of remedies, to individualise the case. One person with a headache, for example, will have a throbbing forehead that feels better for fresh air, while another will have sharp pains in the temples that are better for warmth and lying down. They call for different remedies.

For homeopathic purposes, symptoms are divided into three categories: **general**, **mental/emotional** and **physical complaints**. See pages 227–8 for definitions and checklists to use while note-taking.

Note-taking

It is essential that you write down your patient's symptoms, and also that you record the remedy you give as well as its result. Even if you write only a few words plus the date, the name and the potency of the remedy, that will suffice to remind you should the same problem recur.

I suggest you open a loose-leaf file marked 'Health' and use it for keeping interesting articles as well as for keeping notes on the people for whom you prescribe.

The case-taking questionnaire on page 227 should remind you of the questions to ask to get the information you need. Make your questions general rather than specific. Try not to put words into your patient's mouth.

General	Specific
How are you feeling?	Are you feeling sad?
How painful is it?	Does it hurt a lot?
Can you describe the pain?	Is it throbbing?
Does heat or cold help or aggravate?	Is it better for heat?
Can you tell me some more about what happened?	
Is there anything that makes you or your symptoms feel better or worse?	

Give some attention to your first impressions of what is happening: they are an important and reliable source of information. Say your child wakes up in the night screaming. You go into her room. What do you immediately smell and see? What note do you hear in the scream? Is it one of pain or of fright? Or say your best friend has flu and you have been asked to come and help. You walk into the room and what do you see before she has organised herself to be sociable with you? Is the room tidy or messy? Is it hot or cold? Does she look very sad and tired before she makes an effort

to 'be fine'? Do not ignore first impressions: they can provide you with more information than an hour's case taking.

If remedies do come to mind as you are talking, do not ignore them but write them in the margin: those initial instincts can be inspired. Generally speaking it is better to forget about working out a remedy while you take the case; this analytical part comes later. Concentrate on using your senses to pick up clues and on being receptive to what your patient is telling you.

What do you smell?
The smell is often the first thing you notice on walking into a sick person's room. Smell the head/neck/hands of a feverish or sick child and you will find that perspiration can smell sweet, sour, salty, musty or offensive. Smell the breath, too. Other discharges can also smell 'interesting'; for example, the stools of a teething baby can smell very sour, the urine strong, the vomit offensive. If the smell is strong and you can describe it clearly, write it down and use it as a symptom.

What do you see?
In the case of an illness, note the colour and expression on the face of your patient. In the case of an accident, note whether the colour has drained from the face of a shocked person or if they have become flushed and look anxious.

Look for clues: drinks not drunk; covers piled high or, alternatively, kicked off; restlessness; log-like patients who groan if you sit on the edge of the bed and disturb them; and so on. You will often learn more than the patient herself is aware of.

What do you feel?
Feel the skin to find out whether there is sweat. If so, is it hot or cold, sticky or watery? A dry skin with a fever, for example, is an important symptom. Check the parts of the body to feel if there are temperature variations – hot head and cold hands, for example – or whether some parts of the body are sweaty and others aren't. Perhaps your patient is complaining of an inner, burning heat while the skin feels cold to the touch?

What do you hear?
What noises can you hear? Some sick children moan in their sleep; others might whine for attention if they think you are not listening and stop when you enter the room (or vice versa!). Listen to the tone of the voice. Is it resigned? Anxious? Sad? Angry? Even the grinding of the teeth in a child, either during the day or in sleep, can be a valuable symptom.

Let your patient talk, without any interruption from you if possible. This in itself can be healing, and can also provide you with information. For example, the *Lachesis* patient talks incessantly, jumping from one subject to another, while the *Bryonia* patient will not want to talk at all.

Some people will reply negatively when asked about themselves or their symptoms: 'I'm not well'; 'He's not bad'; 'It isn't much better'; 'It doesn't hurt that much'. These replies do not tell you what is actually happening. Questions like 'How are you, then?', 'What *are* you feeling?' can sometimes help, but people who speak in negatives often need careful questioning to tell you what is wrong. In answer to 'It doesn't hurt that much,' you could ask 'Is the pain stopping you from doing anything?' (that is, 'How serious is it?'). Then you can go on to give a list of different types of pain and if your patient alights on one, saying 'That's it!', then write it down. If they are not sure, go on to another question.

Finally, remember . . .

Do not discount anything! What other information do you have about that person? What has been going on in her life lately that might be part of why she is feeling sick now? What have you been told by her mother/father/son/neighbour? Have you given this person a first-aid remedy before, say for a flu? Did the remedy work well? If that remedy worked marvellously, consider whether it might be indicated again.

I have included a number of checklists (page 227) to help as reminders until you are more familiar with the process of taking a homeopathic case.

WORKING OUT THE REMEDY

Classifying the symptoms

Having taken your case (noted your patient's symptoms), follow these basic steps to select your remedy: choose your symptoms; repertorise; differentiate. (You will develop your own way of working and be able to take short cuts as you become familiar with the processes.)

1 Choose your symptoms

Go through your case and underline all the symptoms that stand out clearly and strongly. It is best to leave vague or unclear symptoms alone for the moment, but they may sway your decision at the end if you can't make up your mind between two or more remedies. However, if you can prescribe a remedy on the strong symptoms of your case, your prescription is more likely to be effective.

Wherever possible, choose at least three strong symptoms, each from a different symptom group. You *can* prescribe on a single symptom but this is rarely successful: to make an effective prescription you need at least one symptom from each of the main groups – general, physical and mental/emotional. If you work out a remedy based on a symptom from each of these groups you can be confident that it has a good chance of working. If you add in a stress symptom you can be even surer of your prescription, and so on. In other words, the more symptoms that fit the remedy picture the better.

Write down the symptoms on a separate sheet of paper or on a blank repertorising chart (see page 230).

2 Repertorise

As you become more and more familiar with the remedy pictures you will learn to recognise the remedy your patient needs without repertorising. In fact, 'repertorising' sounds much more complicated than it is. Simply look up in the Repertory each symptom you have noted and list the remedies that occur under each symptom (or alternatively tick them off on the repertorising chart). When you have completed the list you will be able to see clearly which remedy or remedies occur most often – i.e. which contain all the symptoms on your list.

3 Differentiate

In some cases only one remedy will contain all your symptoms. Go to the Materia Medica and read through the full remedy picture to check that it 'fits'. If it does, then prescribe that remedy, following the potency and dosage guidelines set out on page 27.

Often, however, more than one remedy will contain all your symptoms, or several remedies will have most of your symptoms and none will have all of them. If more than one remedy *is* indicated according to the repertorising chart, choosing between them can be difficult; it is one of the skills that makes a competent homeopath. You need to read through each of the remedies that has all or most of your patient's symptoms and pick the one that fits best.

If you can't find a remedy that fits your patient's picture, then go back to your chart and see if you have missed any remedies. Also check your case for missed symptoms. Add these to your list and repertorise them. Then read through any new remedies that emerge through this process. Repeat these steps until you find a remedy that fits your patient and his or her symptoms. If you are really stuck, you may have to go back to your patient to get new information.

This whole process is brought to life in the sample cases (pages 231–44); make sure you read them before you start prescribing.

NB Your general and emotional/mental symptoms may point to a remedy that does not list the complaint that you are suffering from in its picture. For example, you have flu and are feeling restless, irritable, hot and bothered and extremely thirsty. You find that *Sulphur* comes up strongly for all your symptoms but isn't listed under Flu in the Repertory. The closest remedy is *Bryonia* but *Bryonia* isn't restless. Read through both remedy pictures to see which one fits best; it will probably be *Sulphur* – the one that does not have flu in its picture – in which case *Sulphur* will work more effectively because it covers the whole picture. If the strong general and emotional/mental symptoms point to one remedy then give it even if it doesn't have your physical complaint listed in its picture.

Conversely, certain remedies work well when prescribed on the physical symptoms alone, for example *Natrum muriaticum* for cold sores. However, it will work much better if there are other *Natrum muriaticum* symptoms from the general and/or the emotional/ mental sections.

·5·
PRESCRIBING

WHEN TO PRESCRIBE

Never rush into prescribing, and don't think that you have to give a remedy just because you have the book and someone wants you to. If you don't feel right about prescribing or about giving a remedy to someone (for example, if you don't know the person very well), then don't do it. Let them go to a professional homeopath if they have one, or to their own GP. If, when you have taken the case, you are at all unsure about your choice of remedy – if no remedy is strongly indicated for your patient – then don't prescribe. There are only ninety-six internal remedies in this Materia Medica and, although they cover a very large number of acute conditions, they won't cover them all.

If you are prescribing for an acute illness and your patient is already under the care of a professional homeopath, it is essential that the homeopath is consulted before you prescribe. It is better to give nothing than to interfere with what may be an aggravation of some sort and therefore not fully understood by you.

In an accident or an emergency you should give the indicated remedy (*Arnica*, *Aconite* or *Hypericum*, for example) immediately, but make sure that you write down the remedy and the responses so that you can pass on the information to the professional homeopath.

WHOM TO PRESCRIBE FOR

Babies and children respond very well to homeopathic treatment. If for some reason they do not respond to your first-aid prescriptions, seek the advice of a professional homeopath rather than struggle on with the possibility of making a mess of their case. As children grow up it is always useful to *ask* them if they need a remedy, if they need help to get better. We all have the ability to heal ourselves; the homeopathic remedy taps this resource and puts us in touch with it. Many children have and can develop the ability to heal themselves if they are encouraged to do so. My own child will now always tell me if he needs a remedy after an accident or in an acute illness. Mostly he says to me, 'It's OK, Mum, I don't need anything. I can get better by myself.' If you introduce this concept to a child it will be picked up quite quickly. Adults take a little longer!

When prescribing for adults, however close they may be to you, you should remember this rule: prescribe only if the patient asks you for help. Over-zealousness can be very off-putting and if you force a remedy on to someone the chances of its being sabotaged by antidoting (see page 27) are very high. If there is an improvement, it will be attributed to a coincidence anyway. It is always possible to offer help and leave it at that, but don't get into the way of thinking that you can cure anybody and everybody of their complaints. If someone comes to you, then fine. By all means take the case and see what you can do, but do not impinge on other people's rights to look after their own health in their own way.

If you are self-prescribing, it is always advisable to discuss your remedy with a friend to make sure that you are not deluding yourself about your true state of body and mind.

THE REMEDIES

The forms available

Homeopathic remedies are most commonly available in tablet form. The tablets are made of sugar of cow's milk, or saccharum lactose, commonly known as *sac lac*; this has been found to be the ideal medium for the potentised remedy. *Sac lac* comes in several forms – hard or soft tablets, globules or powders. Most homeopathic pharmacies will automatically make up remedies in the form of hard *sac lac* tablets unless they are specifically asked otherwise.

Listed below are the different forms a homeopathic remedy can take. In each case a few drops of the potentised remedy in alcohol is used to medicate (or moisten) the base substance.

Soft tablets (sac lac). New Era Tissue Salts use these tablets which dissolve quickly and easily under the tongue and are also easily crushed for administering to babies.

Hard tablets (sac lac). Tablets made by Weleda and Nelson's fall into this category and do not dissolve as easily as the soft tablets. They should be chewed and held in the mouth for a few seconds before being swallowed.

Globules (sac lac) are tiny round pills, like poppy seeds. It is usually suggested that a lidful be given as a single dose, though theoretically one grain should suffice.

Sucrose is sometimes used as the medium. Sceptics are always taken aback when a couple of grains of 'sugar' are seen to cure a severely bruised head. I find that a few grains tipped on to the palm of the hand and dissolved on the tongue are enough.

Alcohol. Children or adults known to be allergic to cow's milk may ask for their homeopathic remedies to be made up in liquid form. These remedies come in dropper bottles and the potentised substance has been added to an alcohol base. The dose is either administered neat (although children do not usually like this) or diluted in water. A dose of 6–10 drops is adequate.

Powders (sac lac). Most homeopathic pharmacies can make up remedies in powders. These are wrapped individually in small squares of paper and are convenient if you need only a few doses of an unusual remedy that you are unlikely to want again, or if you need to send small quantities by mail – especially abroad. They should be dissolved under the tongue like soft tablets or added to a small amount of water and sipped as frequently as needed.

Wafers. Selected pharmacies can make up remedies in wafers, which, like powders, are wrapped individually. The wafers are made out of rice paper, which is useful for people sensitive to milk and sugar.

Storing remedies

Homeopathic tablets will keep their strength for years without deteriorating. Remedies made over a hundred years ago still work well. They must be stored in a cool, dark, dry place with their tops screwed on tightly, well away from strong-smelling substances, because strong smells do make the pills lose their potency. It is not a good idea to keep them in a bathroom cabinet alongside perfumes, cough mixtures, etc., or in a spare-room cupboard with the mothballs. A sealed plastic container like an ice-cream tub is good for storing loose bottles. Or you may choose to purchase one of the ready-made kits that are available from many pharmacies, to your own specifications if you wish. The appendix on building up a first-aid kit will help you with this (see page 249).

It is wise to keep all tablets out of reach of children as a matter of course. If your child gets her hands on a bottle of pills and eats the entire first-aid kit in one glorious secret feast, do not panic. Your bank balance is the only thing that will suffer. A single dose at one time is a single dose, whether it it is one pill or one bottle of pills – for example, eating a full bottle of *Chamomilla 6* tablets would have the same effect as taking one single pill.

How to take remedies

When taking a homeopathic tablet, carefully tip one into the lid of the bottle. If you tip more than one out, tip the others back so that only one remains. Tip it out on to the palm of the patient's hand and then replace the lid on the bottle. The patient *can* touch his or her own tablet, but if you are giving the remedy to someone else try to avoid touching it. Never put back tablets that have fallen out on to the floor or anywhere else. In so doing you may contaminate your stock; always throw away any that have been dropped or are unused.

Ideally tablets should be dissolved under the tongue where they are readily absorbed into the body; if they are swallowed whole they become mixed with the stomach acids and are thought to work less effectively.

It is preferable not to eat, drink (except water), smoke or brush your teeth for twenty minutes before and after taking a remedy. This gives it the best possible chance of working. It is sometimes difficult with babies and small children; if you have managed a five-minute gap either side of taking the remedy you are probably OK. The twenty-minute gap makes sure that any residue of food does not affect the action of the remedy. (Homeopaths tend to differ in their opinions on this subject.)

Many of the homeopathic remedies available in the high-street chemist or wholefood shop give dosage instructions on the bottle. They often suggest different doses for adults (two tablets) and children (one tablet). This is illogical, given that there is not a measurable quantity of the medicine in the tablet. The size of the dose is immaterial; it is how often that it is taken that counts. I always instruct my patients to take one tablet, whether they are young or old.

Giving tablets to babies and animals or semi-conscious patients can be difficult. They can be crushed between two spoons and given as a powder which prevents spitting out and also won't cause the patient to choke. If necessary, a little spring water can be added to the crushed powder on the spoon, or the tablet can be dissolved in a very clean glass with a little water. It should be stirred vigorously and then given as needed, a teaspoonful at a time. In these instances, the glass and spoon should be scoured (with boiled water) after use so that the next person to use them doesn't get an inadvertent dose of the remedy.

HOW MANY DOSES AND HOW OFTEN?

Having selected the remedy for your patient, you will need to decide on the dose. This will depend upon the urgency of the case: frequent doses for an acute illness that has come on suddenly and strongly, and less frequent doses for a slowly developing illness. Some earaches with very severely distressed patients need their remedies repeating every five minutes; a head injury may need the remedy repeating every half-hour; and a slowly developing flu may need a remedy every four hours or three times a day. The dosage chart (page 27) will help you to decide how often you should give the remedy you have selected.

Prescribe up to six pills according to the urgency of the case. If you have given six pills and there has been no change whatsoever, then it is probably the wrong remedy.

Once you see that a homeopathic remedy has started to work – once you notice a definite reaction or change resulting from the remedy – then continue with the same remedy but give it less often (that is, increase the gaps between the doses) as the patient continues to improve.

Once there is a *marked* improvement – once a strong positive reaction has occurred – it is essential to stop taking the remedy altogether. This is the absolute opposite of the instructions you receive when taking orthodox medicines (for example, antibiotics), where it is often necessary to finish the whole course of pills. A homeopathic remedy acts as a trigger, a catalyst – it stimulates the body to begin to heal itself, and once that has happened the body's own healing process will take over. In some cases, taking another tablet after this reaction has occurred can actually stop the remedy working and even exaggerate the symptoms (see 'Provings', page 11), and consequently you can be persuaded into thinking that it was a poor prescription.

WHAT POTENCY?

Homeopathic remedies come in different potencies, as we have seen (page 13). The 6X, 6C and the 12C are all safe potencies for the home prescriber. The 6X and 6C are the most widely available; they are fine for first-aid prescribing and are the best potencies to use for less serious complaints. I personally prefer the 12C for first-aid as it is slightly stronger than the 6C. If you are ordering a kit from a pharmacy you can order the remedies in a potency of your choice.

Many people stock remedies in the 30C potency – the highest of the low-potency range. As it is stronger still than the 12C, fewer doses are needed. It tends to work faster and is used for more serious complaints, such as bad burns or head injuries with concussion.

I suggest that first of all you become familiar with the 6X, 6C and 12C potencies in order to understand how they work before trying the 30C.

Dosage guidelines

- Stop on improvement.
- Start again if the same symptoms return – i.e. repeat as needed.
- If you have given six doses and have had no response, stop and reassess the case or seek advice.
- Change the remedy if the symptom picture changes.
- If the patient is already receiving homeopathic treatment, if possible consult the homeopath before prescribing (unless it is an emergency).

ALWAYS SEEK PROFESSIONAL HELP IF YOUR SYMPTOMS RECUR OR DO NOT IMPROVE.

ASSESSING THE RESPONSE TO A REMEDY

I like to think of a homeopathic remedy as a pebble, which when thrown into a pond simply goes 'plop'. It is the ripples that it causes within the body that are the healing responses. The job of the prescriber is to get the pill as close to the middle of the pond as possible.

If you have given six doses and have had no significant response then the remedy you have chosen is likely to be wrong. You need to reassess the case and check your repertorising. Did you have more than one remedy to choose from? How did you make your choice? Check your symptoms. If you are convinced that your choice of remedy was correct, then persevere for another three to six doses – unless your patient is seriously ill, in which case seek immediate professional help.

DOSAGE CHART

Degree of Seriousness	Potency	Dosage
Very serious Symptoms need immediate attention and are usually accompanied by great pain – e.g. earache; head or back injury; second- or third-degree burn; cystitis; etc.	6C, 12C or 30C	one dose every 5–30 minutes
Serious Symptoms need help within about 24 hours and are not necessarily accompanied by pain – e.g. bad cough; abscess; food poisoning; vomiting, etc.	6C or 12C	one dose every 1–2 hours
Less serious Symptoms can wait a day or two to be treated – e.g. sore throat; flu; teething; chicken pox, etc.	6C or 12C	one dose every 4–8 hours
Not serious Symptoms are usually mild and need longer-term treatment – e.g. anaemia; exhaustion, etc.	6X or 6C	one dose 3 times daily for *up to* 10 days

STOP ON IMPROVEMENT. REPEAT AS NEEDED

Having reassessed the symptom picture, you may decide to select another remedy. The same guidelines apply again. Give up to six doses, according to the urgency of the case. If you become unsure, however, it is better to stop prescribing and get professional help or let nature take its course rather than mess up your patient's symptom picture through inaccurate prescribing. It is never dangerous to give the wrong remedy, but it is unwise to continue prescribing if there is no response, especially on a potentially serious illness like an ear infection.

Write down exactly what you have done at each step, with notes to explain your reasons, plus the results of your own prescribing. If you decide to do nothing and your patient gets better, make sure you write that down too. Although it is hard to imagine, it is the easiest thing in the world to forget the one brilliant remedy you gave your daughter for a cough, and here she is with another one six months later . . .

Don't forget that in an acute illness like an earache or a bruised head, one, two or three doses may well be enough to begin the healing process. If your patient feels better in terms of mood and well-being he will get better even if his physical symptoms – the cough, flu or whatever – remain the same or get slightly and temporarily worse. If your patient and/or his symptoms improve for a while and then relapse, a repeat dose of the same remedy may be necessary – but only on return of the symptoms for which the remedy was originally prescribed. If the symptom picture changes, it is likely that you will need a different remedy.

The homeopathic aggravation

This is the term given to the worsening of symptoms that can occur after a constitutional remedy has been taken. This *can* happen during an acute illness. The symptoms a patient complains of may worsen or an old symptom may surface temporarily (see 'Laws of Cure', page 15). There may be a more general clearing out, or 'healing crisis' as it is often called, in the form of a streaming cold or diarrhoea. The aggravation can occur on a mental/emotional level with some patients feeling very weepy if, for example, it is suppressed grief that has caused the general lowering of their health and/or the complaint.

The higher potencies (200C and above) are especially renowned for their ability to cause aggravations and that is one of the main reasons why a first-aid prescriber should stick to the lower potencies.

ANTIDOTES

The subject of antidotes always arouses heated discussion among homeopaths. There are those who believe that coffee strongly counteracts the effects of a homeopathic remedy, while others believe that it has no effect whatsoever.

I have taken a position somewhere in between. I believe that some people are sensitive to the effects of coffee. These people are often generally sensitive and find coffee extremely enervating, giving them palpitations. In such cases, remedies may well be antidoted by coffee and it is wise to stop drinking it while the remedies are being taken and for a short time afterwards. If you are sensitive to coffee and stop drinking it while you are taking your remedy, then note whether your symptoms return when you start drinking coffee again. If they do, you may have to stop drinking it and take another short course of the remedy to clear your symptoms once more.

The following all counteract the effects of a homeopathic remedy to some extent. They are not necessarily 'bad', but as the action of a remedy can last for as little as a few days or for as long as a few months, they are strong enough to stop it working and should be avoided while it is being taken and for several weeks afterwards.

Camphor. In mothballs, tiger balms, deep-heat ointments and most lipsalves.

Coffee. See above.

Menthol/eucalyptus. In cough mixtures, Karvol capsules, tiger balms, Fisherman's Friend, Vick, Olbas Oil, etc.

Peppermint. In regular toothpaste, peppermint teas and strong peppermint sweets (natural, fresh mint in cooking is fine). As alternatives to ordinary, minty toothpaste, use fennel toothpaste (available at most health-food shops), salt water or bicarbonate of soda. A solution of *Calendula* will act as an efficient mouthwash, both at home and at the dentist (see External Materia Medica).

Recreational drugs. Cannabis and other, stronger drugs counteract the effect of homeopathic remedies and should be avoided.

The dentist. Dentist's mouthwash, toothpaste for cleaning the teeth and oil of cloves all counteract the effect of homeopathic remedies, so it is wise not to visit the dentist if you are taking a remedy. It is sensible to avoid having X-rays (unless they are essential).

Basically, any strong-smelling or strong-acting substance will affect a homeopathic remedy. Some people have found that a very strongly spiced curry will have an adverse effect, as might a night of heavy drinking.

An emotional or physical shock can also stop a remedy working. For some people this can mean a bad piece of news; for others a visit to the dentist with the stress and strain of treatment can quite easily counteract the action of a remedy taken a short time before.

If your remedy has 'stopped working' (you took it and your symptoms cleared for a period of time and now they have returned), always ask yourself if you have antidoted the remedy in any way. If you think you have, then repeat your last remedy – sometimes a single repeat dose is enough.

AND FINALLY . . .

I would encourage anyone who is taking first-aid homeopathic prescribing seriously to enrol for a short homeopathic first-aid course. Many adult education colleges run courses and many homeopathic practitioners also run their own on a private basis. Being signed on with a local homeopath is also important as there is then someone who knows your case (or that of your family) with whom you can check whether the steps you wish to take are appropriate. I encourage my patients to ring in with a list of symptoms if, for example, their child has flu, and make sure that it is all right to give, say, *Gelsemium*, or whether it will interfere with the child's long-term constitutional treatment. This also enables them to confirm their choice of remedy in the early stages of getting to know the remedy pictures.

Last but not least, I hope that this book will demystify homeopathy for you and that in understanding the homeopathic process you will also start to become familiar with your *own* processes of falling ill and will therefore be able to use homeopathic medicines appropriately and effectively.

BEFORE PRESCRIBING TURN TO PART III FOR FURTHER INFORMATION ON WHEN AND HOW TO PRESCRIBE.

PART II

THE MATERIA MEDICAS AND REPERTORIES

In this part of the book you will find one section listing remedies to be taken internally and one for those to be used externally. Each of these sections is divided into two: a Materia Medica, listing the remedy pictures, and a Repertory (index) of all the symptoms listed in these remedy pictures.

EXTERNAL MATERIA MEDICA AND REPERTORY

INTRODUCTION

External remedies are not true homeopathic remedies; they have not been proved, or tested, on healthy individuals in order to establish their symptom pictures, and they have not been potentised. They are basically plant extracts and the indications for their use have developed out of herbal lore over thousands of years. I have chosen the remedies I have found most effective from my own experience.

The remedies are listed in alphabetical order, and precise instructions are given for using each one. The symptoms, or complaints, for each remedy are also listed alphabetically within each entry.

External remedies come in various forms (see below) and next to each symptom are instructions for the most appropriate form to use. In the entry for *Arnica*, for example, I suggest you use *Arnica* oil or ointment for bruised muscles and *Arnica* tincture for a wasp sting.

Tinctures, oils, ointments and creams are sold by homeopathic pharmacies (and sometimes stocked by ordinary chemists). Lotions are usually made up at home by diluting tinctures, and instructions for this are given below.

Tinctures

A tincture is a solution of the plant in alcohol – usually a one in ten dilution. It is prepared by homeopathic pharmacies.

Lotions

A lotion is simply a dilution of tincture in water, used for burns, gargling or douching. Lotions do not keep so you should keep a stock of tinctures and make up lotions as and when you need them.

Basic lotion:
Dilute 5 drops of tincture with 1 tablespoon of cooled, boiled water, or for a larger quantity use 40 drops to ¼ pint (40 drops = approximately ½ teaspoon).
Strong lotion:
Use only where indicated in the External Materia Medica.
Dilute 10 drops of tincture with 1 tablespoon of cooled, boiled water, or 40 drops to ⅛ pint.

Eyebaths

Add 2 drops of tincture to an eyebath of cooled, boiled water and use in the normal way.

Ointments

To make an ointment, the tincture is incorporated into a lanolin base, which serves to seal cuts from dirt. Ointments are not water soluble and so do not wash off easily. Some people are allergic to lanolin (particularly those sensitive to wool), so it's worth testing it overnight on a small patch of skin. If this produces any redness or irritation, avoid using ointment where possible.

Creams

A cream is a remedy tincture in an aqueous (water-soluble) base, which washes off easily and isn't sticky. It is easily absorbed by the skin and is good for areas that are not going to get wet, and for people who don't like sticky ointments.

Oils

To make an oil, the plant material is crushed and macerated in oil and allowed to stand for a period of time before being strained ready for use. I have indicated in each instance where an oil might be more useful than, say, a cream or a lotion.

NB   SEE ALSO PAGES 203–26 FOR GENERAL ADVICE, DOS AND DON'TS.

NB BEFORE PRESCRIBING FOR ANY
COMPLAINT IT IS ESSENTIAL TO READ THE
GENERAL ADVICE AND DOS AND DON'TS
LISTED ON PAGES 203–26.

AESCULUS AND HAMAMELIS
(Aesc./Ham.)

Piles

A combination of these two herbs in an ointment or
cream provides relief from painful piles, but you
should seek professional help so that they can be
treated 'from the inside' to prevent their recurrence
(see page 222).

ARNICA (Arn.)

Warning: *never* apply *Arnica* externally to open
wounds, cuts or grazes – that is, to broken skin – as it
can cause a nasty rash.

Bed sores

Use for the first stage of pressure sores caused by a
long confinement in bed.

Bruises

Apply the ointment, cream or lotion directly to the
affected part (remembering to use it only on *unbroken*
skin) as soon as possible. If you can do this before the
bruise has started to discolour (even if it has already
swollen), it will simply be re-absorbed by the body,
especially if you take *Arnica* internally as well. Rub
ointment or cream in gently, or if you are using lotion
apply it on a piece of lint or gauze and keep in place
until the swelling has subsided – usually a matter of
several hours.

Corns

Apply the ointment two or three times a day for relief.

Sore muscles

Rub *Arnica* ointment or oil into sore, bruised muscles
after exertion (such as gardening or skiing) and take
the appropriate internal remedy if your symptoms are
severe.

Sprains/strains (first stage)

Rub in *Arnica* ointment or cream, or wrap the sprained
joint in a lotion-soaked bandage. This will deal with
the initial swelling.

Wasp stings

Dab the wound with neat tincture immediately after
being stung.

CALENDULA (Calen.)

Warning: *Calendula* helps the layers of the skin (the
epithelium) to 'knit' back together and will mend a
clean wound in a matter of hours. It heals so rapidly
that it can seal dirt *into* the body, so always clean the
wound very carefully before applying *Calendula*.

Burns/scalds (second degree)

Use *Calendula* cream or lotion for the later stages of a
burn once the pain has passed. *Calendula* will promote
new skin growth and is especially useful where
blisters have broken.

Childbirth

Massage *Calendula* oil into the perineum during labour
to soften the area and to help make an episiotomy
unnecessary.

Cracked nipples

If *Phytolacca* has failed to help, apply *Calendula* ointment, or cream if sensitive to lanolin, to heal cracked,
painful nipples.

Cuts/wounds

Apply ointment or cream to minor cuts, and bandage
if necessary. For serious wounds apply lotion on a
piece of lint or gauze and keep in place. Use a plant
spray filled with lotion to keep the dressing damp but
do *not* remove the dressing until the bleeding has
stopped and healing is well under way.

Eczema/rashes

Calendula lotion or cream is especially useful for soothing eczema or rashes where the skin has cracked or
been scratched raw. It will not treat the underlying
cause of the eczema; you should seek professional
help for this.

Handcream

Calendula cream makes a marvellous handcream after
gardening or working on the car when there may be
little cuts in the skin.

Mouthwash

Use a strong lotion after tooth extractions or after any
sort of dental work where the gums have been cut.

Nappy rash

Use ointment or cream several times daily, making
sure that the whole area is clean and dry first (wash
with water and a mild, unscented soap). See also
Symphytum.

Sunburn

Use the lotion or cream (see Burns above).

Thrush

For vaginal thrush douche with the following mixture to relieve soreness and itching: make one pint of chamomile tea (one pint of boiling water to one table-spoon of dried chamomile leaves or one chamomile teabag). Leave to cool, strain, add 40 drops of *Calendula* tincture and douche twice daily for up to a week only. You can buy a re-usable douche from larger chemists (not the disposable type which comes with its own solution). Douching will not cure the com-plaint; it will only help during the acute phase (see page 225), and you should seek professional help.

EUPHRASIA (Euphr.)

Eye infections/inflammations/injuries

Use *Euphrasia* whenever the eye needs bathing – whether it is sore after the removal of dirt or grit, after swimming in a chlorinated pool, when irritated by hayfever or when actually infected or inflamed.

If *Euphrasia* doesn't help, use *Hypercal* tincture (see opposite). Some people find it more effective, especially in the case of infection.

It is essential to use cooled, boiled water in an eyebath, and to clean the eyebath itself with boiling water after *each* eye is bathed to prevent the spread of infection.

HAMAMELIS (Ham.)

Hamamelis, or witch hazel, is widely sold in chemists as distilled witch hazel, but it is neither as astringent nor as effective as the tincture available from homeopathic pharmacies. Use the distilled form if this is all you can find.

Bruises

Hamamelis is useful for bruises where the skin has been broken (*Arnica* is for use on *un*broken skin and is therefore inappropriate). Use *Hamamelis* in the same way as *Arnica*, as an ointment, cream or lotion.

Piles

Apply a compress of the lotion (you can use a small sanitary towel or a strip of cotton wool) to provide instant relief from pain. Keep in place for a while (up to an hour, twice daily) to reduce inflammation.

Alternatively, *Aesculus* and *Hamamelis* ointment or cream may be applied as often as necessary. It is essential that the correct internal homeopathic remedy is given so that the piles are treated from the inside and real healing can take place.

Varicose veins

Apply the lotion to varicose veins, especially painful ones, by wrapping the leg in lotion-soaked bandages. Leave in place for as long as possible, until the discom-fort eases and then use only when needed. An elastic (tube) bandage over the top will keep bandages in place.

HYPERCAL®

This is a mixture of *Calendula* and *Hypericum*; the combined healing qualities of the two plants make it especially effective in soothing and healing wounds.

Childbirth

After childbirth *Hypercal*® will help to heal a cut or torn perineum. Apply a strong lotion on a small pad or compress to the affected area, keeping it in place for up to an hour at a time, and repeating every four hours for several days.

Cold sores

Dilute one part tincture to three parts cooled, boiled water and apply this strong lotion frequently to cold sores as soon as they appear, or use ointment. Take the appropriate internal remedy at the same time.

Cuts/wounds

Use ointment, cream or lotion to heal wounds just as you would use *Calendula* or *Hypericum* on their own.

Soak cut fingers, toes or elbows in a basin of water into which a teaspoon of *Hypercal*® tincture has been added and gently remove any bits of dirt. The clean wound can then be dressed with a smear of the cream or ointment.

Eye infections/inflammations/injuries

As an alternative to *Euphrasia*, use 2 drops in an eyebath to help clear inflammation caused by dust, foreign bodies, infection or injury. Seek professional help if the soreness persists.

Mouth ulcers

Use the mouthwash below frequently, as well as taking the appropriate internal remedy.

Mouthwash

This mouthwash is good for mouth ulcers, inflamed, sore or spongy gums. Make a strong lotion by diluting 40 drops of tincture in ⅛ pint and swoosh it well around the mouth after brushing your teeth, then massage it into the gums with your fingers.

Sore throat

Dissolve one teaspoon of sea salt in ¼ pint of hot water. Add 40 drops of *Hypercal* tincture and gargle as frequently as necessary.

HYPERICUM (Hyp.)

Hypericum soothes and heals wounds, especially where nerves have been damaged and the injury is painful. The pains of a '*Hypericum wound*' are typically shooting and/or severe.

Boils

Apply the lotion externally as a compress (on lint or gauze) and renew it every four to six hours to relieve pain and encourage healing. It is important to treat a tendency to boils from the inside so seek professional help if you have a recurring problem.

Burns (second degree, with blistering)

Soak gauze strips or lint in *Hypericum* lotion, wring out and lay over the burned area. Keep the bandages damp by spraying the area with the lotion. Do not remove the cloth until the pain has ceased. *Hypericum* is also useful in the first stage of a burn on a nerve-rich and therefore very painful part. Give the appropriate internal remedy.

Cuts/wounds

Use lotion to bathe and clean dirty cuts/wounds, and apply ointment before bandaging. *Hypericum* is especially good where there are shooting pains in or around the wound and for injuries to nerve-rich parts (crushed fingers and toes). If a compress is applied to a crushed finger or toe and kept damp for a few days, a damaged nail can be prevented from taking an odd shape once healed.

Insect bites

Use neat *Hypericum* tincture on any insect bite. If swelling persists, apply the lotion as a compress, and keep in place for as long as it takes for the swelling to diminish.

Piles

Use a compress of *Hypericum* lotion (or ointment if preferred) for bleeding piles with severe shooting pains. Repeat as necessary, but seek professional help.

Sunburn

See Burns above.

LEDUM (Led.)

Insect bites/stings

Use *Ledum* tincture neat on insect bites and stings to prevent swelling and itching.

Many homeopathic pharmacies have their own preparations for relieving bites and stings. These are generally mixtures of a number of remedies and are applied neat as above.

If you are often bitten and are sensitive to insect bites, you will benefit from constitutional homeopathic treatment (see page 205), especially if your response is extremely severe.

PHYTOLACCA (Phyt.)

Cracked nipples

Apply the tincture neat for speedy healing of nipples that are sore and/or cracked through breastfeeding.

Sore throat

Use a strong lotion as a gargle (40 drops to ⅛ pint of cooled, boiled water to which a teaspoon of sea salt can also be added). Take the appropriate internal remedy.

PLANTAGO (Plant.)

Earache

Dilute a few drops of tincture with equal quantities of warm almond oil (or cooled, boiled water) and drop into the painful ear. Follow these guidelines:

1 Heat a spoon by dipping it in boiling water, then pour the oil and the tincture into it and wait 30 seconds for the spoon to cool and the oil to warm.
2 Tip the head on one side.
3 Drop the liquid into the ear.
4 Pull the lobe of the ear down and round and out very gently so that the liquid goes right into the ear.

Some children will not allow anything to be put into their ears when they are in pain. Do not force this on them. Offer instead a warm hot water bottle wrapped in a soft towel for them to lie on; if that doesn't help try an ice pack (crushed ice in a plastic bag in a thin, soft towel). Or wrap the head tightly with a scarf. One of these measures might offer temporary relief and also guide you to the correct internal remedy.

NB   SEEK PROFESSIONAL HELP IF PAIN IS SEVERE.

Toothache

Apply neat tincture to the affected tooth or swoosh the mouth out frequently with a strong lotion (40 drops tincture with ⅛ pint cooled, boiled water).

PYRETHRUM (Pyr.)

Insect repellent

Apply the lotion to all exposed areas of skin, and carry a spray bottle of the lotion with you to renew the applications. Some pharmacies sell *Pyrethrum* in a spray, otherwise buy the tincture and make a fresh batch of lotion daily. Some homeopathic pharmacies also produce their own 'anti-bite lotion' which can be diluted and used as above. Experiment to see which suits you best.

RESCUE REMEDY (RR)

This wonderful all-purpose 'remedy' is based on flowers and comes in a cream or as a tincture. It has been known to help anything from bruises, cold sores, cracked nipples, eczema, insect bites and stings, nappy rash and piles to sunburn. If Rescue Remedy is all you have then use it. (See page 250.)

RHUS TOXICODENDRON (Rhus-t.)

Joint pain

Rhus toxicodendron ointment rubbed into joints can provide relief for sufferers from rheumatism and arthritis.

Sprains (second stage)

After the swelling has subsided (with applications of *Arnica* ointment or cream), apply *Rhus toxicodendron* ointment twice daily to the sprained joint, and bandage tightly. Use the joint/limb as little as possible and keep it elevated to give it a chance to heal. *Rhus-t.* is especially useful where ligaments are torn.

Strains

After lifting or over-exertion, the ointment can help enormously, especially if you have the typical *Rhus* symptoms: stiffness on beginning to move (on getting up, for example), improvement with continued movement, but a return of the painful stiffness if you overdo it or sit down again.

RUTA GRAVEOLENS (Ruta.)

Bunions/corns

Apply the ointment twice daily to ease pain.

Bruises

This is for when bony parts of the body are sore after a knock, after *Arnica* has reduced the swelling, but the soreness persists. Shinbones, elbows and kneecaps are all parts that have little protective muscle and the covering to the bone can take longer to heal. *Ruta* can speed up the process. Apply the ointment two or three times daily until the pain eases.

Eye strain

Dilute two drops of *Ruta* tincture with an eyebath of cooled, boiled water, to help eyes strained by too much study, reading, or working at a VDU.

Sprains

Use *Ruta* where *Rhus-t.* hasn't helped and the covering to the bone may have been damaged. I have found a mixture of *Rhus-t.* and *Ruta* in an ointment wonderful for sprains and strains.

Tennis elbow

Apply ointment or cream as necessary to relieve the pain. Do not further stress the joint by more strenuous activity.

SYMPHYTUM (Symph.)

Cuts/wounds

Symphytum is a good all-purpose ointment or cream. Use on minor cuts once you have cleaned them.

Nappy rash

Where *Calendula* hasn't helped, *Symphytum* ointment often will. If it doesn't, your baby will need constitutional treatment from a professional homeopath.

It is worth asking your midwife or health visitor for simple practical measures to help this complaint. For instance, drying a baby's bottom with a warm hairdryer (at a safe distance) before applying ointments helps to clear a stubborn rash. *Caution* Test the hairdryer on your own inner forearm first and take *great* care.

Sprains

Apply *Symphytum* ointment to sprains that don't respond to *Ruta* or *Rhus-t.* within 48 hours. Also take *Symphytum* internally, as there may be damage to the bone itself.

NB   SEE ALSO PAGES 203–26 FOR GENERAL ADVICE, DOS AND DON'TS.

TAMUS (Tam.)

Chilblains

Apply the ointment two to three times daily *before the chilblains break* to stop itching and to speed up healing. **Warning:** *never* apply to a chilblain where the skin has broken.

THIOSINAMINUM (Thios.)

Scars

Thiosinaminum reduces the swelling of a badly healed scar – where there are lumps and bumps (keloids) – as long as it is used soon after the event (within three months), but it is still worth trying on older scars. It is useful for lumpy scars following appendicectomies, episiotomies, and so on. A professional homeopath will also treat these with internal remedies.

THUJA (Thu.)

Warts/verrucas

Neat *Thuja* tincture can be applied twice daily and *Thuja 6* taken orally for up to ten days.
Warning: if this remedy has no effect seek the advice of a professional homeopath. The continued use of *Thuja* is not advisable as the symptoms from the proving are unpleasant and difficult to get rid of. It is a deep-acting remedy that should not generally be used in a first-aid kit for self-prescribing. However, since it is part of the range stocked by many chemists I have included the minimum indications for safe administration.

It is now accepted that you do not 'catch' verrucas in swimming pools as was commonly believed until recently. Homeopaths believe that warts and verrucas are part of an overall symptom picture and need to be treated with respect. They are cured successfully with constitutional homeopathic treatment, so do not suppress them with acids from the chemist or have them cut out. Homeopaths have found again and again that suppressing warts in this way can lead to the development of more serious complaints.

URTICA URENS (Urt-u.)

Bee sting

Dab on neat tincture and take the appropriate internal remedy.

Burns (minor)

For minor burns with redness but no blistering, apply cream, ointment, or a compress soaked in lotion. Take the appropriate internal remedy if needed.

Eczema/rashes

Urtica cream or lotion can relieve the itching of eczema or any rash, especially if it itches *and* stings and then burns. It is essential to seek professional help for this condition.

Sunburn

Apply lotion or cream to sunburned areas, repeating according to the severity. Use a mixture of *Hypericum* and *Urtica* tinctures in the lotion if there are severe shooting pains (20 drops of each tincture in ¼ pint of water) and take the appropriate internal remedy.

VERBASCUM OIL (Verb.)

Earache

Drop the warmed oil into the ear to relieve pain and promote healing. Follow the instructions under *Plantago* (page 34).

EXTERNAL REPERTORY

The External Repertory is an index of the symptoms listed in the External Materia Medica.

Bed sores   *Arn.*
Bee stings   see **Stings**
Boils   *Hyp.*
Bruises
  on unbroken skin   *Arn.*, RR
  on broken skin   *Ham.*
  on bones   *Ruta*
Bunions/corns   *Ruta*
Burns/scalds
  minor   *Urt-u.*
  second degree (with blistering)   *Calen.*, *Hyp.*
Chilblains   *Tamus*
Childbirth   *Calen.*, *Hypercal*®
Cold Sores   *Hypercal*®, RR
Conjunctivitis   see **Eye infections**
Corns   *Arn.*
Cracked nipples   *Calen.*, *Phyt.*, RR
Cuts/wounds   *Calen.*, *Hyp.*, *Hypercal*®, RR, *Symph.*
Earache   *Plant.*, *Verb.*
Eczema/rashes   *Calen.*, RR, *Urt-u.*
Eye infections/inflammations/injuries   *Euphr.*, *Hypercal*®
Eye strain   *Ruta*
Gargle   see **Sore throat**

Handcream   *Calen.*
Herpes   see **Cold sores**
Insect bites   *Hyp.*, *Led.*, RR
Insect repellent   *Pyr.*
Joint pain   *Rhus-t.*
Mouth ulcers   *Hypercal*®
Mouthwash   *Calen.*, *Hypercal*®
Nappy rash   *Calen.*, RR, *Symph.*
Piles   *Aesc./Ham.*, *Ham.*, *Hyp.*
Pink eye   see **Eye infections**
Scars   *Thios.*
Sore muscles   *Arn.*
Sore throat   *Hypercal*®, *Phyt.*
Sprains
  first stage (with swelling)   *Arn.*
  second stage   *Rhus-t.*, *Ruta*, *Symph.*
Stings
  bee   *Led.*, RR, *Urt-u.*
  wasp   *Arn.*, *Led.*, RR
Strains   *Arn.*, *Rhus-t.*
Sunburn   *Calen.*, *Hyp.*, RR, *Urt-u.*
Tennis elbow   *Ruta*
Thrush   *Calen.*
Toothache   *Plant.*
Ulcers   see **Mouth ulcers**
Varicose veins   *Ham.*
Warts/verrucas   *Thu.*
Wasp stings   see **Stings**

INTERNAL MATERIA MEDICA

ACONITUM NAPELLUS (Aco.)

Family name: *Ranunculaceae*
Other names: monk's-hood; wolf's-bane; common aconite

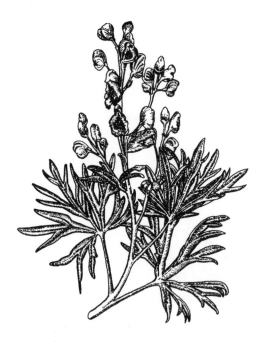

This plant grows in moist pastures and wastelands in the mountainous districts of Europe, Russia and Central Asia. It grows to a height of between two and six feet and has bluish-violet hooded flowers.

Aconite contains a deadly poison (the root possesses 90 per cent more than the leaf), which is said to be more potent even than prussic acid and is the poison that was used by the ancient Greeks – in fact throughout history it has been renowned more for its power to kill than to heal. It is said that the huntsmen of the Alps dipped their arrows in it when hunting wolves – hence the name wolf's-bane.

According to Mrs Grieve (*A Modern Herbal*), *Aconite* and *Belladonna* were the ingredients of witches' 'flying ointments', with their combined actions (palpitations and delirium) producing a sensation of flying!

Hahnemann published his provings of *Aconite* in 1805, and it soon became a widely used remedy, especially for fevers and inflammations, which until then had been largely 'cured' by bloodletting. And so it became known as the 'homeopathic lancet'.

The homeopathic remedy is prepared from the whole plant (except the root), which is taken at flowering time in June/July and chopped, pounded to a pulp and the juice expressed, mixed with alcohol, and then succussed.

GENERAL SYMPTOMS

Complaints from: cold dry wind; fear; getting chilled; shock. **Face** red. **Onset of complaint** sudden. **Likes** cold drinks. **Pains** unbearable. **Palpitations. Sweat:** hot; on covered parts of the body. **Thirsty. Taste:** mouth tastes bitter.
Better for fresh air.
Worse at night; for touch.

This remedy will work only at the very beginning of an illness – within the first twenty-four to forty-eight hours. The symptoms are often a result of fright, shock or being chilled. Someone who has been very angry can also bring on an *Aconite* state. Exposure to a draught, or a cold, dry wind, can cause a wide range of symptoms (colds, coughs, cystitis, etc.). If in pain, the pains – in the head, throat, teeth, or wherever – are intolerable, and will drive these people to despair. Generally, people who need *Aconite* will be worse at night; though they are usually OK on going to bed, they wake up around midnight (usually before midnight) with the cough, croup, earache, etc. They will not want to be touched (examined or interfered with) and will be better for some fresh air.

EMOTIONAL/MENTAL SYMPTOMS

Anxious: when chilled; generally; during a fever. **Expression:** anxious; frightened. **Fearful:** in a crowd; of death during pregnancy/labour. **Screaming** with pain. **Sensitive** to noise. **Tearful** during a fever.

Someone who needs *Aconite* looks anxious, and has shocked, staring, glassy eyes (the pupils may be dilated). '*Aconite* shock' is the opposite of '*Arnica* shock' in that a person needing *Aconite* will be extremely distressed (anxious and fearful). They may well be inconsolable. They are scared of going out into a situation where there will be lots of people. Their pains may be severe, especially in childbirth, for example, and patients may say, 'I want to die'. *Aconite* types may also scream with the pain.

PHYSICAL COMPLAINTS

Chicken pox

Symptoms With *Aconite* general and emotional/mental symptoms, and fever.

Common cold

Symptoms With HEADACHE (see below).
Causes shock; getting chilled; cold, dry wind.
Give *Aconite* at the first sign of a cold if the stress is as above.

Cough

Symptoms COUGH: barking; dry; hoarse; irritating; short; tickling. BREATHING fast.
Worse at night; during fever; dry, cold air.
Causes cold, dry wind.
All the air passages are irritated. It is often worse at night after being out in a cold, dry wind (especially a north or an east wind).

Croup

Symptoms Symptoms of COUGH (above).
Unless you have strong indications for another remedy, this is the first remedy to think of giving for croup.

Cystitis

Symptoms PAINS pressing.
Causes getting chilled.

Earache

Symptoms PAINS unbearable.
Causes getting chilled; cold, dry wind.

Eye inflammation

Symptoms EYES sensitive to light; whites of eyes red. PAINS: aching; burning. With a COMMON COLD.
Causes getting chilled; foreign body in eye.
Worse for cold, dry wind.

Fever

Symptoms HEAT: alternating with chills at night; burning; dry at night. PULSE: fast; strong. With ANXIETY.
Better for uncovering.
Worse at night; in the evening.
Causes getting chilled.
The person feels hot inside and chilly externally. The cheeks may alternate between hot and red and pale and ghostly (the colour may drain from the face on getting up); or one cheek will be hot and red and the other pale and cold, especially in teething children. Those parts of the body that are covered with clothing become sweaty; the person may kick off the covers. There is a burning, unquenchable thirst; everything tastes bitter except water, and even that tastes bad.

Headache

Symptoms PAINS: burning; bursting; throbbing.
Causes fright; shock; getting chilled.

Injuries

Symptoms CUTS/WOUNDS bleed freely. With SHOCK (see below).
Aconite helps with wounds that are bleeding excessively where the characteristic shock is present.

Insomnia

Symptoms Restless SLEEP. Anxious DREAMS.

Measles

Symptoms ONSET sudden. SKIN RASH: itches; burns. With FEVER; COUGH.
Sudden onset with restlessness, fever, cough and thirst.

NB   SEE ALSO PAGES 203–26 FOR GENERAL ADVICE, DOS AND DON'TS.

Mumps

Symptoms ONSET sudden. With FEVER.

Period problems

Symptoms PERIOD late.
Causes fright; shock; getting chilled; pregnancy.

Shock

Causes injuries; surgery; childbirth.
This is accompanied by the extreme *Aconite*-type fear and anxiety. It is useful during or following operations, and for shocked mothers and/or babies either during or after labour, especially a fast labour. The mother may experience some shaking with the shock, whereas the baby may just be very still, with an anxious or fearful look in its eyes.

Sore throat

Symptoms PAINS: burning; stitching.
Causes getting chilled.

Teething

Symptoms CHEEKS hot and red. With symptoms of FEVER (see above). PAINFUL IN CHILDREN with restless sleep.
Children toss and turn in their sleep and bite their fists and scream. The teething may well be accompanied by fever.

Toothache

Symptoms PAINS: tearing; in good teeth.
Causes cold, dry wind.

Retention of urine

Symptoms IN NEWBORN BABIES; IN CHILDREN who catch cold.
This is especially useful for newborn babies who don't pee, who have been shocked by the birth (especially a fast labour).

AGARICUS MUSCARIUS (Agar.)

Natural order: fungi
Common names: fly agaric; bug agaric; toadstool

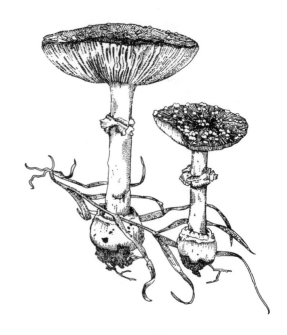

This poisonous toadstool grows in dry places, especially in dry pine woods, in Europe, Asia and the USA. It is uncommon in England but abundant in some parts of Scotland.

Agaricus is thought to be the oldest of hallucinogens used for ritualistic purposes. Medicine men ate this toadstool to achieve ecstatic states (although these periods of great animation, which were often accompanied by dancing, singing and talking to imagined persons, alternated with times of deep depression). It was also employed at one time in the making of alcoholic beverages but this practice was beset with dangers in view of the terrible deaths that sometimes occurred from the poisonings.

For the homeopathic preparation, the mushroom is well washed, mashed in a mortar, then equal parts of alcohol are added to it. This is left to stand for three days before being strained and succussed.

GENERAL SYMPTOMS

Clumsy: trips easily while walking. **Trembling**. **Twitchy**.
Worse for cold.

This remedy is a specific cure for chilblains, especially of the feet and toes, and, used with *Tamus* ointment, will cure most cases of straightforward chilblains where no other strong symptoms would lead you to prescribe a more 'important' remedy.

General symptoms of people needing *Agaricus* are trembling and twitchiness, which may be so bad that they drop things or stumble when walking. They are generally very sensitive to cold, damp weather.

There are no marked emotional/mental symptoms.

PHYSICAL COMPLAINTS
Chilblains

Symptoms CHILBLAINS: burning; itching; red.
Worse for cold.

Chilblains are on the hands and feet, or very occasionally on the ears, but which are worse on the feet. They are terribly painful when the hands or feet become cold.

Headache

Symptoms EYES/EYELIDS twitching.
Worse in the morning.
Causes alcohol; nerves.

ALLIUM CEPA (All-c.)

Family name: Liliaceae
Common name: common red onion

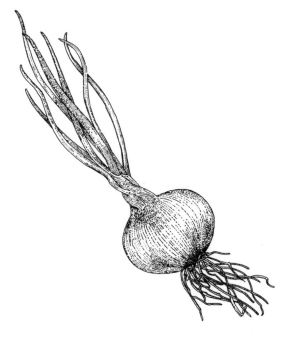

This plant is universally cultivated as a garden vegetable, and it has been renowned for hundreds of years among country folk and herbalists for its healing properties. It has been used in a variety of ways: externally as a poultice for acne, chilblains and arthritis (to draw out inflammation), and internally as a blood purifier and to clear the intestines of worms. The juice has been sniffed up the nostrils, dropped into the ears or applied to 'blemished' skin; onion wine has been brewed for those with weak chests; and the whole onion has been roasted with honey or sugar for stubborn coughs.

The ancient Egyptians swore by the onion, and consumed vast quantities. They have even worshipped it. In it they saw symbolised the universe, since they believed the various spheres of heaven, earth and hell were concentric, like the onion's layers; and therefore Egyptian priests were forbidden to eat it.

For the homeopathic preparation the fresh bulb is gathered in July/August and chopped, then pounded to a pulp before it is mixed with alcohol and succussed.

GENERAL SYMPTOMS

Homeopathically, the common red onion is used only for those symptoms that it is capable of producing in a healthy individual, that is, streaming eyes and nose. Any illness that produces these symptoms – be it a cold or hayfever – can be cured by *Allium cepa*.

Euphrasia is very similar in that it too produces streaming head colds or hayfever, but there is an important difference: in *Allium cepa* the nasal catarrh burns and the eye discharge doesn't. The reverse is true of *Euphrasia*, where the nasal catarrh doesn't burn and the discharge from the eyes does.

There are no marked emotional/mental symptoms.

PHYSICAL COMPLAINTS
Common cold

Symptoms NASAL CATARRH: burning; one sided; profuse; watery. With EYE INFLAMMATION; HEADACHE; SNEEZING; SORE THROAT.
Better for fresh air.
Worse in a stuffy room.
Causes cold wind; getting wet feet.
The nasal discharge may be one sided, that is, only one nostril may stream. The cold symptoms, especially the sneezing, will be generally worse in a warm room.

Cough

Symptoms COUGH: hacking; irritating; painful. Tickling in LARYNX. VOICE hoarse.
Worse for cold air.
The cough is generally better for being in a warm room (this is the opposite of the cold symptoms).

Eye inflammation

Symptoms of a COMMON COLD (see above). DISCHARGE: bland, non-irritating; profuse. EYES watering.

Hayfever

Symptoms of a COMMON COLD (see above) and EYE INFLAMMATION (see above).
Worse in the spring; in August.

ANTIMONIUM CRUDUM (Ant-c.)

Other names: antimonii sulphuratum; sulphuret of antimony; native sulphide of antimony

Black antimony occurs both as a chemical compound and in crystalline form as the mineral stibnite which is found in many parts of Europe and the United States.

It has been used as a veterinary medicine to cure horses with sore heels and to fatten pigs and lean, scabby cattle. Tradition in fact relates that a German monk threw some antimony to his pigs and observed that, after purging them violently, it immediately fattened them. This made him think that by giving his fellow monks a dose they would likewise be the better for it. The experiment failed, however; they all died and the 'medicine' henceforth was called antimony or anti-monk.

It is used as an alloy with other metals for lining brasses, in bell metals to make their sound clearer, and for purifying and heightening the colour of gold. Stibnite (or kohl) was used in the Middle East as a powder to darken the eyebrows, to protect the eyes from the heat of the sun and make them more beautiful. Nowadays, matches are tipped with stibnite, which causes ignition when rubbed against the red phosphorus.

The homeopathic remedy is made from the native sulphide of antimony by trituration.

GENERAL SYMPTOMS

Complaints from over-eating. **Cracks** on corners of mouth/nostrils. **Eyes:** sunken; dull. **Lips** dry.
Sluggish. Thirstless. White-coated **Tongue.**
Worse for getting overheated; for sun; swimming in cold water.

People who need *Antimonium crudum* are often gluttons who eat more than they need; they consequently become fat, sluggish, irritable and sick. They develop weak stomachs and their digestive systems complain frequently. This remedy can in fact be used for any digestive upsets arising from having overloaded the stomach. Thirstlessness is another general symptom to look out for; it is often present with the nausea or indigestion. A key symptom of this remedy is a thick white coating (like whitewash) on the tongue, which must be present in any complaint if the remedy is to work. The nostrils and the corners of the mouth may have cracks.

Antimonium crudum has similar effects to those of *Carbo vegetabilis* with regard to overloaded stomachs, but a *Carbo vegetabilis* person has much more flatulence and doesn't have the white tongue of *Antimonium crudum*.

Antimonium crudum types are very sensitive to the sun, or being overheated in any way, which can exhaust them and cause them to lose their voices or in fact aggravate any symptom, though swimming in cold water can bring on a cold.

EMOTIONAL/MENTAL SYMPTOMS

Dislikes being looked at; being touched. **Irritable. Sentimental. Sulky.**

Sick children needing this remedy are foul; they can't bear to be touched or looked at and may even shout 'Go away!' if you go anywhere near them. They don't want to speak or be spoken to, and are angry if you give them any attention. They can be as angry as *Chamomilla* types (but *Chamomilla* will be demanding and will want to be touched or carried at least for a short while). Adults may also behave in a sulky, irritable way, not wanting to speak or be spoken to, especially if they are suffering from gastric problems. This can be a useful remedy for sentimental, lovesick teenagers who 'moon' over lost loves, who become sluggish and difficult to live with.

PHYSICAL COMPLAINTS

Chicken pox
Symptoms with COUGH.

With typical emotional/mental and general symptoms (see above).

Corns

Symptoms CORNS: on soles of feet; under nails; inflamed; horny. PAINS pressing.
Corns or horny patches may be inflamed and sore and will usually be situated on the soles of the feet, at the tips of the toes or under the nails, especially of the big toes, although fingernails, especially damaged nails, can have these horny growths under them. They can look like warts.

Diarrhoea

Symptoms Alternating with CONSTIPATION in elderly persons. STOOLS: with small, hard lumps; watery.
Worse for getting overheated.
Causes over-eating; sour wine.

Exhaustion

Symptoms With SLEEPINESS.
Worse in hot weather.

Fingernails split

Causes injury to the nail.
This is for injured or crushed fingernails that grow in splits (*Silica* is the other remedy that has this).

Indigestion

Symptoms BELCHING: empty; tasting of food just eaten. BELLY/STOMACH: bloated; feels empty; feels full.

Nausea

Symptoms NAUSEA: constant; during pregnancy. BELCHING: empty; tasting of food just eaten.
Worse after eating acidic and/or starchy foods.
The nausea may be accompanied by a headache.

Toothache

Symptoms PAIN: gnawing; in decayed teeth; spreading to head.
Better fresh air (walking in).
Worse after eating; cold drinks/food; at night in bed; touch of tongue.

Vomiting

Symptoms VOMITING: of bile; of curdled milk; during pregnancy. Occurs in breastfed babies.
Worse after drinking milk/sour wine.
Caused by measles; sour wine.
This is a remedy for nausea and vomiting during pregnancy where there is the characteristic white tongue and an intolerance of milk and/or bread. Babies who vomit up their breastmilk after a feed, who get cross and refuse the breast the next time it is offered will also benefit.

ANTIMONIUM TARTARICUM (Ant-t.)

Other names: tartus emeticus; antimonii potasii-tartras; tartar emetic

Antimony is a powerful poison used in the sixteenth century as a fast (and painful) way of cleaning an open, festering wound; it was not known that toxic substances are easily absorbed in this way into the bloodstream, and side effects were often fatal.

It was also the favourite emetic (drug to cause vomiting) of olden times and was called 'the Prince of Evacuants' because even very small doses caused severe purging with violent vomiting and profuse sweating. Everlasting emetic cups or 'pocula emetica' were made of antimony, and wine left standing in them for a day or two acquired emetic properties. Unfortunately, vomiting did not always take place and the poisonous preparation then remained in the stomach and bowels, with sometimes fatal results. It is because of this that it fell into disrepute and has not been used in orthodox medicine for many years. As Paracelsus wrote, 'It depends only upon the dose whether a poison is a poison or not.'

The homeopathic preparation is made by mixing and then heating together oxide of antimon and acid potassium tartrate. Once cooled and dried, crystals form and it is this pure tartar emetic that is dissolved in distilled water and succussed.

GENERAL SYMPTOMS

Exhaustion. Face: pale. **Sweat:** cold. **Thirstless. Tongue** white coated.

Antimonium tartaricum and *Antimonium crudum* are similar in that they are both effective at dealing with gastric upsets. Patients are generally thirstless and their complaints are often accompanied by profuse cold sweat, mostly during the night. The face looks very pale and sunken and may go blue around the lips. It is a particularly useful remedy for children and may be called for during chicken pox or measles if a chest infection sets in. It is also a remedy that is often indicated in chest infections in the elderly, where the patients feel incredibly weak, especially with the cough.

EMOTIONAL/MENTAL SYMPTOMS

The emotional/mental symptoms from the provings of *Antimonium tartaricum* are not very strong and the character is thus not very marked. Typically, the children are irritable, they whine and complain and want to be carried by their mothers, but they do not want to be touched or examined. They will be less angry than those needing *Antimonium crudum*. Adults may be apathetic, anxious and despondent.

PHYSICAL COMPLAINTS
Chicken pox

Symptoms SKIN RASH slow in coming out. With symptoms of COUGH (see below). The child will be bad

NB   SEE ALSO PAGES 203–26 FOR GENERAL ADVICE, DOS AND DON'TS.

tempered, with the typical white-coated tongue. If *Antimonium tartaricum* is indicated but doesn't work, and the child is *very* bad tempered, give *Antimonium crudum*. The rash is slow to appear or starts to come out and disappears again. There is drowsiness and nausea.

Cough

Symptoms Cough: loud; rattling; whooping. Breathing: asthmatic; abdominal; difficult; fast, rattling. Difficult expectoration. With sleepiness; vomiting.
Antimonium tartaricum has a marked action on chest complaints. For it to work well in a chest complaint, the difficult expectoration and characteristic loud rattling in the chest must be present; this can usually be heard before entering the room, whether the patient has pneumonia, bronchitis, whooping cough, or any chest infection. Bringing up phlegm only temporarily relieves the complaints. The cough is made worse in children by their getting angry. They may cough and yawn alternately. There may be tickling in the larynx which aggravates the cough. Vomiting is also difficult – the patient may retch ineffectually and may have to sit up to cough.

Nausea

Symptoms Nausea intermittent.
Better for belching; for vomiting.
The nausea is felt in the chest or a weight on the chest, and is as intense as that associated with *Ipecacuanha* but not so persistent. Vomiting and belching provide only temporary relief. Sometimes the desire to vomit may be accompanied by ineffectual retching (it does not produce vomiting).

Vomiting

Symptoms Vomit sour. Vomiting: difficult. With fever.
Worse for coughing.
The vomiting may be aggravated by eating and drinking, and may be worse if the patient has a fever (the higher the temperature the stronger the vomiting).

APIS MELLIFICA (Ap.)

Family name: Hymenoptera
Other name: honey bee

The bee provides us with honey, which contains enzymes and vitamins that make it both nutritious and delicious, and beeswax which is used in polishes, candles and cosmetics.

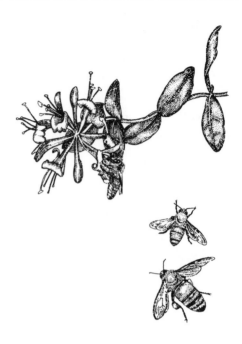

The bee's behaviour gives us some clues to the emotional symptoms of the homeopathic remedy. It is an incredibly restless insect, and is extremely irritable, reacting instantly and angrily to any interference from the outside. It is sensitive to heat and has an elaborate system of cooling down a hive which involves dropping water onto the top of the hive.

Medicinally, bee stings have been observed by country folk to cure rheumatism, and the venom transmitted by the stings has consequently been used to treat this complaint in allopathic and homeopathic medicines. Allopathic doctors have also used the venom to desensitise patients to strong reactions from insect bites.

Apis is prepared from the sting of the live common hive bee.

GENERAL SYMPTOMS

Clumsy: drops things. **Face:** red; puffy. **Pains:** burning; stinging. **Symptoms:** right-sided; move from right to left. **Thirstless. Tongue** fiery red.
Worse for heat; for touch; at 3–5 p.m.

People needing *Apis* have burning, stinging pains that are always better for cold and worse for heat. Their symptoms are either right-sided or start on the right and move or spread to the left. If there is a fever or any localised inflammation, the surface of the body may be generally sore and sensitive, as if bruised, and worse for touch (patients will not want the pressure of heavy blankets, for example). These are warm-blooded people who are better for being out in the fresh air, and are worse for heat generally as well as for hot baths, beds and drinks, and so on. They are generally thirstless but are better for cold drinks, and having the painful part bathed in cold water.

EMOTIONAL/MENTAL SYMPTOMS

Apathetic. Fearful: of being alone; of death. **Irritable. Jealous. Restless. Tearful. Whiny.**

In a fever the person is weepy for no apparent reason, and may also be fearful and restless, with a fear of death, and/or a fear of being alone. Generally, an *Apis* character will be a jealous one; this may be seen in a child who is not getting the attention he is used to, in a family where there is a new baby, for example, who may develop an *Apis* 'picture' as a result. In some ways the *Apis* character is similar to that of *Pulsatilla*, but where *Apis* is worse for touch *Pulsatilla* is much better for it – craves it even! They are both better in the open air.

PHYSICAL COMPLAINTS

Bites/stings

Symptoms BITES: burning; itching; red; stinging; swollen.
Better for cold.
Worse for heat.
Causes insects.
Apis will benefit any bite that reacts very badly, leaving a large, shiny swollen red lump that itches and/or burns and/or stings.
NB *Apis* can be used for the severe allergic reaction that can occur not just from a bee or wasp sting but from certain foods (like nuts) or even penicillin. This reaction is called anaphylactic shock and is always an emergency situation as it can be fatal. But it is worthwhile giving *Apis* while you get emergency help. The classic symptoms are swollen eyelids, lips, tongue, urticaria and difficulty breathing.

Cystitis

Symptoms DESIRE TO URINATE: constant; frequent. PAINS: burning; pressing; stinging. URINATION: constant; frequent.
There may be blood in the urine (it will look red); if this is the case, and if the symptoms agree, take *Apis* but seek professional help immediately. There will be a constant urge to urinate but only small amounts will be passed each time.

Diarrhoea

Symptoms DIARRHOEA painless.
Although this diarrhoea is painless, the anus may be sore after passing a stool.

Earache

Symptoms PAINS stinging. With typical *Apis* general symptoms (worse for heat, pains starting on the right side, etc.) and SORE THROAT.

Eye inflammation

Symptoms IN BABIES. EYES: burning; red; sore; stinging. EYELIDS swollen.
Worse for heat.
The whites of the eyes are red with bright red blood vessels visible in them. The lower lids may be more swollen than the upper ones.

Fever

Symptoms HEAT burning. With CHILLINESS; SENSITIVE SKIN.
Better for uncovering.
Worse for heat; for being in a stuffy room; for warm covers; afternoon; morning; for washing.
The patient feels hot, finds heat intolerable, has a high fever and feels very sleepy. This type of fever will accompany most acute complaints that call for *Apis*. The patient kicks off the covers and then shivers but keeps the covers off.

Headache

Symptoms HEAD: feels full; hot. PAINS: stabbing; sudden.
The scalp feels tight and sore.

Hives

Symptoms With FEVER (see above); SWEATING.
Worse at night.

Joint pain

Symptoms PAINS: burning; stinging. With SWELLING.
The joint is red, swollen and shiny.

Measles

Symptoms SKIN RASH slow to appear. With *Apis* general and emotional/mental symptoms; EYE INFLAMMATION (see above); FEVER (see above); puffy face and eyelids, and thirstlessness.

Mumps

Apis general and emotional/mental symptoms will be present.

Retention of Urine

Symptoms IN CHILDREN.
Sometimes children just can't pee, and often there seems to be no reason for this. If you notice that it has been a long time since your child urinated, and he has been drinking normally, half-hourly doses of *Apis* will encourage this function back to normal.

Sore throat

Symptoms MOUTH dry. Burning PAINS.
The person will have no thirst even though the mouth is very dry. The throat is as red as the tongue.

ARGENTUM NITRICUM (Arg-n.)

Other names: argenti nitras; silver nitrate; lunar caustic

Silver nitrate solutions are used as fungicides and as a starting point for making materials such as silver for photographic film and plates, and for mirrors. It is used in marking inks (in solution it is a powerful black stain, and in the nineteenth century many hair dyes used it), and today certain wart preparations employ it.

Weak solutions of silver nitrate have also been used as an antiseptic for cauterising wounds and for applying to the eyes of newborn infants in certain countries to 'insure' against blindness from gonorrhoea. Chronic poisoning from the long-term ingestion of small amounts of silver nitrate is not common but includes symptoms of nervousness and anxiety (especially after the 'successful' treatment of warts) and skin discolouration (grey to blue to black). Acute poisoning is very rare (usually after accidental ingestion) and, following symptoms of violent vomiting, diarrhoea, paralysis and convulsions, is usually fatal.

The homeopathic preparation is made from the pure crystals which are dissolved in distilled water and then succussed.

GENERAL SYMPTOMS

Complaints from mental strain. **Exhaustion** with trembling. **Cravings:** for sugar/sweets. **Face** sallow. **Pains** needle-like. **Palpitations. Taste:** mouth tastes sour. **Tongue** red-tipped.
Better for fresh air.
Worse for heat; after eating sugar/sweets.

The exhaustion of someone who needs *Argentum nitricum* will be accompanied by trembling. It often follows a period of intense mental work where the mind has become exhausted to the point that the brain feels worn out and the memory starts to give out. Students swotting for exams become inefficient through anxiety so that additional mental exertion only makes things worse, and they may actually forget everything when the exam starts. These are warm people who are generally worse for heat and suffer in warm stuffy rooms. They feel much better for some fresh air. They have very sweet tooths and crave sugar and sweets but these make them sick.

EMOTIONAL/MENTAL SYMPTOMS

Anxious: anticipatory; general. **Desires** company. **Exam nerves. Excitable. Fearful** of being alone; of public speaking. **Hurried:** while speaking; while walking, while waiting. **Impulsive.** Weak **memory.** Feeling of **panic. Restless.**
Better for company.

Argentum nitricum types dread ordeals. They tremble with nervous excitement and suffer from diarrhoea when, for example, they are about to take an exam, or perform in a play. Anxious and impulsive thoughts torment them. They become fidgety and walk hurriedly around to calm themselves and time seems to pass inexorably slowly. They feel hurried (speedy) and they hate to queue or be kept waiting, and doubt their ability to succeed – their lack of confidence may be well founded in that their anxiety can prevent them from doing well. They are not happy alone and are better for company.

PHYSICAL COMPLAINTS

Diarrhoea

Symptoms STOOLS: green; smelly; watery. With FLATULENCE (see below); VOMITING.
Worse immediately after drinking; at night; after eating sugar.
Causes anticipatory anxiety; excitement; sugar; after weaning.
Liquids consumed pass straight through the body (as soon as they are drunk there is diarrhoea), and the diarrhoea is green, like chopped spinach. There may be vomiting at the same time. Newly weaned infants can produce this picture; or someone who has been on a sugar binge; or someone suffering from acute anxiety and/or panics.

Eye inflammation

Symptoms IN BABIES. DISCHARGE: purulent; smelly; yellow. EYELIDS: glued together; red. EYES: red; sensitive to light.

Better for cold; for cold compresses.
For newborn babies who develop an eye infection shortly after birth. The eyelids and the corners of the eyes are red and inflamed.

Flatulence

Symptoms BELLY/STOMACH: bloated; intolerant of tight clothing. WIND: loud; obstructed.
Worse after eating.
This is wind at both ends that is difficult to expel. The noisy, explosive burps provide relief from the bloating and the pain.

Headache

Better for binding up the head.
These headaches are usually a result of too much studying. The sufferer may ease the pain by wrapping her head with a scarf or headband.

Hoarseness

Causes over-using voice.

Indigestion

Symptoms BELLY/STOMACH bloated; painful. BELCHES: loud, difficult; empty. With FLATULENCE (see above); NAUSEA.
Better for belching.
Worse after eating.
The painful bloating of indigestion is usually worse for eating, though it may be slightly better, and the whole belly is as tight as a drum.

Sore throat

Symptoms THROAT: irritated; raw. PAIN splinter-like. VOICE: hoarse; lost.
Causes singing; talking.
These are the sore throats of singers and public speakers who suffer from anxiety.

Voice lost

Symptoms IN SINGERS.

ARNICA MONTANA (Arn.)

Family name: Compositae
Common names: leopard's bane; fall-kraut; mountain tobacco; sneezewort

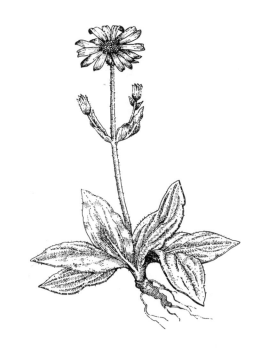

Arnica montana is a perennial herb that grows to a height of ten to twelve inches and has yellow flowers rather like those of a daisy or a marigold. It is found in moist, cool upland meadows throughout Europe, and on mountain slopes in the Andes, in Northern Asia and Siberia, and in certain north-eastern parts of the United States. It grows in the rarefied atmosphere of high altitudes, near snow level – at an altitude of between 4000 and 9000 feet.

The plant's virtues are well known to country folk, and *Arnica* has long been valued by Swiss mountain climbers who seek it out and chew it to relieve muscular aching after a day's hard climbing. In nineteenth century Europe, 'Flowers of *Arnica*' was a popular household remedy, used externally as a soothing compress for bruises and sprains. *Arnica*'s dried leaves have been smoked as a kind of tobacco in various parts of the world, and its flowers, if inhaled when freshly crushed, cause sneezing – hence one of its nicknames, sneezewort.

The whole fresh plant including the root is commonly used in the homeopathic tincture. The plant is gathered when the flowers are blooming and the root, leaves and flowers are pounded together to a pulp and mixed with alcohol, then left to stand for eight days before being strained.

GENERAL SYMPTOMS

Breath smelly. **Complaints from:** accident/injury.
Pains: sore, bruised; glands.

NB   SEE ALSO PAGES 203–26 FOR GENERAL ADVICE, DOS AND DON'TS.

Worse for jarring movement; for lying on injured part; for touch.

Arnica promotes healing, controls bleeding, reduces swelling and prevents pus forming and is therefore an essential ingredient of your first-aid kit. It is the first remedy to think of after an accident that has caused an injury, or any other trauma where there is shock, such as surgery or childbirth. People needing *Arnica* will usually feel sore and bruised and will not want to be touched or jarred. When lying down the bed feels hard and in trying to find a comfortable position to lie in they appear restless.

EMOTIONAL SYMPTOMS

Complaints from: shock. **Denial:** of illness; of suffering. **Fearful:** generally; of being touched. **Forgetful:** following injury. **Shock.**

People needing *Arnica* will deny that they are ill and will say they are well when in fact they are (sometimes very) sick. They may moan and complain about their pains, but more usually they will deny that they are suffering, especially after an injury accompanied by delayed shock. After being knocked down by a car, for example, a person might stand up demanding to be left alone, maintaining that nothing is the matter, whilst blood pours from a gaping wound in his head. He'll say, 'I'm OK. Leave me alone' that is, 'Don't touch me'. He may even ask for a taxi to be called so that he can go home. This is extremely dangerous after a head injury because of the possibility of delayed concussion. Actual concussion following a head injury may leave the person hopeless and indifferent and in a sort of stupor. On coming round he will forget words while speaking and will not want anyone to come near him in case he is touched and caused pain.

PHYSICAL COMPLAINTS

Bleeding gums

Causes dental treatment.
Give *Arnica* after dental treatment to control bleeding and to speed up healing, especially where shock and bruised soreness are present (for example after a tooth has been pulled out).

Blood blisters

Causes a blow or injury.

Boils

Symptoms BOILS: small/sore.
A succession of small, painful boils will often clear up with a short course of *Arnica*.

Broken bones

Symptoms With SWELLING/BRUISING.
Give in the first stage of a fracture where there is swelling and bruising. Move on to *Symphytum* once the swelling has gone right down.

Bruises

Symptoms With SWELLING. Without discolouration.
Causes childbirth; injury; surgery.
Arnica is the number one remedy for bruising. It speeds up healing and controls bleeding both externally and internally, thus preventing bruising from occurring. It is best given before the skin begins to discolour – if it is given soon enough, even if there is already some swelling, the bruise will not materialise. Given after the bruise has formed, *Arnica* will speed the healing and quickly reduce any swelling.

The bruised soreness that often accompanies and nearly always follows childbirth is greatly alleviated by *Arnica*. If it is very severe and persistent, *Bellis perennis* may be needed.

For bruises to the shins see *Ruta*.

Cough

Symptoms COUGH whooping. EYES bloodshot. PAIN IN CHEST: sore, bruised; must hold chest to cough. With NOSEBLEEDS.
Worse for crying.
Children cry before coughing in anticipation of the pain, and the crying itself may set off the cough.

Eye injuries

Symptoms BRUISING: to eyeball; to surrounding area.
Give *Arnica* before discolouration if possible, even if the eye is swollen.

Head injuries

Give *Arnica* as a routine after a fall or bang to the head, whether or not there is concussion. For maximum effect, wait for an egg to appear on the head (before it has discoloured), and then give *Arnica*; you will be able to watch the lump disappear in front of your eyes!

Injuries

Symptoms CUTS/WOUNDS with bruising. PAINS: sore, bruised.
Give *Arnica* in any injury to the soft tissues, i.e. muscles, where there is swelling and bruising.

Joint pain

Symptoms PAINS: sore, bruised.
Worse for touch.

Arnica may be useful for joint pain (rheumatism) where the joints are sore, bruised and very sensitive to touch.

Nosebleeds

Causes injury.

Sprains

Symptoms SPRAINS of ankle; of foot; of wrist; in first stage. With BRUISING (see above); SWELLING.
Use *Arnica* first in all sprains to bring down the swelling, to prevent bruising from occurring, and to speed up healing.

Strains

Symptoms PAINS: sore, bruised.
Causes childbirth; over-exertion.
Arnica is for strained muscles caused by over-exertion – or from some unusual or unexpected exercise. The pains are a bruised feeling and sore and are not better for moving about. (If the pains are stiff and *are* better for moving about, albeit temporarily, then *Rhus toxicodendron* is called for.) Jetlag can produce this feeling and if it does *Arnica* will help.

Toothache

Causes concussion; after a filling.
These are pains in the teeth after a head injury, or dental work.

ARSENICUM ALBUM (Ars.)

Common names: arsenic trioxide; white oxide of metallic arsenic; arsenius acid; arsenic

Arsenic is a greyish-white metallic element. Although minute traces are found in many vegetables and animal forms of life, arsenic in its crude form is a deadly poison.

It is used in the manufacture of some dyes and medicines, and many household and garden pesticides contain various forms of arsenic.

Applied externally, it burns and causes actual destruction of the skin tissue, and has consequently been incorporated into external ointments for cancerous affections.

Weak compounds of arsenic have also been used until recently as tonics to increase physical strength and endurance, and for anaemia. Animal breeders used preparations with arsenic to improve the skin and fur of animals. But a slow accumulation of small quantities of arsenic will, over a period of time, cause chronic poisoning: disorders of the digestive tract, nausea, vomiting, diarrhoea, dehydration and some paralysis. In cases of acute poisoning, the first signs are a metallic taste in the mouth and the smell of garlic on the breath. This is followed by violent burning pains throughout the entire gastro-intestinal tract, vomiting and purging, dehydration, shock syndrome, coma, convulsions, paralysis and death.

Arsenic cannot be destroyed, even by fire. Attempts have been made to destroy the evidence of deliberate arsenic poisoning by cremation, but evidence survives in the very bone ash that is left. It may change in form, and combine into an infinite variety of compounds, but the element itself, like the other metallic poisons (mercury, lead, etc.), remains immutable and indestructible.

The homeopathic preparation is obtained by roasting natural arsenides of iron, nickel and cobalt. These are diluted by trituration.

GENERAL SYMPTOMS

Catches colds easily. Discharges: burning; smelly; watery. **Dryness** generally. **Face** pale. **Likes** hot food/drinks. **Lips:** cracked; dry; licks. **Mouth:** burning; dry. **Pains** burning. **Palpitations. Restless. Sweat:** absent during fever; clammy; profuse; sour; cold. **Taste:** mouth tastes bitter. **Thirsty** for large quantities or frequent small quantities; sips. **Tongue** red-edged or red-tipped.
Better for heat; for hot drinks; for warmth of bed; for lying down.
Worse for change of temperature; for cold; for damp; for exertion; after midnight; on waking; for wet weather; at 1 a.m.

People needing *Arsenicum* look pale and anxious, and feel chilly to the touch. They are weak and exhausted, sometimes to the point of collapse in an acute illness, and often out of proportion to the severity of their complaints. The weakness will often come on suddenly, especially after any physical exertion (even walking). Although they are generally better for lying down, many of their symptoms are worse for doing so, and they become restless, and will toss and turn until driven out of bed by their pains.

The pains are characteristically burning and, with the exception of the headaches, are better for heat in general and for warm drinks, food, or compresses. *Arsenicum* is one of the few remedies with burning pains that are better for heat. Cold drinks and food will only aggravate, especially in gastric symptoms. They may well have dry, burning mouths and unquenchable thirsts, but they will drink only sips, albeit at frequent intervals. *Arsenicum* types are extremely sensitive to cold, and they have a need for fresh air so would ideally love to live in a house with the heating turned right up and the windows open. In particular, the *Arsenicum* headache benefits from fresh air and, unlike other *Arsenicum* pains, also benefits from cold in general (or a cold compress).

EMOTIONAL/MENTAL SYMPTOMS

Angry. Anxious: generally; on waking; at night; after midnight; during a fever; when alone; at 3 a.m. **Complaints from** anger with anxiety. **Critical. Depressed. Desires** company. **Despair** of getting well. **Expression:** haggard; sickly; suffering. **Fearful:** generally; of being alone; of death. **Forgetful. Irritable. Restless:** in bed; with anxiety. **Tidy.**

Arsenicum characters are more restless and anxious than virtually any other remedy type. They are frightened of being alone (as they think they will die), and want desperately to be looked after. They need people around them and are very demanding. They are difficult patients, who criticise what is being done for them and make a fuss. They may well clear up for visitors or for the doctor in spite of being too weak to get out of bed to make a cup of tea! Even an *Arsenicum* child will want his room to be tidied and feel better for it. Babies in need of *Arsenicum* may want to be carried around, but briskly, rather than gently (which is the case with *Pulsatilla*).

PHYSICAL COMPLAINTS

Boils

Symptoms PAINS burning.

Burns

Symptoms PAINS burning. With BLISTERS.
Better for heat.

Common cold

Symptoms EYES: burning; dry. EYELIDS: puffy; red. NASAL CATARRH: burning; profuse; watery. With frequent SNEEZING.
Worse during the evening; on right side.
Causes getting chilled when overheated.
This is an acute cold with violent symptoms that can move to the chest (see COUGH). The burning nasal discharge makes the area under the nostrils red and sore. The right nostril may be more affected initially, and the burning discharge may be blood streaked. The lips may become so badly cracked that they bleed.

Cough

Symptoms COUGH: dry at night; exhausting; hacking; loose. BREATHING: difficult; fast; wheezing. LARYNX: tickling. MUCUS: copious; frothy; tastes salty. With SWEATING.
Better for hot drinks.
Worse for cold; for cold drinks; fresh air; during the evening; for lying down; after midnight; at night; during fever.
The cough may be loose or dry but it is more likely to be dry at night. The person will want to lie down, propped up with lots of pillows. May wake up coughing around 1 or 2 a.m.

Cystitis

Symptoms DESIRE TO URINATE ineffectual. PAINS burning. URINATION with unfinished feeling.
Better for heat; for sitting in a hot bath.

Diarrhoea

Symptoms IN ELDERLY PEOPLE. Burning PAIN after passing stools. STOOLS: smelly; watery. With EXHAUSTION (see below); SWEATING; ICY-COLD HANDS AND FEET.
Worse for cold; after drinking; after eating fruit and any cold food; after midnight.
Causes food poisoning; ice-cream; fruit.
This is the exhausting diarrhoea that can accompany acute food poisoning.

Exhaustion

Symptoms EXHAUSTION: extreme; paralytic; sudden. With FAINT FEELING; FEVER (see below); RESTLESSNESS.
Worse in the morning; for movement.
Causes food poisoning; pain.
This exhaustion can come on suddenly, especially after diarrhoea, and will be worse for the slightest exertion. The unusual symptom that accompanies this tiredness is the restlessness.

Eye inflammation

Symptoms IN BABIES. EYELIDS burning. EYES: burning; gritty; sensitive to light.

Fever

Symptoms HEAT: burning; dry; dry at night; alternating with chills. With ANXIETY; DELIRIUM; EXHAUSTION (see above).
Worse at night; after midnight.
The feverishness or feeling hot may alternate with feeling chilly, causing the patient to sweat. The head

and face may feel hot to touch whilst the body feels cold; or the body may feel hot to touch whilst the patient feels chilled inside. At other times the patient will feel heat internally – as though the blood were burning in her veins. The characteristic *Arsenicum* thirst will be present.

Flatulence

Symptoms BELLY/STOMACH bloated. WIND smelly.

Flu

Symptoms With symptoms of COMMON COLD (see above); FEVER (see above); RESTLESSNESS.
Causes change of temperature.
The cold and fever symptoms should be accompanied by the *Arsenicum* general symptoms.

Food poisoning

Symptoms With DIARRHOEA (see above); NAUSEA; VOMITING (see below).
Causes rotten meat.
The nausea is so intense that the person cannot bear the sight, smell or thought of food.

Gastric flu

Symptoms of FLU (see above).
This type of flu is often accompanied by diarrhoea.

Hayfever

Symptoms With symptoms of COMMON COLD (see above).

Headache

Symptoms PAINS: burning; throbbing; in forehead; recurring at regular intervals.
Better for fresh air.
Worse for heat.
The patient will want to lie down with the head held high on lots of pillows. The pains may start at the bridge of the nose and spread to the whole head. The only pains that are better for cold air are the head pains. An *Arsenicum* patient with a headache may be seen wrapped in a duvet from the neck down, sitting next to an open window.

Indigestion

Symptoms Burning PAINS. With HEARTBURN.
Better for hot drinks.
Warm milk may be particularly soothing. The pains may be accompanied by a headache.

Insomnia

Symptoms DREAMS anxious; Nightmares. Restless SLEEP.
Worse after midnight.
Causes anxiety; over-active mind; shock.
Even though the person is completely exhausted, his anxiety prevents him from sleeping. When he does sleep he dreams frightful dreams, of danger, of the dead.

Measles

With *Arsenicum* general and emotional/mental symptoms.

Mumps

With *Arsenicum* general and emotional/mental symptoms.

Retention of urine

Causes childbirth.
For women who find it difficult to urinate after childbirth.

Sore throat

Symptoms Burning PAINS. ULCERS in throat.
Better for hot drinks.
Worse for cold drinks; for swallowing.

Vomiting

Symptoms VOMIT: of bile; food; smelly; watery. VOMITING: easy; frequent; violent. With DIARRHOEA (see above); FAINTNESS after vomiting; SWEATING while vomiting.
Worse after eating/drinking; for movement.
Causes ice-cream.
This is the acute vomiting (and diarrhoea) of nasty food poisoning. Everything is vomited immediately – even the smallest quantity of water (unlike *Phosphorus*, where vomiting occurs after a few minutes). Eventually there will be nothing left in the stomach to vomit, and it may then be foul-smelling bile that is vomited up.

BAPTISIA TINCTORIA (Bapt.)

Family name: Leguminosae
Other names: wild indigo; horsefly weed; yellow broom; false indigo; dyer's baptisia

NB   SEE ALSO PAGES 203–26 FOR GENERAL ADVICE, DOS AND DON'TS.

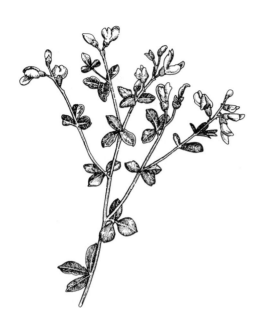

Wild indigo is indigenous to the United States and to Canada, where it is found growing in the dry soil of woods and clearings. It is a perennial plant that grows up to four feet high, with bright yellow flowers and a warty, bitter-tasting misshapen root.

It was used by the American Indians as an antiseptic and as a dressing for gangrenous wounds, especially when these wounds were accompanied by fever. They also used it as a remedy for typhoid and typhoid-like fevers.

The name 'dyer's baptisia' originates from the plant's use in America as a source of the famous blue-violet dye that the name indigo is famous for. This is now made synthetically.

The homeopathic preparation is made from the fresh root including its bark. It is pounded to a pulp and mixed with alcohol, stirred vigorously and left to stand for eight days in a cool dark place, then strained and succussed.

GENERAL SYMPTOMS

Face, mouth, tongue dark red. **Discharges**: smelly (breath, urine, sweat, etc.). **Exhaustion.**
Worse for fresh air.

This is a small remedy with a limited range of action, but it is important for a certain type of flu and sore throat. The face and tongue are a dark, dusky red colour in both the flu and the sore throat. There may be ulcers on the tongue and it may be so dark that it looks brown rather than red. The flu and sore throat are usually accompanied by total exhaustion. There may also be a fever and the person will become easily chilled in fresh air.

EMOTIONAL/MENTAL SYMPTOMS

Drowsy. Expression besotted. **Restless. Scattered sensation. Stupor.**

These patients are drowsy and weak and sink into a sort of confused stupor where they look as if they are drunk. They will answer a question when spoken to but will drift back into a comatose state as soon as they have stopped talking. They may even fall asleep whilst talking. They are usually too exhausted to move but the awful feeling of 'being scattered in bits' about the bed will cause them to toss about in order to try to gather the pieces together again. Children in particular have described this to me as being 'all in bits' or as their legs or arms not feeling connected to their body. Thoughts may be scattered also and difficult to pull together.

PHYSICAL COMPLAINTS
Flu

Symptoms Body feels bruised. Muscles: feel heavy; sore; stiff. Nightmares. With fever.
Muscles feel sore, stiff and heavy. The patient curls up tightly in bed to try to get some relief from the pain, but the bed feels too hard (as in *Arnica*) and any part of the body lain on feels sore and bruised. This constant restlessness is interspersed with a comatose nightmare-filled sleep. The fever is accompanied by chills.

Gastric flu

Symptoms Painless DIARRHOEA. With FEVER and symptoms of FLU (see above).

Sore throat

Symptoms THROAT dark red. TONSILS dark red; swollen.
Worse for eating solid food; for swallowing.
Though the throat may not be very painful, there is a feeling of constriction that makes the person gag on solid foods and only able to swallow liquids.

BARYTA CARBONICA (Bar-c.)

Other names: barium carbonate; carbonate of barium; solution of acetate; trituration of carbonate

Barium is a metallic element that constitutes about 0.05 per cent of the earth's crust. In the seventeenth century it was known to alchemists as *lapis solaris* because it is luminous in the dark after heating. The mineral *Baryta carbonica* is a naturally occurring compound, also called 'witherite' after W. Withering who discovered it in 1783 in Scotland. It is a brilliant yellowish-grey colour and is comparatively rare except in Northumberland and in Durham where it is found in faults in the coal seams.

It is used commercially in the manufacture of glass and porcelain, in optical glass, in the ceramic industry and as a pottery glaze. It is not soluble in water but dissolves in the hydrochloric acid of the stomach and thus was used in the preparation of rat poison.

The homeopathic preparation is made from the pure chemical barium carbonate by trituration.

GENERAL SYMPTOMS

Catches cold easily. Concentration poor. **Exhaustion:** after eating; in the elderly. **Glands:** swollen; sensitive. **Slowness** of children to learn. **Sweat** one-sided.
Worse for cold; for pressure; for getting feet wet.

The young and the old benefit most from this remedy. *Baryta carbonica* babies and children are slow in their development and may appear to be stuck, to have difficulty reaching the next stage. Children may lag behind in their schoolwork or may be unable to concentrate or take in new concepts (and bright children may suddenly come up against a learning 'block'). Elderly people may be going through a second childhood and appear to those around them to be surprisingly scatty, and they become very difficult to live with.

The classic *Baryta carbonica* body shape is a big round belly with disproportionately skinny arms and legs. These people are very sensitive to the cold and need to wrap up warmly because they have a tendency to 'catch' colds. They are prone to endless coughs and colds and swollen glands, and are weak both mentally and physically.

EMOTIONAL/MENTAL SYMPTOMS

Anxious during a fever. **Childish. Desires** to be alone. **Dislikes** company (strangers). **Fearful** of strangers. **Forgetful. Indecisive. Jumpy. Lack of self-confidence. Shy. Sluggish** in children.

These children are shy and nervous of strangers. They hide behind their mothers or the furniture and peer through their fingers. They are whiny and prefer to sit around at home rather than play with other children. They take teasing very badly and may be very serious at times, although at others they talk in a babyish way and clown around.

Elderly *Baryta carbonica* types may appear scatty and childish; they prefer to spend their time alone and become confused and anxious in company.

PHYSICAL COMPLAINTS
Common cold

Symptoms GLANDS swollen. NOSE dry.
The person will feel the cold and catch colds easily and often. These may be the winter colds of old people who are tired and anxious.

Cough

Symptoms IN ELDERLY PEOPLE.
Worse at night.

Exhaustion

Worse after eating.

Mumps

With *Baryta carbonica* general and emotional/mental symptoms.

Sore throat

Symptoms THROAT: inflamed; raw. Roaring noises in EARS on swallowing. PAINS burning. TONSILS swollen. With INCREASED SALIVA.
Better for swallowing liquids.
Worse at night; for swallowing saliva; for swallowing food.
A person with this sore throat can only swallow liquids; he will gag and choke when swallowing food. There is a lot of mucus in the throat and increased saliva in the mouth.

BELLADONNA (Bell.)

Family name: Solanaceae
Common names: deadly nightshade; common dwale; Atropa belladonna; Solanum furiosum; sorcerer's cherry; witches' berry

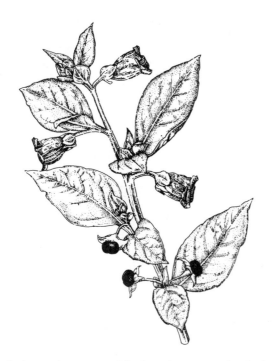

Belladonna is a perennial plant that grows in shady places throughout Europe. It flowers in July and produces bright red berries in September.

Its poisonous properties have been well known throughout history and even though every part of the plant is poisonous it has been used in many herbal preparations, external and internal. Culpeper cites its use in the form of ointments and extracts to heal inflammatory swellings, ulcers and even cancers, and in Chaucer's time it was used internally as a sleeping potion.

Belladonna eyedrops were used in the sixteenth century by Italian women to dilate their pupils and make their eyes sparkle (*belladonna* is the Italian for 'beautiful woman'). Its generic name, *Atropa*, comes from the Greek fate Atropos, 'the inflexible one', who cuts the thread of life, although another ancient belief states that this plant is the earthly form of a fatal enchantress or witch called Atropa. It was also said to be connected with the devil and was known to some as devil's berry. Belladonna was at its height of usage in witchcraft and magic in the Middle Ages in Europe, when it was used as a hallucinogen and in ritualistic practices.

It is the poisonings, though, that have been of interest to the homeopath over the years; the symptoms of the poisoning – dry mouth, fever, constricted throat with difficulty swallowing, nausea (and sometimes vomiting), red face, dilated pupils, dim vision, difficulty thinking, giddiness and delirium – were seen to be almost identical to the symptoms of scarlet fever, thus creating a classic homeopathic remedy picture.

The homeopathic preparation is made from the entire plant which is gathered when coming into flower, then chopped and pounded to a fine pulp. The juice is expressed, mixed with alcohol and left to stand for eight days before being filtered and succussed.

GENERAL SYMPTOMS

Complaints from: cold, dry wind; getting head wet. **Eyes** shining. **Face:** red; with toothache red in spots; dark red. **Glands:** swollen; sensitive. **Onset of complaint** sudden. **Pains:** appear suddenly; appear and disappear suddenly; in glands; shooting; throbbing. **Pupils** dilated. **Sweat:** absent during fever; on covered parts. **Symptoms** right-sided. **Thirsty. Tongue** red or white; 'strawberry'. *Better* for lying down.
Worse for jarring movement; for touch; for cold wind; at 3 p.m.; getting head wet.

Think of *Belladonna* as the first remedy to give someone where one part of the body becomes inflamed or infected and the inflamed part reddens and throbs painfully, radiating heat. (*Aconite* is more useful if there is a general inflammation and where the patient is much more thirsty.) The violent, throbbing pains are intensified by moving or being moved or touched, or jarred (for example during a car journey).

The eyes sparkle or shine, and pupils are usually dilated. The tongue may be red, coated with white dots, or have a uniform white coating, or be uniformly red. The face is red/flushed, and burns. Pain/fever may cause the blood vessels in the neck to throb visibly.

A *Belladonna* illness – be it a sore throat, earache or sunstroke – comes on suddenly and strongly (as it does with an *Aconite* illness). By the same token, pains disappear as rapidly as they arrive. *Belladonna* types can catch cold easily if their heads get cold, especially after having their hair cut and then becoming chilled. Generally, their symptoms are often worse at 3 p.m., although 3 a.m. may also be a bad time. These people will want to lie in quiet, darkened rooms, and their symptoms are better if they lie down, or they may be better for standing.

EMOTIONAL/MENTAL SYMPTOMS

Angry. Anxious. Confused. Delirious. Excitable. Expression fierce. **Restless. Screaming** with pain. **Sensitive:** to light; to noise. **Tearful** during a fever.

Belladonna suits happy, easy-going children who become difficult and obstinate when ill, and are then prone to tantrums. The *Belladonna* person is in a turmoil. Patients become wildly agitated, restless and delirious with a fever. May lie in bed moaning and jump up from time to time. They are hypersensitive to light and noise.

Patients tend to be angry rather than fearful although children may want to run away and hide, may hit out at those around them.

PHYSICAL COMPLAINTS

Bedwetting
Children sleep deeply and are difficult to wake up.

Breastfeeding problems

Symptoms BREASTS: engorged; hard; hot; inflamed; painful; with red streaks. PAINS throbbing. MILK SUPPLY over-abundant.
When the milk 'comes in', in the first week after the baby's birth, the breasts sometimes become hard and painful, and they may throb. If *Belladonna* is called for they may also be red with red streaks radiating out from the nipples.

Chicken pox
With *Belladonna* general and emotional/mental symptoms; FEVER; HEADACHE (see below).

Common cold

Symptoms With FEVER (see below); HEADACHE (see below); LOSS OF SMELL/TASTE.
Causes getting chilled; getting head wet.
Give *Belladonna* in the early stages of a cold that has come on suddenly and fiercely.

Convulsions

Symptoms IN CHILDREN.
Causes teething.
The typical *Belladonna* general and emotional symptoms will accompany these convulsions.
Seek professional advice immediately (see page 211).

Cough

Symptoms COUGH: barking; dry; exhausting; hard; hollow; in fits; irritating; racking; tickling; tormenting; violent. BREATHING fast. PAINS sharp; in chest. With HOARSE VOICE.
Worse at night; deep breathing.
Children may cry before the cough in anticipation of the pain. After midnight the coughing usually comes in fits.

Earache

Symptoms PAIN: spreading down into neck; stitching; tearing; throbbing. With FACE-ACHE; NOISES IN THE EAR.
Worse on right side.
The pain will often be very violent and the child will be in a great state of anguish. The radiating pains may travel towards the face.

Eye inflammation

Symptoms EYES: bloodshot; burning; dry; sensitive to light; watering. With symptoms of COMMON COLD (see above).
Worse for light; for heat.
This may accompany a cold.

Fever

Symptoms HEAT: alternating with chills; burning, dry at night; radiant. With GRINDING OF TEETH; DELIRIUM. Without sweating.
Worse for light; for being uncovered; in the afternoon; in the evening; at night.
The patient radiates heat, especially from the head, although she may feel that her limbs are cold. The skin may be alternately dry and moist and if there is sweat it will be on those parts of the body covered with clothes. There will often be no thirst with the fever. The person may hallucinate, 'seeing' ghosts and hideous faces. She will look wild, and have raging tantrums, hitting and biting those around, and jumping out of bed.

Headache

Symptoms PAINS: in back of head; in eyes; in forehead; in temples; bursting; hammering; pulsating; throbbing; violent; start and stop suddenly.
Better for resting head; for lying in a darkened room; for pressure.
Worse for bending down; for cold; for heat; for light; during menstrual period; for exposure to sun; for tying up hair; for walking.
Causes cold air; getting head wet (haircut); over-exposure to sun.

Hoarseness

Symptoms WHEN CRYING. PAINFUL.
This often accompanies a fever.

Insomnia

Symptoms SLEEP restless. With SLEEPINESS; GRINDING OF TEETH.
The person may have frightful nightmares or dreams

NB   SEE ALSO PAGES 203–26 FOR GENERAL ADVICE, DOS AND DON'TS.

of falling, and may moan in sleep. Feels sleepy but is unable to sleep.

Measles

Symptoms ONSET sudden. SKIN RASH: burns; hot; itches; red. With FEVER (see above); COUGH (see above); EYE INFLAMMATION (see above).
With *Belladonna* general and emotional/mental symptoms.

Mumps

Symptoms GLANDS: painful; swollen; worse right side. ONSET sudden. With FEVER (see above); HEADACHE (see above); SORE THROAT (see below).
The glands are swollen and painful to touch.

Period problems

Symptoms PERIODS: heavy; painful. BLOOD: bright red; clotted. PAINS violent.
Worse before and during period.
Periods are very painful; they may be delayed or interrupted after getting chilled.

Sore throat

Symptoms THROAT: constricted; irritated; raw. Swollen GLANDS. PAINS: severe; stitching.
Worse on right side; for swallowing liquids.
Causes getting cold.
The patient's neck is tender to touch, and talking is difficult. Has a constant desire to swallow despite the extreme pain; pains may radiate from the throat up into the right ear on swallowing. Will drink sips with head bent forward.

Sunstroke

Symptoms FEVER (see above). HEADACHE (see above).
Belladonna will cure sunstroke if *Glonoine* is indicated and fails (the pictures are very similar and are in fact difficult to differentiate).

Teething

Symptoms PAINFUL IN CHILDREN. CHEEKS: hot and red; swollen. SLEEP restless.
The pains are severe and there is a lot of the typical *Belladonna* thrashing about (restlessness).

BELLIS PERENNIS (Bell-p.)

Family name: Compositae
Other names: English daisy; garden daisy; eye of the daisy; bruisewort

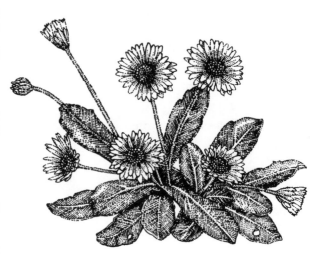

Bellis perennis is the well-loved common daisy found growing in pastures, meadows, parks and gardens throughout Europe and New England. Its flowers open up only during the day; when the daylight goes, the petals close so that only their pink-tipped undersides show. It is thought that the name '*Bellis perennis*' comes from the Latin meaning 'perennial beauty', for the daisy flowers throughout the summer.

Traditionally the daisy has a great reputation with country people as a cure for fresh wounds, and it is still known in some areas as 'bruisewort'. It was used mainly in ointment form as an external remedy for fresh wounds. It was also used for all kinds of aches and pains. As a herbal remedy Culpeper says 'an infusion of it just boiled in ass's milk is very effectual in consumptions of the lungs', and in Pliny's time it was used as a solvent of tubercular tumours.

In the homeopathic preparation the fresh plant in flower is chopped and pounded to a pulp. The expressed juice is mixed with equal parts of alcohol, and allowed to stand for eight days before being filtered and succussed.

GENERAL AND EMOTIONAL/MENTAL SYMPTOMS

Complaints from: getting chilled when overheated; accident/injury; surgery.

Bellis perennis is a small but important remedy for the first-aider. It has no general or emotional/mental symptoms, but it does have a number of specific indications for its use. It is indicated for any illness that follows a plunge into cold water while the person is overheated, that is, sudden chilling either externally by bathing in cold water, or internally by drinking ice-cold drinks or eating ice-cream on a very hot day.

PHYSICAL COMPLAINTS

Bruises

Symptoms With BUMPS AND LUMPS remaining. PAINS sore, bruised. MUSCLES sore, bruised.
Causes childbirth; injury; over-exertion; surgery.
Sometimes a bump or lump remains after bruising has disappeared, following a blow, knock or accident, or after a period of over-exertion, even if the injury occurred a long time ago. *Bellis* is particularly useful where *Arnica* has cleared the bruising but the lump remains. It is a deeper-acting remedy than *Arnica* and it may relieve bruised soreness after childbirth where *Arnica* has not helped. It is specifically useful for injuries to the breast.

Insomnia

Symptoms SLEEPLESSNESS after 3 a.m.
The person falls asleep easily and sleeps well before 3 a.m., but after this time cannot get back to sleep.

Joint pain

Causes getting chilled after being very hot.
This joint pain may be that of a gardener who is accustomed to becoming hot while working outside and then taking very cold drinks.

Pregnancy problems

Symptoms PAIN: in groin; while walking; severe.
Worse for movement.
The pain is caused by a trapped nerve during the last few months of pregnancy, when the baby is pressing down in the womb. It comes on suddenly while walking and may last for only a few minutes.

BORAX VENETA (Bor.)

Other names: Natrum biboracicum; sodium biborate; sodium tetraborate; tincal

Borax is a white mineral found in crystal form in alkaline soils and salt deposits in Tibet, Canada, Peru, Transylvania and California.
    Borax is used mainly in the manufacture of a tough and durable glass, but its many other commercial applications include its use in porcelain enamels, pottery glazes, paints, starch, adhesives, and detergents; it is also used in textile dyeing, printing, leather processing and as a glaze for linen, silk and paper, to which it gives a sheen.
    Medicinally, it was formerly an ingredient of a powder for inducing childbirth.
    The homeopathic preparation is made by fusing boracic acid with sodium carbonate, and dissolving out the borax with warm water; the borax is then diluted by trituration.

EMOTIONAL/MENTAL SYMPTOMS

Anxious of downward motion. **Dislikes** strangers. **Expression** anxious. **Fearful:** generally; of downward movement; of sudden noises (sneezing, etc.). **Irritable** before stools. **Jumpy. Screaming:** in children during sleep.

Borax babies hate downward motion and will scream on being rocked, or on being put down in their cots. If they are already asleep when they are put down they may well waken because of this sensitivity. They do not like to be thrown up (and then down) in the air as do many babies and small children. Adults will have an aversion to going down in lifts.
    These are serious, nervous youngsters who are easily startled by sudden noises such as sneezing or the hoover being turned on. They may wake up screaming following the slightest noise, or they may scream during their sleep and then wake up as if from a bad dream. They may even wake up screaming from a peaceful sleep for no apparent reason. They are particularly irritable leading up to passing a stool, and change dramatically to being cheerful directly afterwards.
    There are no marked general symptoms.

PHYSICAL COMPLAINTS

Breastfeeding problems

Symptoms BREASTS: painful during nursing; aching after nursing.
The pain is in the breast that the infant is not nursing on. After nursing, when the breasts are empty, there is an aching in both breasts.

Diarrhoea

Symptoms DIARRHOEA painless. STOOLS with mucus.
This diarrhoea may occur in teething infants. It may also accompany thrush (see below).

Thrush (genital)

Symptoms DISCHARGE like egg white; burning; white.
Worse between menstrual periods.

Thrush (oral)

Symptoms THRUSH: of mouth; of tongue. Occurs in CHILDREN. MOUTH: bleeds easily; hot; dry. With EXCESS SALIVA.
Worse for breastfeeding; for touch.
A nursing infant will cry with pain whilst feeding or refuse the breast altogether. The baby's mouth will feel hot to the mother's nipple. Elderly people whose false teeth are the cause of thrush can be helped with *Borax*, especially if the patches are sensitive and bleed easily.

Travel sickness

Symptoms With NAUSEA; VOMITING.
Worse for downward movement.
The nausea and vomiting are worse for downward movement, that is, when the ship dips or when the aeroplane lands.

BRYONIA ALBA (Bry.)

Family name: Cucurbitaceae
Common names: white bryony; wild hops; vitis alba

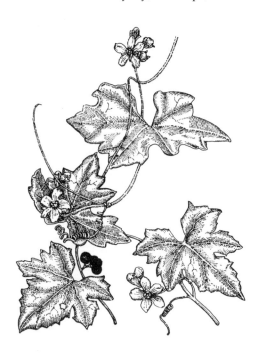

The *Bryonia alba* is a climbing perennial that grows wild in vineyards and woods in southern England and central and southern Europe. It has bright green leaves and black berries (unlike the red berries of the white bryony (*Bryonia dioica*) so common in the hedges and thickets in many parts of Britain).

The root has a very unpleasant, bitter taste and smell, and is poisonous to man and animals alike, causing severe inflammation and such violent vomiting and diarrhoea that death usually follows an accidental poisoning, often within a matter of hours.

Bryony has been used medicinally for thousands of years. Culpeper states, 'when mixed with honey, it doth mightily cleanse the chest of rotten phlegm and wonderfully helps any old and long cough, to those that are troubled by shortness of breath'.

The homeopathic remedy is made from the fresh root, gathered before the plant is in bloom, and chopped and pounded into a fine pulp. The expressed juice is mixed with equal parts of alcohol and left to stand for several weeks before it is filtered and then succussed.

GENERAL SYMPTOMS

Complaints from: change of weather from cold to warm; getting chilled. **Dryness** generally. **Face** dark red. **Likes** cold drinks; hot food. **Lips** dry. **Mouth** dry with thirst. **Onset of complaint** slow. **Pains:** sore, bruised; stitching. **Sweat** absent during fever. **Taste:** mouth tastes bitter. **Thirsty:** for large quantities; at infrequent intervals. **Tongue:** coated brown; dirty white.
Better for lying still; for firm pressure.
Worse for slightest movement; at 9 p.m.; for flatulent food (beans, cabbage, etc.).

Many complaints needing *Bryonia* come on in the first warm weather as spring turns to summer, or from getting chilled when overheated, like swimming in very cold water on a hot day. A *Bryonia* illness will develop slowly over days, like *Gelsemium* (and unlike *Aconite* and *Belladonna*, where complaints come on very quickly). Many of the acute complaints needing *Bryonia*, such as flu, fevers and coughs, are accompanied by headaches. The patients characteristically suffer from dryness everywhere (mouth, lips, tongue, chest, eyes, etc.). They are usually very thirsty and will drink large quantities at frequent intervals, gulping the drinks straight down, or at infrequent intervals if they are in a great deal of pain and do not wish to move. They will probably not disturb themselves to ask for drinks as the movement and the talking will make the pains worse, but they will drink drinks left by the bedside. Generally, the pains will be 'stitching'. They feel especially bad in the evening around 9 p.m. although their symptoms may also be bad on waking in the morning. The keynote of a *Bryonia* state is that the slightest movement aggravates the pains. The head will ache even from rolling the eyeballs around in their sockets. Patients want to stay still without moving at all. Firm pressure helps, so they will lie on their backs and/or apply pressure to the bits that hurt, or will actually lie on the side that hurts (in a cough where one lung is painful, for example) to keep it as compressed and as still as possible. *Bryonia* types like fresh air and are generally worse in hot stuffy rooms (that is, from being over-heated), although they are better for being kept warm and covered, especially if very ill.

EMOTIONAL/MENTAL SYMPTOMS

Angry. Anxious. Capricious. Irritable. Morose. Sluggish.

Bryonia has been nicknamed 'the bear' because of *Bryonia* types' irritability. They are especially irritable when disturbed, and they may lie like logs and pretend to be asleep to avoid having to respond. They resent any intrusion, and want to be left alone when they are ill. Someone in a fever needing *Bryonia* may say, 'I want to go home', even though he is already at home. They are touchy, and do not want to be questioned, examined or interfered with in any way.

Children do not want to be carried or moved about. They are capricious and reject things – toys, food, etc. – they have just asked for.

PHYSICAL COMPLAINTS
Backache

Symptoms Pains: in lower back; stitching.
Worse for coughing; during a menstrual period; for slightest movement.

Breastfeeding problems

Symptoms Breasts: engorged; hard; hot; inflamed; pale; painful. Milk supply over-abundant.
Worse for slightest movement.
The breasts look pale, compared with *Belladonna* breasts which are red; and with *Belladonna* the pains are more likely to be throbbing whereas with *Bryonia* they will be stitching. Any movement is painful and the inflammation may be accompanied by fever and some depression.

Broken bones

Symptoms Pain stitching.
Worse for slightest movement.
Bryonia can be given after a fracture where *Arnica* and *Symphytum* have been given and there is still tremendous pain with the characteristic *Bryonia* general symptoms.

Common cold

Symptoms With headache; sneezing.
Nose may feel stuffed up after the watery discharge ceases; the cold then quickly settles on the chest.

Cough

Symptoms Cough: dry; in fits; irritating; racking; vomiting; disturbs sleep. Breathing fast. Pain in chest: stitching; holds chest with hands. Pain in stomach from coughing. With headache (see below).
Better for fresh air; for lying on painful side.
Worse for deep breathing; for slightest movement of the chest; in the right lung.
The cough is accompanied by little or no expectoration. Eating or drinking can make the cough worse, because of the movement involved.

Diarrhoea

Worse after getting up; during the morning; for movement.
Causes hot weather; excess of fruit.
This 'summer diarrhoea' is always worse in the mornings after getting up and moving about a bit.

Exhaustion

Symptoms Exhaustion extreme.
Worse for slightest exertion.

Eye inflammation

Symptoms Eyes: dry; sore.
Worse for moving the eyes.

Fever

Symptoms Heat: burning; dry; alternating with chills; one-sided; without sweating.
Better for complete rest.
Worse in the autumn; around 9 p.m.
The patient will feel hot internally and externally, and often the right side of the body will be hotter than the left. If there are chills, they will generally be present during the day.

Flu

Symptoms With *Bryonia* general and emotional/ mental symptoms.

Gastric flu

Symptoms Biliousness. Taste: mouth tastes bitter. Pains aching; in stomach. With symptoms of fever (see above).
Better for belching.

Worse for coughing; after eating bread; for movement; for walking; in the evening; after lying down in bed.
All food and drink (except water) tastes bitter. There is a sensation of a stone lying in the stomach, and the pains in the stomach are often better for belching.

Headache

Symptoms PAIN: behind eyeballs; in forehead; bursting; violent.
Better for cold compresses; for pressure.
Worse for coughing; after getting up.
Causes change of weather; cold, damp weather; ironing; over-exposure to sun.
These are headaches that last all day, from the moment of getting out of bed.

Joint pain

Symptoms PAINS stitching. With SWELLING.
Better for pressure; for rest.
Worse for cold; for slightest movement.
Joints look either pale or red, and they are better for resting on the painful parts, that is, for pressure. Tight bandaging will also help.

Measles

Symptoms ONSET slow. SKIN RASH slow to appear. With COUGH; FEVER; HEADACHE (see above).
There will be the characteristic *Bryonia* dryness and dislike of movement.

Mumps

With *Bryonia* general and emotional/mental symptoms.

Sore throat

Symptoms PAINS stitching. VOICE hoarse. With symptoms of FEVER (see above).
Worse for swallowing.

Vomiting

Symptoms VOMIT: tastes bitter; watery.
Worse for movement; for coughing.

CALCAREA CARBONICA (Calc-c.)

Other names: calcium carbonate; carbonate of lime; calcii carbonas; calcarea ostorearum; oystershell

The most familiar form of calcium carbonate is limestone, which is found in all parts of the world and originates mainly from the shells of sea creatures worn away over the years. Other forms include chalk, marble, pearls and coral. Calcium is the fifth most abundant element in the human body, and is a vital agent in the structure of cells.

Calcium carbonate is used to build macadam roads, in cement and plaster, polishes, pigments and putty, and in dental powders and pastes. It is also widely used in the chemical industry.

Before Hahnemann introduced *Calcarea* into homeopathic practice, it had been used, with limited success, as a common antacid.

The homeopathic preparation is made from thick oyster shells which are cleaned and broken into small pieces. The pure white portions of the shell between the interior and exterior surfaces are selected carefully and ground to a powder.

GENERAL SYMPTOMS

Anaemia. Catches colds easily. Clumsy. Complaints from: getting wet; sprains. **Cravings** for boiled eggs. **Discharges** thick. **Dislikes:** coffee; meat. **Face** pale. **Glands:** swollen; painless. **Pains** cramping. **Palpitations. Slowness:** of children to teethe/to walk. **Sweat:** on head; sour; profuse; from slightest physical exertion; from mental exertion. **Symptoms** right-sided. **Taste:** mouth tastes bad; sour. **Tongue** white-coated.

Better for being constipated; for heat; for lying down.
Worse for cold; for damp; for draughts; for exertion; for fresh air; after drinking milk; tight clothes.

People needing this remedy tend to be sluggish, to move slowly and to look white and pasty. There is a spineless feel to them – adults have a limp handshake and may slump down in their chairs when talking to you. Exertion of any sort leaves them weak, sweaty and breathless – even climbing the stairs – and they feel better for lying down. The children are slow to learn to walk, slow to produce teeth and their fontanelles are slow to close. They have large heads and bellies.

This is a chilly remedy and people who need it will be worse for cold and damp although they can overheat easily and then be subject to hot flushes. Their feet and hands are always cold and often clammy, even in bed. They hate draughts or fresh air and they can catch cold easily after swimming or getting wet. Being warm relieves their symptoms.

The children especially sweat on their heads and at the back of the neck whilst asleep – so profusely that they may wet their pillows. Adults sweat when they exert themselves. Their sweat smells sour, as do their stools, their vomit and their urine. They have a sour taste in their mouths.

Calcarea is a remedy that affects the assimilation of food – the metabolism is slow and everything turns to fat. Milk may turn sour in their stomachs and may aggravate them and make them feel nauseous. They crave eggs, especially boiled eggs, especially when ill, and may also want to eat strange, indigestible things like chalk or pencils. They have one unusual symptom and that is that constipation makes them feel generally better.

EMOTIONAL/MENTAL SYMPTOMS

Anxious during the evening. **Confused. Depressed. Despair** of getting well. **Fearful** generally; of death; in the evening. **Melancholic. Sluggish. Stubborn. Tearful.**
Worse for thinking.

Calcarea carbonica babies are usually happy and content and will sit and watch the world go by. They may even seem lethargic at times although they will usually be more difficult to handle if they are teething or unwell as their stubborn side will come out more strongly then. Older children are sluggish and sensitive to being teased or criticised. Adults are sensitive and melancholic; full of self-pity, they weep easily about their problems and feel they are failures. They talk repeatedly about their anxieties and worries and bore close relatives and friends away. Their memories are weak and they become easily confused because thinking is difficult for them.

PHYSICAL COMPLAINTS

Backache

Symptoms PAINS: aching; in lower back; sprained feeling.
Worse for damp; on getting up after sitting.
Causes lifting.
   The back feels weak; the person cannot easily sit straight and soon slumps down in the chair.

Breastfeeding problems

Symptoms MILK SUPPLY over-abundant.
The breasts may also be very large and uncomfortable.

Broken bones

Symptoms BONES slow to mend.
If a fracture is not healing well after *Symphytum* has been given, *Calcarea carbonica* or *Calcarea phosphorica* can be given (one week on, one week off, until it has healed). Give *Calcarea phosphorica* unless there are strong general symptoms that would indicate *Calcarea carbonica*.

Common cold

Symptoms NASAL CATARRH: dry; smelly; yellow. NOSE blocked. With: LOSS OF SMELL; PAINLESS HOARSENESS.
Worse during the morning.

Constipation

Symptoms STOOLS: hard at first; large; pale; sour smelling.
Better for being constipated.
The initial large, hard stool (which may be clay-like, or like lumps of chalk) is followed by diarrhoea (see below). The person does not suffer with this constipation – in fact he feels better for it.

Cough

Symptoms COUGH: dry at night; loose during the morning. MUCUS: copious; smelly; yellow; sour; tough; tastes sweet. With symptoms of FEVER (see below).
Worse playing the piano; morning; evening in bed; during fever.
The person coughs up mucus with difficulty. Infants especially are prone to coughs during bouts of teething and the cough may then last all winter if not treated.

Cramp

Symptoms CRAMP: in calves; hands; soles of feet; toes.
Worse at night; during pregnancy; stretching leg in bed.
These are the cramps that come on when stretching limbs on waking up in bed (during the night or first thing in the morning).

Diarrhoea

Symptoms IN TEETHING CHILDREN. STOOLS: containing undigested food; sour; watery.
Worse after drinking milk.
Causes drinking milk; teething.
The diarrhoea follows a formed stool, is full of undigested food and smells sour.

Earache

Symptoms PAINS throbbing. With NOISES IN THE EAR.
The typical *Calc-carb* general and emotional symptoms will be present.

Exhaustion

Symptoms With BREATHLESSNESS. DIZZINESS.
Worse for mental exertion; for slightest physical exertion; for walking; walking upstairs.
The person is particularly worse for walking uphill or upstairs.

Eye inflammation

Symptoms IN BABIES. DISCHARGE purulent. EYES: sensitive to light; watering. EYELIDS: glued together; gritty. With symptoms of COMMON COLD.

NB   SEE ALSO PAGES 203–26 FOR GENERAL ADVICE, DOS AND DON'TS.

This is the inflammation that accompanies a common cold, and the eyes may well ooze a nasty-smelling discharge.

Flatulence

Symptoms BELLY/STOMACH: bloated; intolerant of tight clothing.

Headache

Symptoms PAINS: burning; bursting; maddening.
Better for lying down.
Worse for light; for noise; on right side of head.
Causes cold, damp weather; getting wet; mental exertion.
The head pains are worst in the back of the head and spread up to the top of the head. They are often worse whilst reading and for any jarring upward movement. The person feels better for lying down with his eyes closed.

Hoarseness

Symptoms PAINLESS.
Worse in the morning.

Indigestion

Symptoms BELCHES sour. BELLY/STOMACH: bloated; hard. PAINS pressing. With FLATULENCE; HEARTBURN.

Insomnia

Symptoms Anxious DREAMS.
Worse before midnight.
Causes over-active mind; worry.
These people become sleepless from worry and they have persistently anxious thoughts. Their anxious dreams may be interspersed with pleasant ones.

Joint pain

Symptoms PAINS: cramping.
Worse for wet weather.
Causes wet weather.
Pains are worse for the cold. When *Rhus toxicodendron* has worked well but has stopped having any effect, *Calcarea* will often help if the typical general and emotional/mental symptoms are present.

Sore throat

Symptoms THROAT dry.
Causes change of weather.

Sprains

Symptoms SPRAINS: of ankle; of hand; of wrist.
Worse for lifting.
Causes lifting heavy weights.

This remedy is useful for clumsy people (adults or children) who stumble frequently while walking and sprain their ankles easily as a result. Also for sprains from lifting heavy weights that do not clear up with *Rhus toxicodendron* and/or *Ruta graveolens*.

Stiff neck

Causes lifting.

Teething

Symptoms PAINFUL IN CHILDREN. SLOW. DIFFICULT. With DIARRHOEA (see above).
Babies may make a chewing motion with their jaws in their sleep and grind their teeth, or rather their gums!

Toothache

Symptoms PAINS gnawing.
Worse for cold air; drawing in cold air between teeth; hot drinks/food.
Causes draughts; cold, damp weather.

Vomiting

Symptoms VOMIT: curdled milk; sour.

CALCAREA FLUORICA (Calc-f.)

Other names: calcium fluoride; fluorspar; fluoride of lime; fluorite

Calcium fluoride is found worldwide, in the form of the mineral fluorspar, which occurs as beautiful-coloured crystals. The most common of these crystals is violet coloured and when this is exposed to ultra-violet radiation it emits a beautiful blue light (it is from this that we derive the term 'fluorescence').

The largest single use of fluorspar is in the steel industry as a flux – an agent to increase the fluidity of certain metals in the refining processes – and it is also used in the smelting of gold, silver, copper and lead. The word 'fluor' comes in fact from the Latin meaning 'a flowing'.

Calcium fluoride is present in the enamel of the teeth, the surface of the bones and in the elastic fibres of the skin, the muscles and the blood vessels.

The homeopathic preparation is made from selected pieces of crystal fluorspar, which are prepared by trituration.

GENERAL AND EMOTIONAL/ MENTAL SYMPTOMS

There are no strong general or emotional/mental symptoms for *Calcarea fluorica*, although as with the other *Calcarea* salts people needing this remedy are generally worse for cold, damp weather. It is especially useful as a tonic for any tissues that have become worn out, flabby and lax, in the same way that *Calcarea phosphorica* can be used as a tonic for worn-out *nervous* systems. For example, during pregnancy this may be indicated for women whose skin is dry and out of condition; and varicose veins is another example of elastic tissue that has lost its tone. Those with firm, elastic skin and no worry of stretch marks will not need this remedy. Short courses of *Calcarea fluorica* can be repeated if it is found to be of benefit.

PHYSICAL COMPLAINTS

Backache

Symptoms PAINS in lower back.
Better for continued movement.
Worse on beginning to move.
If *Rhus toxicodendron* was indicated and only partially relieves the pain, or if it fails, then *Calcarea fluorica* will usually help.

Common cold

Symptoms NASAL CATARRH dry. SNEEZING with difficulty.
Better for sneezing.
This is for stuffy colds in the head with dry catarrh.

Tooth decay

Symptoms CRUMBLING; DECAYING.
This remedy used as a tonic will help to build strong healthy teeth in children. It is a safer option than fluoride tablets, whose potential side effects continue to cause concern.

CALCAREA PHOSPHORICA (Calc-p.)

Other names: calcium phosphate; calcii phosphas precipitata; phosphate of lime

Calcium phosphate is a mineral salt and is the principal mineral constituent of bones and teeth. It accounts for about 60 per cent of the average human skeleton.

Commercially, the most important of the calcium phosphates is primary calcium phosphate, or 'superphosphate'. This is used as a fertiliser ingredient, as a leavening agent in baking powders, as a stabiliser for plastics, and in the manufacture of glass. Other forms of calcium phosphate are also widely used in commercial products.

The homeopathic preparation is obtained by dropping dilute phosphoric acid into lime water. The particles which form as a result of this process are washed in distilled water and dried, and then triturated.

GENERAL SYMPTOMS

Catches colds easily. Complaints from: loss of body fluids. **Face** pale. **Slowness** of children to learn/to teethe. **Thin**.
Worse for cold; for damp; for draughts; for fresh air; for wet weather.

Calcarea phosphorica is of vital importance in the growth and maintenance of healthy cells. It nourishes blood cells, bones, teeth and all connective tissue and it is therefore a remedy that may be indicated in young children who develop slowly. Young children are slow learning to walk and slow to learn. Because their food is not well assimilated they tend to be anaemic, grow slowly and their teeth decay easily. They develop slowly, babies' fontanelles close slowly and they are slow to teethe. This is a wonderful tonic to give to children who have had a growth spurt and have become pale and exhausted as a result. Adults and children who are weak and tired while convalescing from an illness will likewise benefit from this remedy – it will help them to regain their strength. The typical *calcarea phosphorica* type is thin with long, dark eyelashes and dark hair. They are sensitive to the cold and the damp, and have cold extremities.

EMOTIONAL/MENTAL SYMPTOMS

Anxious. Discontented. Restless. Sighing. Sluggish in children.
Worse for mental exertion.

Adults complain and grumble about many things. Thinking of their complaints often makes them feel worse. They sigh a lot while talking and are generally restless. Children are peevish and lifeless and have no 'go' in them. They want something but they don't know what.

PHYSICAL COMPLAINTS

Anaemia

Symptoms With EXHAUSTION.
Causes acute illness.
This is for the convalescent stage of an illness, or post-childbirth, where regaining strength is proving difficult.

Broken bones

Symptoms BONES slow to mend.
This remedy is indicated for fractures that are taking longer than expected to heal. It can be given routinely after *Symphytum* has dealt with the pain of the fracture, as it will speed up the healing of the fracture and ensure that the bone is good and strong.

Cough

Symptoms Yellow MUCUS.
Worse when teething.
Calcarea phosphorica may be useful in clearing obstinate coughs (or whooping cough) in children. These are coughs that tend to be worse in the cold-weather months. Teething may also make this cough worse.

Cramp

Symptoms CRAMP in calves.
Worse for walking.

Headache

Symptoms IN SCHOOLCHILDREN.
Causes mental exertion; overworking; anaemia.
The headache is often worse for a cold wind, but cold bathing can relieve it.

Insomnia

Symptoms WAKING: difficult; late.
Worse before midnight.
Mornings are an awful time when waking is difficult.

Joint pain

Worse for cold weather.
The joints of the feet in particular are often affected. The feet are always cold and there is a cramping and aching numbness.

Period problems

Symptoms PERIOD: painful; heavy. BLOOD: dark red; clotted.
Women become anaemic after these heavy painful periods. *Calcarea phosphorica* will work as an effective tonic.

Stiff neck

Symptoms IN ADULTS.
Causes draughts.

Teething

Symptoms PAINFUL IN CHILDREN. SLOW. DIFFICULT. STOOLS green.
Calcarea phosphorica is helpful for either first or second teeth that are proving slow and difficult in cutting through the gums. Teething children may develop diarrhoea, colds and coughs; these complaints plus the teething difficulties will be helped by this remedy.

The teeth are also inclined to decay easily and prematurely. *Calcarea* will ensure a better assimilation of calcium and so encourage healthy dentine formation.

CALCAREA SULPHURICA (Calc-s.)

Other names: calcium sulphate; sulphate of lime; gypsum; plaster of Paris; selenite

Calcarea sulphurica is a chemical compound found most commonly either in the form of crystals, as selenite, or in earthy masses, when it is known as gypsum. It is one of the first minerals to crystallise as seawater evaporates, and beds of gypsum frequently underlie deposits of rock salt formed by the evaporation of ancient seas.

Raw gypsum (mined from pits and cliffs) is used mainly as a retarder in Portland cement (it slows down the rate of setting). It is also used as an agricultural fertiliser, and in the manufacture of paints, pharmaceuticals and insecticides. When partially dehydrated and mixed with water, calcium sulphate forms plaster of Paris, which is used for surgical casts, for models, moulds, statues and to cover interior walls of buildings.

The homeopathic preparation is made from plaster of Paris by trituration.

GENERAL SYMPTOMS

Abscesses discharging pus.   **Discharges** blood-streaked.
Worse for heat; for milk; for physical exertion; in stuffy rooms.

Calcarea sulphurica's sphere of action is that of curing discharging abscesses or long-standing catarrhs. People needing this remedy are prone to thick, lumpy, yellow or bloody discharges. Patients are generally worse for warmth and overheating, unlike the other *Calcarea* remedies which are chilly, and unlike *Hepar sulphuris*, another important remedy for abscesses and catarrhs, which is also chilly. They like to be uncovered (if feverish) and are usually better for some fresh air, though they are not fond of draughts.

EMOTIONAL/MENTAL SYMPTOMS

Anxious during the evening. **Dull. Sluggish. Tearful.**

These people are anxious types, weepy and sluggish, like *Calcarea carbonica* types.

PHYSICAL COMPLAINTS

Abscesses

Symptoms ABSCESS discharging pus; of glands.
Heals discharging abscesses, that is, ones that have burst or broken and are discharging – usually a thick, yellow, lumpy and possibly bloody matter. It is often when an abscess is at this stage that one is told to let it drain and let nature take its course. This can be interminable in some cases and this remedy will help to speed up the healing process.

Common cold

Symptoms NASAL CATARRH: blood-streaked; smelly; thick; yellow. With HEADACHE; LOSS OF SMELL.
Worse after drinking milk.
This is for post-nasal catarrh (where mucus drips down the back of the throat) or for catarrh that is one-sided (only one nostril is blocked). Patients dislike milk and it aggravates their condition.

Cough

Symptoms COUGH dry. MUCUS: copious; lumpy; yellow.

Croup

Symptoms COUGH occurs only on waking.
In croup where *Hepar sulphuris* is indicated but fails, *calcarea sulphurica* will cure, especially if the child is warm and wants to be uncovered and/or if the croupy cough is only there on waking.

Earache

Symptoms DISCHARGE: blood-streaked; smelly; thick.

Eye inflammation

Symptoms DISCHARGE: thick; yellow.
This remedy is especially indicated if both the nose and the eyes are discharging thick, yellow mucus.

Injuries

Symptoms CUTS/WOUNDS: slow to heal; suppurating.
Where a wound has become inflamed and has started to discharge a thick yellow pus, *Calcarea sulphurica* is indicated to complete the healing. (*Hepar sulphuris* is for the stage before this, where there is redness and inflammation but not necessarily a discharge.)

CALENDULA OFFICINALIS (Calen.)

Family name: Compositae
Common names: marigold; pot marigold; marygold; caltha officinalis

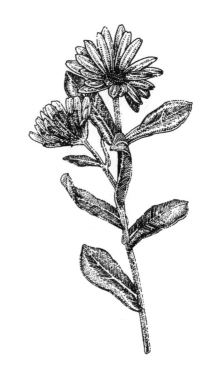

The marigold is an annual flowering plant which originally grew wild in Egypt and throughout the Mediterranean. It grows to a height of one to two feet and has deep orange flowers that open with the rising sun and close with the setting sun, like *Bellis perennis* (common daisy).

It has been known for hundreds of years for both its use in cookery and in medicine. In the kitchen a dye extracted from the flowers was used to give cheese a yellow colour, and in Elizabethan times the blossoms were sprinkled on salads to cheer them up. The old herbalists advised that the dried flowers be added to broths in order to comfort 'the heart and the spirits, and to expel any malignant or pestilential quality which might annoy them'.

Calendula has always been a highly respected healer of diseases of the skin, and has been used by herbalists for extremely serious diseases such as cancer and smallpox.

In the homeopathic preparation, the leaves, blossoms and buds are chopped and pounded to a pulp, then the expressed juice is mixed with alcohol and succussed.

GENERAL SYMPTOMS

There are no general symptoms to look out for with this remedy. It is used as a great healer of wounds and cuts, both externally in ointment form (see the External Materia Medica) and internally in potentised form (which makes the wound heal even more quickly).

Use *Calendula* in the case of a straightforward injury where the skin is broken but where there are no other noteworthy symptoms. It seems to work especially well where the pains are stronger than you would expect in relation to the size of the injury.

PHYSICAL COMPLAINTS
Injuries

Symptoms CUTS/WOUNDS: lacerated; suppurating. PAINFUL out of proportion to injury.

CANTHARIS VESICATORIA (Canth.)

Family name: Caleoptera
Other names: Spanish fly; fabricus; de geer

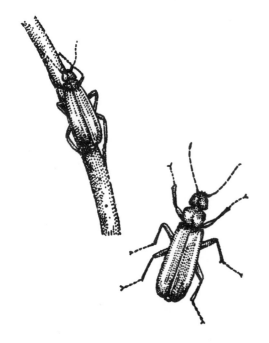

The Spanish fly is a handsome green beetle found in southern France and Spain where it feeds on the leaves of white poplar, privet, ash, elder and lilac trees. If touched, the beetles produce unpleasant blisters on the skin.

Spanish fly is one of the most ancient (and least reputable) drugs known to man. Hippocrates described its value in treating dropsy 2000 years ago, and it has been used as an external application in the form of blistering plasters for various rheumatic conditions. It has also had a reputation as an aphrodisiac because it causes an irritation of the kidneys and bladder and consequently an increased awareness of the genital area. Those who took it were supposed to be driven into a sexual frenzy (which the Marquis de Sade apparently made full use of according to many accounts). The poisonings from increased doses produce various terrible symptoms ranging from appalling abdominal cramps, vomiting of blood, intolerable burning pains in the mouth and throat, diarrhoea, blood in the urine, and kidney damage.

To make the homeopathic remedy, the flies are collected at dawn when they are still sleepy after the cold night. They are killed by being heated in the steam of boiling vinegar. They are then crushed and the homeopathic remedy is prepared by trituration.

GENERAL AND EMOTIONAL/ MENTAL SYMPTOMS

Cantharis is easily confused with *Apis* and *Arsenicum* because all have restlessness and burning pains. Inflammations come on rapidly and violently. Patients may have a burning, unquenchable thirst, but their complaints are often aggravated by drinking cold liquids or the smallest amount of coffee. They feel worse for urinating.

There are few strong emotional symptoms. The pains may drive a person to moan and complain loudly.

PHYSICAL COMPLAINTS
Burns

Symptoms BURNS: second degree; with blisters. PAINS burning.
Better for cold compresses.
Scalds, sunburn or second-degree burns with blisters (or just before the blisters form). The pain is better for cold compresses.

Cystitis

Symptoms DESIRE TO URINATE: constant; frequent; ineffectual; urgent. PAINS: before, during and after urination; burning; cutting. URINATION frequent. URINE: hot; red; scanty.
Worse for cold drinks; before, during and after urination.
Pains are violent and spasmodic. There may be a constant desire to pass water, and the bladder never feels empty.

CARBO ANIMALIS (Carb-a.)

Other names: animal charcoal; leather charcoal

Carbo animalis is a soft charcoal that has all the properties of wood charcoal with the difference that it produces a brownish tinge when used as a pigment in artists' colours.

For the homeopathic preparation ox leather is placed on red-hot coals and left there for as long as it burns in the flame. As soon as the flame dies the leather is placed between two flat stones and the flame extinguished.

GENERAL SYMPTOMS

Ankles weak. **Sweat:** exhausting; profuse; smelly.

This is a small remedy which has few general indications. The sweating is profuse and will be worse at night, or during/after eating. The ankles of children learning to walk are weak and they sprain easily.

EMOTIONAL/MENTAL SYMPTOMS

Depressed. Desires to be alone. **Dislikes** company. **Uncommunicative.**

This remedy is for anyone who has become debilitated by illness, but it is especially suited to elderly people who have become withdrawn and worn out because of long-term illness.

PHYSICAL SYMPTOMS

Exhaustion

Worse for walking; during a menstrual period.
Causes breastfeeding; after an acute illness; lifting; sweating.
The typical *Carbo animalis* sweat accompanies this exhaustion, which occurs in people recovering from an illness and also in nursing mothers who become exhausted, and are weepy whilst eating because they feel too tired to even eat. Walking across the room seems too much. They may also have painful, lumpy breasts which hurt whilst their baby nurses. Tiredness can be caused by bouts of sweating (see general symptoms).

Flatulence

Symptoms BELLY distended.
Causes abdominal surgery.
Carbo animalis will provide some relief where the belly is blown up with wind that is very difficult to pass after an operation on the abdomen (such as an appendicectomy or a laparoscopy).

Food poisoning

Causes bad fish.

Strains

Symptoms STRAINS: of muscles; of tendons; of wrist. The person strains muscles easily – of the wrist especially, although the back can also be pulled – from lifting even small weights; the strained muscle is then made worse by the slightest exertion, and the person will not be able to lift anything at all.

CARBO VEGETABILIS (Carb-v.)

Common name: wood charcoal

Charcoal is half-burnt wood or artificial coal, a black amorphous (lacking a crystalline structure) form of carbon made by heating wood in the absence of air. Carbon as an element is found in all living matter, from the hard crystalline form of diamonds to the softer form of graphite and the amorphous form of charcoal. There are so many carbon compounds that their study forms a separate branch of chemistry.

Charcoal is so hard that it is insoluble in acids and it doesn't rot like ordinary wood. Because of this it was used in ancient times by landowners to stake out the boundaries of their property. Nowadays, it is used commercially as a polish for brass and copper plates, as a black pigment in artists' paints and as artists' charcoal pencils amongst other things.

Charcoal is a great purifier and is capable of rendering a rancid oil clear and sweet smelling; and it is said to have the same property with regard to putrid-smelling meat and vegetables! In fact, *Carbo vegetabilis* illustrates well how the properties of the natural product are similar to the characteristics and symptoms of the classic *Carbo vegetabilis* picture (or person): wood charcoal absorbs air and continues to do so for a long time after it is made, and its vapour on burning is harmful; the classic picture is of a person prone to incarcerated wind which, once released, is also noxious!

Different woods make charcoals with different properties; the homeopathic preparation is made from the finest beech, which is stripped of bark, cut into pieces the size of a fist, then heated until red hot and rapidly smothered in an earthen jar with a tightly fitting lid.

NB   SEE ALSO PAGES 203–26 FOR GENERAL ADVICE, DOS AND DON'TS.

GENERAL SYMPTOMS

Breath smells. **Complaints from:** measles; loss of body fluids. **Discharges** smelly. **Face** pale; sallow or blue. Feels **faint** on getting up; on waking. **Sweat** cold; profuse. **Taste:** mouth tastes bitter.
Better for fanning; for fresh air.
Worse for exertion; after eating rich/fatty foods; for humidity.

Carbo vegetabilis is indicated for children who have not fully recovered from a serious illness such as whooping cough or measles. They are sluggish and low in vitality afterwards and want to lie down and sleep. The slightest exertion exhausts them; they have to force themselves to get going.

People recovering from chest infections, particularly the elderly, often benefit from the remedy. Patients are chilly and their legs especially are cold to the touch, but they feel much better out in the cool, fresh air, especially if there is a breeze, and they ask to be fanned. Becoming overheated makes them feel worse as does humidity (warm, damp weather). They may feel worse for lying down in spite of being too weak to do otherwise. Mornings and evenings are their worst times of day.

The other main use of this remedy is for dealing with acute indigestion, in which case the other mental and general characteristics may not be present.

EMOTIONAL/MENTAL SYMPTOMS

Anxious during the evening; in bed. **Confused.** **Indifferent** to everything. **Irritable. Sluggish.**

This is a remedy for inactive, sluggish folk who find it difficult to rouse themselves to do anything. It is more of a mental than a physical state. They may become indifferent to the point that they do not care if they live or die. They suffer from anxiety, however, in the late afternoon through to the evening, and this intensifies when they go to bed and shut their eyes.

PHYSICAL SYMPTOMS

Common cold

Symptoms Nose blocked. Sneezing: frequent; with difficulty. With hoarseness; itching throat.
The tickling in the throat may be acute and the patient may not be able to sneeze at times in spite of wanting to.

Cough

Symptoms Cough: racking; in fits; suffocative; violent; whooping. Breathing: fast; wheezing. Mucus green. Voice hoarse. With retching.

Worse at night; evening; before midnight.
The coughing fits are worse at night, especially before midnight, and are often accompanied by the characteristic cold perspiration.

Exhaustion

Symptoms Breath cold. Breathing difficult.
Better for being fanned.
Causes carbon monoxide poisoning; food poisoning; accident/injury; acute illness; loss of body fluids; diarrhoea; vomiting; breastfeeding; surgery.
Carbo vegetabilis is useful for extreme weakness, a state which most commonly occurs as a result of an accident or an operation, after severe vomiting, or during convalescence from a serious illness. This weakness may be so acute that 'collapse' would be a more accurate label. The characteristic *Carbo vegetabilis* general symptoms are present, the breath is cold, the body feels icy-cold to touch and the sweat is also cold. The person may feel hot inside. The face, which is cold and sweaty, may be deathly pale or even blue, with bluish lips. The head feels very heavy. I do not suggest that you treat people who are this seriously ill without help, but if you are the only person available and this remedy fits the case, give it.

Carbo vegetabilis may also be indicated to treat forms of poisoning: food; North Sea gas, or poisoning from car exhausts that may come on after sitting in a traffic jam on a hot, windless day for a period of time.

Flatulence

Symptoms Stomach/belly: bloated; rumbling. Wind smelly. With diarrhoea.
Better for passing wind.
The belly (below the navel) is bloated, as it is with *Lycopodium* flatulence. Passing wind affords much relief.

Food poisoning

Causes rotten fish/meat.

Hair loss

Symptoms hair falls out.
Causes an acute illness.

Headache

Symptoms Pains: in back of head; heavy; pressing.
The head feels heavy, like lead.

Hoarseness

Symptoms Painless.
Worse morning and evening.

Indigestion

Symptoms BELLY/STOMACH bloated. BELCHES: empty; sour. PAINS: burning; cramping. With FLATULENCE (see above); NAUSEA.
Better for belching; for passing wind.
Worse after eating rich/fatty food.
The *Carbo vegetabilis* digestion is easily upset, especially by eating fatty, rich foods. The stomach feels full and becomes bloated after eating, to the extent that the skin is stretched as tight as a drum. Tight clothes feel extremely uncomfortable then. The nausea is worse in the mornings. Burping may only relieve the bloatedness for a while, and it builds up quite quickly again.

Mumps

Symptoms GLANDS: swollen/painful. PAINS: spread to breasts, ovaries or testicles.
With typical *Carbo vegetabilis* pale face and cold sweat.

Nosebleeds

Symptoms BLOOD dark.
Worse at night.
This is specially for children who are in a weakened state after an acute illness (such as measles) and who start having these night-time nosebleeds for no apparent reason.

Voice lost

Worse in the evening.

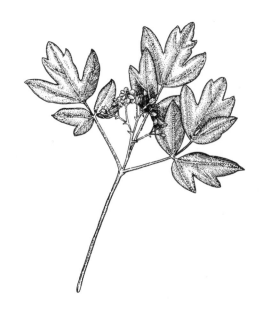

CAULOPHYLLUM (Caul.)

Family name: Berberidaceae
Common names: caulophyllum thalictroides; blue cohosh; papoose root; squaw root; blueberry root

This perennial herb grows in moist, swampy places or near running streams throughout the USA. It produces yellowish-green flowers in May and June and a few seeds the size of large peas which can be roasted and made into a coffee-like drink.

The American Indians used *Caulophyllum* as their chief remedy for expectant mothers. Drunk as a tea for two weeks before delivery it was said to render the birth painless and rapid. It was also used for rheumatism, dropsy, inflammation of the womb and colic.

The homeopathic preparation is made from the knotty root, which is gathered early in the year when new growth is beginning. It is chopped, ground to a pulp and mixed with alcohol, and then left to steep.

GENERAL SYMPTOMS

There are no strong general or emotional symptoms. *Caulophyllum*'s major use as a homeopathic remedy is in childbirth. It is also useful for a very specific type of rheumatism and I have given the indications below. Many homeopathic books advise that pregnant women take *Caulophyllum* during the last weeks or months of their pregnancies in order to prepare them for an easy labour. This needs careful thought as I have seen women who have had short, violent labours after taking *Caulophyllum* during their pregnancies. If this is not your first baby and you have a history of easy labours then do not take this remedy. If this *is* your first baby and you are worried about the birth then find a homeopath who can properly advise you on the remedies that *you* will need.

PHYSICAL SYMPTOMS

Joint pain

Symptoms PAIN: in the small joints; flying around; irregular.
The pains occur in the small joints of the fingers and hands and move around frequently.

Labour pains

Symptoms EXHAUSTION with trembling. PAINS: irregular; stop altogether; ineffectual.

The labour pains are short and ineffectual. They can appear in the groin, bladder and legs, and fly from one place to another. The cervix is rigid and does not dilate. There is chilliness in labour, with internal trembling or shivering, even when covered up.

CAUSTICUM (Caust.)

Other names: Causticum Hahnemanni; potassium hydrate; tinctura acris sine kali

Causticum is a substance invented by Hahnemann. He made it from burnt or slaked lime (calcium hydroxide) which he mixed with bisulphate of potash. *Causticum* smells like the lye obtained from potash, and has an astringent and burning taste on the back of the tongue. Its freezing point is below that of water. It promotes the putrefaction of animal substances which are placed in it.

Slaked lime is used extensively in the making of mortars, plasters and cements and is simply the reaction of quick lime with water, and in agriculture to add calcium to the soil.

The caustic element to this remedy – its ability to burn – gives us one of the major indications for its use as a homeopathic remedy, that is, for serious burns that blister.

The homeopathic remedy is prepared by succussion.

GENERAL SYMPTOMS

Blisters: on tip of tongue; painful. **Clumsy:** trips easily while walking. **Complaints from:** change of weather to dry; getting wet. **Discharges** watery. **Exhaustion** during evening. **Eyelids** heavy. **Likes** smoked foods. **Restless** during evening. **Tongue:** red stripe down centre (white edges).
Better for cold drinks; for heat; for warmth of bed.
Worse for changes in weather; for coffee; for cold; for draughts; during the evening; for fresh air; for walking; for getting wet.

These are chilly people who are affected badly by getting wet, by draughts, by changes in the weather and especially by clear, dry, cold weather. Their symptoms are aggravated by walking out in the fresh air and also by drinking coffee. Mild, wet weather makes them feel better, especially their 'rheumatics' and their 'chests'; when everyone else is complaining about the damp they will be enjoying some relief from their pains. The weakness of a person needing *Causticum* comes on in the evenings and is overwhelming. Blisters are a useful guiding symptom as they often

accompany a cough or sore throat in someone who needs *Causticum*.

Causticum is one of the first-aid remedies for burns and scalds, but it is only for very serious burns, and these must also receive expert attention. It is possible, however, to prescribe *Causticum* on the way to the hospital to provide some relief from the terrible pains of a third-degree burn.

EMOTIONAL/MENTAL SYMPTOMS

Absent-minded. Anxious. Concentration: poor. **Complaints from** grief. **Depressed. Fearful** during the evening. **Irritable. Memory** weak. **Sympathetic. Tearful.**

These are sensitive souls who suffer when those close to them are hurting – either emotionally or physically. They are very sensitive to injustice in any shape or form, wherever it may be. Being pessimistic by nature, they tend to look on the dark side of things and become gloomy and full of anxious forebodings. They become great worriers and they despair of getting well. Irritability sets in, and then depression. They cry easily, especially if they see a sad news item in the paper or on television. The children also cry easily and are frightened of the dark, of ghosts, of going to bed on their own.

Another indication for *Causticum* can be grief, where someone has suffered a loss of someone close to them (this could even be a favourite pet); they sink into a negative state and start to develop some of the general symptoms listed above. If the picture is very clear then prescribe but if you are at all uncertain it is better to seek the help of a professional homeopath than make a mess of the case.

PHYSICAL COMPLAINTS

Bedwetting

Symptoms BEDWETTING during first sleep.
For whiny children who cry easily, don't want to go to bed alone and who sleep restlessly.

Burns

Symptoms BURNS third degree. PAINS burning. With BLISTERS.
For serious, third-degree burns, chemical burns, or scalds, with the characteristic *Causticum* pains. *Causticum* can also help to cure soreness that remains at the site of old burns.

Constipation

Symptoms DESIRE TO PASS STOOL ineffectual.
The stool may be soft despite the person being consti-

pated and unable to pass it. May have to stand up to pass a stool.

Cough

Symptoms COUGH: constant; distressing; exhausting; hollow; racking; rattling; tormenting; violent; wakens from cough at night. MUCUS: difficult to cough up; must swallow what comes up. PAINS: raw in chest. With HOARSE VOICE.
Better for sips of cold water.
Worse for breathing in; for cold air; in bed; bending head forward; lying down.
The hoarseness that accompanies this cough is worse in the mornings. Coughing up mucus is especially difficult as it comes up to the throat and then slips back again. Small sips of water are about the only thing that eases the cough and stops it, albeit temporarily.

Cramp

Symptoms CRAMP: in feet; in toes; in sole of foot.
Worse at night.

Cystitis

Symptoms DESIRE TO URINATE: frequent, ineffectual. PAINS: burning; during urination. URINATION: difficult; frequent; involuntary; slow to start; with unfinished feeling.
Worse while urinating.
This is a cystitis where there is a frequent urging to urinate but on attempting to do so the person suddenly has difficulty actually passing water or can't pass water at all. May in fact pee involuntarily when coughing, sneezing or blowing the nose.

Hoarseness

Symptoms Loss of VOICE.
Worse during the morning; during the evening.
Causes over-using voice.
Singers often experience a sudden, temporary loss of voice or a painless hoarseness.

Indigestion

Symptoms BELCHES: empty; tasting of food just eaten. BELLY/STOMACH feels full. PAINS cramping; pressing.
The burps taste of food just eaten.

Joint pain

Symptoms PAINS: in back; in joints; in neck; burning; gnawing; pressing; stitching; tearing. With STIFFNESS.
Better for heat; for warmth of bed.
Worse for dry cold; getting up from sitting.
The pains cease on getting warm in bed and begin again on getting up in the morning. Sufferers are very restless at night.

Sore throat

Symptoms THROAT: burning; dry; raw. CHOKING sensation; constant DESIRE TO SWALLOW.
Worse for talking.
Swallowing is difficult as the throat feels too narrow, and the person can't expectorate. Hoarseness remains after the sore throat has cleared up (see above).

Retention of urine

Causes childbirth.
Women find it difficult to urinate after childbirth.

Voice lost

Symptoms In SINGERS. SUDDEN.

CHAMOMILLA (Cham.)

Family name: Compositae
Common names: corn feverfew; matricaria chamomilla; German chamomile

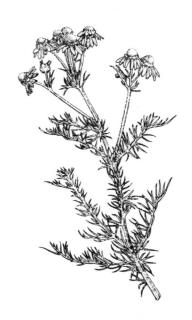

This is an annual plant that grows in uncultivated fields among wheat and corn, especially in the sandy regions of Europe.

In ancient medicine *Chamomilla* was used only occasionally for treating consumption (tuberculosis). Culpeper mentions it in his *First Complete English Physician* and recommends it as a strengthener of the womb, as a remedy for the after effects of the 'careless midwife' and as an antidote for opium poisoning.

It is worth mentioning that it is not too difficult to conduct your own proving, unintentionally. The recent fashion of drinking herbal teas has meant that some poor souls are drinking upwards of two cups of chamomile tea a day (1–2 pints). I have found that many patients suffering from irritability and sleeplessness have been cured simply by the removal of chamomile tea from their diets. By all means have the odd cup of herbal tea but do bear in mind that they have medicinal properties and that large amounts drunk on a daily basis can produce the symptoms they were supposed to cure.

The homeopathic preparation is made from the whole fresh plant when it is in full flower. It is chopped and pounded to a fine pulp, the juice is expressed, mixed with equal parts of alcohol and then allowed to stand for eight days before it is succussed.

GENERAL SYMPTOMS

Complaints from: coffee; teething. **Face** red; one-sided – in spots; with toothache (teething). **Likes** cold drinks. **Pains** unbearable. **Sweat:** clammy; hot; better for uncovering.
Worse during the evening; for fresh air; for coffee; for wind.

Chamomilla pains are often brought on or associated with teething, anger or too much tea or coffee. It is especially suited to teething children and women in labour, and anyone who has been in a highly emotional state (especially angry) for a long period of time and who has become over-sensitive, mentally or physically, as a result. Hahnemann said of this remedy, 'It ought not to be given to those who bear pain with patience and resignation,' as its keynote is unbearable pain. There may be sweating with the pains, especially on the scalp and face – along with a high fever. The sweating may make them feel better. *Chamomilla* patients are generally worse in the evening before midnight (teething, cough, fever, etc.). The typical *Chamomilla* patient feels hot and doesn't like it, will kick off the bedclothes or stick the burning soles of her feet out of bed. They sweat easily and feel better for it. They are sensitive to wind and to being chilled by cold, damp air.

EMOTIONAL/MENTAL SYMPTOMS

Violently **angry. Complaints from** anger. **Depressed. Desires:** to be carried; to be alone. **Dislikes** company; being spoken to; being looked at; being touched. **Excitable. Impatient. Irritable** children. **Screaming** with pain. **Sensitive** to pain. **Stubborn.**

People who need *Chamomilla* will be angry and excitable and will tolerate nothing and nobody. They are incredibly sensitive to pain and are enraged by it. They may snap and snarl and demand relief from their pain, but nothing helps. A *Chamomilla* patient will often say, 'I can't bear the pain any longer.'

Children can be spiteful and hit their parents. They whine and scream and cannot be comforted. They ask for things which they may immediately hurl across the room (drinks, toys, etc.). Babies insist on being carried around and cry loudly when they are held still or put down. Even after being carried for a short while they may start to cry. The parents of a 'Chamomilla baby' will be at their wits' end and may talk of adoption!

PHYSICAL COMPLAINTS

Cough

Symptoms Cough: dry during sleep; irritating; tickling. Mucus tastes bitter.
Worse at night.
The cough is often worse at night when the child is asleep but it does not waken him/her.

Diarrhoea

Symptoms Stools: green; hot; smelling of rotten eggs; painful. In teething children.

Earache

Symptoms Pains: aching; pressing; stitching; tearing; unbearable.
Worse for wind; bending down.

Fever

Symptoms Heat: burning; one-sided. With Thirstiness; Shivering.
Worse mid morning.
Causes anger.
The face and breath are hot whilst the body is chilly and cold. The face may sweat after eating.

Flatulence

Symptoms Belly/stomach bloated.

Insomnia

Symptoms With Sleepiness.
This insomnia results from pain, anger or stimulants (coffee, etc.), or it can be caused by too much chamomile tea – even in babies. The person may be restless.

Joint pain

Symptoms Pains violent. With numbness.
The pains drive the patient out of bed at night – walking about helps a bit.

Labour pains

Symptoms PAINS: distressing; severe; unbearable.
The woman may say that she can't bear the pain and
that she wants to die. She isn't anxious like *Aconite*, but
she is usually very angry and impatient as the cervix
may be slow to dilate.

Period problems

Symptoms PERIOD painful. BLOOD clotted.
Causes anger.
The periods may be more frequent or earlier than
normal after getting very angry.

Teething

Symptoms PAINFUL IN CHILDREN. CHEEKS: hot and
red; pale and cold; red spot on one cheek. PAINS:
unbearable; cries out in sleep. With RESTLESS SLEEP;
DIARRHOEA; GREEN STOOLS.
Worse for heat of bed; warm food/drinks; for pressure.
An infant may have at the same time one hot, red
cheek, or a red patch on one cheek, and one pale and
cold cheek.

Toothache

Symptoms IN CHILDREN. PAINS unbearable.
Worse for hot drinks/food; for pressure; for warmth of
bed.
These pains are truly terrible and are worse for
warmth and pressure (chewing anything hurts). It is
often accompanied by diarrhoea and/or a cough.

Vomiting

Symptoms VOMITING easy. VOMIT bile.
Causes anger.

CHINA OFFICINALIS (Chin.)

Family name: Rubiaceae
Common names: cinchona officinalis; Peruvian bark;
calisaya bark; yellow cinchona; loxa bark; red bark

This beautiful evergreen tree is indigenous to tropical
forests of South America, although they are now
cultivated in India, Sri Lanka and South-east Asia.
The bark has a deep red lining, and is spongy and
extremely bitter tasting.
   The history of the discovery and use of Cinchona
bark as a medicine is not fully known. It was first
introduced into Europe around the middle of the
seventeenth century by the Jesuits, who brought it
back from Peru where they had used it to treat malaria.

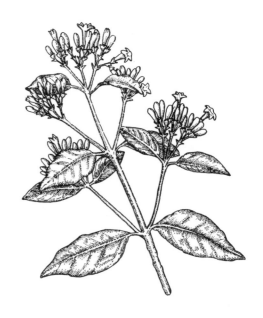

(Its first authentic cure is said to have been that of the
Countess of Chinchon, wife of the Viceroy of Peru,
whence it acquired the name of Cinchona bark.) For
nearly two centuries it was used in medicine in the
form of powders, extracts and infusions, for malaria
and all manner of fevers, as well as for general debility.
   After 1820, when pure quinine was isolated from the
bark, the use of the drug spread rapidly. Excessive
quinine use causes a set of symptoms known as cin-
chonism: nausea, headache, ear and eye disturbances,
widespread effects on the heart, nerves, circulation,
kidneys and respiration. Skin rashes, asthma and
swelling are common in people who are actually
allergic to the drug.
   Cinchona was the first substance that Hahnemann
was inspired to test on himself, and it was to lead to his
discovery of the homeopathic law of similars (see
page 4 for an account of his first provings). For the
homeopathic preparation the bark is collected between May and November and then dried and
powdered. It is mixed with five parts (by weight)
alcohol, and then left to stand for eight days and
strained and filtered.

GENERAL SYMPTOMS

Anaemia. Appetite lost. **Complaints from:** loss of
body fluids. **Dislikes:** bread; rich, fatty food; meat.
Eyes sunken. **Face** pasty. **Likes** cold drinks; spicy
foods. **Pains:** sore, bruised. **Sweat:** cold; on covered

NB   SEE ALSO PAGES 203–26 FOR GENERAL ADVICE, DOS AND DON'TS.

parts of the body, profuse; on single parts of the body; worse for slightest exertion. **Taste:** mouth tastes bitter.
Better for firm pressure.
Worse for cold; for fresh air; for light touch; for movement; at night.

The *China* picture often emerges when people are anaemic, weak and depleted following conditions with prolonged, exhausting discharges or loss of body fluids, such as diarrhoea, vomiting, perspiring, breastfeeding; or from prolonged mental or physical strain. The anaemia is temporary, but causes them to look pale and have dark blue rings around their eyes. The homeopathic remedy will, if indicated, speed up the convalescing time dramatically.

A curious symptom is that they have no appetites whatsoever, but eating just one mouthful will cause their appetites to return in full and they will then eat voraciously. The skin over the whole body feels sore, but whereas it is aggravated by light touch, hard pressure is soothing. They are persistently chilly, are worse for cold weather and are sensitive to draughts and fresh air. Their symptoms may recur at regular intervals or be worse, say, every other day. They sleep restlessly and with difficulty, and will sweat then also; they feel sluggish on waking.

EMOTIONAL/MENTAL SYMPTOMS

Anxious. Apathetic. Depressed. Despondent. Fearful: of animals; of dogs. **Sensitive:** generally; to noise.

People needing *China* feel utterly exhausted and may seem confused and taciturn. When talking, they use the wrong words or mix them up. Apart from their physical tiredness they seem emotionally weary, as if they really have had enough. Formerly, they may have been quite lively and active, both mentally and physically, but the acute illness or stress that has caused the tiredness has brought them right down. Children for whom this remedy will work exceptionally well may also have a fear of animals, especially dogs.

PHYSICAL COMPLAINTS

Diarrhoea

Symptoms PAINLESS. STOOLS containing undigested food. With INDIGESTION (see below).
Worse after eating; during the afternoon; on alternate days; at night.
Causes after an acute illness; fruit; hot weather; after weaning.

This diarrhoea is accompanied by slow digestion and often follows an indigestible fruit meal, or comes on in babies who have been newly weaned and are not taking well to solids.

Exhaustion

Symptoms EXHAUSTION nervous. Profuse SWEATING.
Causes loss of body fluids (breastfeeding, diarrhoea, haemorrhage, vomiting).
This weakness is characteristic during the convalescent stage of an illness where the patient has lost a lot of body fluids (see general symptoms). He may feel faint and have ringing in the ears as well as a lot of sweating, especially on exertion and during sleep.

Flatulence

Symptoms BELLY/STOMACH: bloated; obstructed (wind difficult to expel); rumbling.
Causes eating fruit; abdominal surgery.
The stomach (above the navel) is distended (bloated), and the wind stays stuck, causing much discomfort and pain.

Headache

Symptoms NERVOUS. PAINS: sore, bruised; pressing; throbbing. SCALP sensitive.
Better for firm pressure.
Causes mental strain.
May feel as if the brain is beating against the skull. The pains are relieved by hard pressure although the scalp may be so sensitive that even the individual hairs in their follicles feel sore.

Indigestion

Symptoms BELCHES: bitter; tasting of food eaten; ineffectual, incomplete; sour. BELLY/STOMACH: bloated. FLATULENCE: obstructed. PAINS pressing.
Worse after drinking; after eating; after eating fruit; after belching.
Causes operation on abdomen.
The digestion is slow, and it feels as if all food turns to gas; much like *Carbo vegetabilis*, but in the case of *China* burping does *not* relieve the discomfort or the bloating. The abdomen is swollen tight like a drum, and it seems as if the wind is blocked. Fruit ferments in the stomach and turns to wind. The condition may have been caused by an operation to the abdomen.

Vomiting

Symptoms VOMIT: food; sour. VOMITING frequent.
Worse after eating.

CIMICIFUGA (Cimi.)

Family name: Ranunculaceae
Common names: actea racemosa; bugbane; black snake root; macrotys racemosa; rattle root; black cohosh

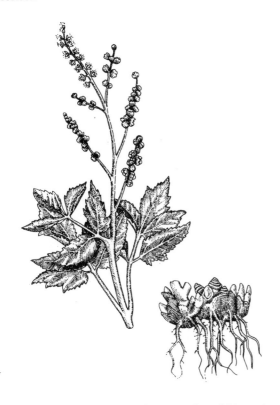

This hardy perennial plant thrives in the wild in moist, shady woods in the USA and Canada. It is a tall plant that grows up to a height of eight feet, and in June produces long feathery blossoms measuring up to three feet.

The root of the plant has been used by American Indian tribes for many complaints. A tincture was made from the fresh root (dug up in October) and given for rheumatism, diarrhoea (overdoses produce this symptom), tuberculosis, whooping cough, menstrual problems and slow labours. It was also said to be an antidote against the poisonous bite of the rattlesnake, hence its nickname rattle root. The root has also been chewed to alleviate depression and calm the nerves. Evil spirits were prevented from entering a room by sprinkling it with tea prepared from this herb.

The homeopathic preparation is made from the knotty, black roots, which are pounded to a pulp, mixed with alcohol, left to stand and then strained, filtered, and succussed.

GENERAL SYMPTOMS

Pains: sore, bruised. **Trembling.**
Worse for cold.

Cimicifuga is used mostly for women and is often needed in pregnancy. Chilliness is marked, and, with the exception of the headaches, the symptoms are worse in the cold. Physical symptoms may alternate with depression.

EMOTIONAL/MENTAL SYMPTOMS

Depressed. Fearful of death. **Restless. Sighing.**

Cimicifuga is useful in women who have bouts of gloominess, of depression, as if a black cloud has settled over them. This can be common during pregnancy or after childbirth. The woman may be afraid of death (like *Aconite*), and scared of losing her reason. During the gloomy phase she will sit silently sighing and then when her dejection lifts she may become excitable and talkative, jumping from one subject to another.

PHYSICAL COMPLAINTS

Headache

Symptoms PAINS: in back of head; top of head; pressing out; pressing up.
Better for fresh air.
The pains radiate from the back of the head to the top of the head which feels as if it will fly off. Or it can start in the forehead and extend to the back of the head. The pains are severe and are better for cool, fresh air.

Labour pains

Symptoms PAINS: flying around; stop altogether; weak.
Pains fly about the belly from one side to the other and the whole body feels sore and bruised and sensitive to touch.

Pregnancy problems

Symptoms PAINS: flying about belly.
Shooting pains can occur during the later months; these are distressing but there is usually no serious cause – it is just the body's way of accommodating the growing foetus. Sore, bruised pains in the joints and heaviness in the lower back may also occur.

CINA

Family name: Compositae
Common names: European wormseed; tartarian southernwood; artemisa cina

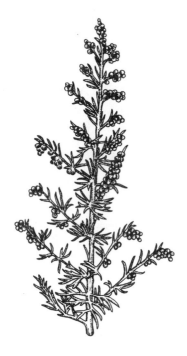

Cina is a herb that is found mostly in Europe and Russia. Since the time of Hippocrates it has been an important medicine for fever-reducing, as an aid to digestion and as a remedy for removing worms.

When first proven by Hahnemann, it was found in the main to affect the nervous system and the digestive tract, and it has since become an important remedy for intestinal complaints in children.

The dried flowers are used for the homeopathic preparation. They are first coarsely powdered, and then mixed with alcohol and left to steep.

GENERAL SYMPTOMS

Eyes sunken. **Face** pale. **Likes** cold drinks.
Expression sickly. **Nose**: child picks constantly.
Worse at night; for pressure.

The general picture of Cina occurs most commonly in children, where it is often an indication of worms. If Cina fits the overall state, the patient will be cured and the worms will usually cease (see below). It is useful for other complaints too, however, if the whole picture fits.

Cina types may be very pale and sickly looking, especially around the mouth, with red, hot cheeks, and they are always picking and rubbing their itchy noses. The symptoms are generally worse at night.

EMOTIONAL/MENTAL SYMPTOMS

Capricious. Dislike of being hugged; being looked at. **Irritable** children.

The Cina character is an angry, touchy and stubborn one. Cina children dislike being looked at, touched, examined or interfered with in any way; they may demand to be carried or rocked but are no better for it and will kick and scream when picked up and cuddled (rather like Antimonium crudum and Chamomilla). They ask for things which they then reject or throw away.

PHYSICAL COMPLAINTS

Convulsions

Symptoms IN CHILDREN.
Causes worms; teething in children.
Seek professional advice immediately.

Cough

Symptoms COUGH: in fits; suffocative. With RETCHING.
Worse after getting up.
The body goes stiff before a coughing fit, and there is a gurgling in the throat after coughing. There may be almost constant (involuntary) swallowing with the cough.

Fever

Symptoms THIRSTLESS. With HUNGER.
Worse at night.
There may be frequent high fevers that recur daily at the same time.

Restless sleep

Symptoms BODY twitching. LIMBS jerking. With GRINDING OF TEETH.
Children scream out at night and lie on their backs kicking their legs.

Worms

Symptoms ANUS itching. APPETITE: changeable; lost; ravenous. NOSE itching. With symptoms of FEVER (see above).
This remedy is for worms in children who are forever picking their noses; who grind their teeth at night in their sleep; who have enormous appetites and will ask for food soon after a big meal, or who conversely want

to eat nothing but sweet things, and who are generally very irritable.

COCCULUS INDICUS (Cocc.)

Family name: Menispermaceae
Other names: India berry; Levant nut; fish berry; anamirta paniculata

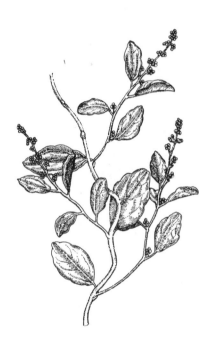

This strong climbing shrub is found in eastern parts of India, Bangladesh and Malaysia. It has a corky bark and berries, rather like those of a bay tree, which contain an active poison.

The poisonous berries were used by Asians to stupefy fish by throwing the berries on to the water for the fish to eat, which would knock them out and make them easier to catch. The poison has also been used by thieves to stupefy their victims before robbing them. In America and Europe the berries were imported for the illegal adulteration of beer in low public houses to give it an additional bitterness, to increase its alcoholic content artificially and to prevent it from fermenting a second time and bursting the bottles in warm weather.

Cocculus has rarely been used medicinally except as an external preparation for scabies and ringworm.

In the homeopathic preparation the powdered seeds are mixed with alcohol and heated gently for twenty-four hours, then strained and succussed as normal.

GENERAL SYMPTOMS

Dislikes fresh air. **Hot flushes. Sweat** on single parts of the body; cold. **Taste:** mouth tastes metallic. **Trembling:** from emotion.
Better for lying down in bed.
Worse for exertion; for loss of sleep; for movement; for touch; for walking in the fresh air.

This is a remedy for people who are utterly worn out and exhausted, usually from lack of sleep or irregular sleeping from working night shifts, from looking after sick patients through the night, or nursing babies, etc. They become trembly with tiredness and feel much worse out in the fresh air; physical exertion of any sort is tiring. There is a general feeling of numbness as well as a feeling that specific parts of the body have gone to sleep. The only thing they want to do is to lie quietly in bed and try to sleep, but this will be difficult because they are out of the habit of sleeping and so are in a dreadful vicious circle of exhaustion.

EMOTIONAL/MENTAL SYMPTOMS

Anxious. Complaints from: anger; grief. **Confused. Dazed. Forgetful. Introspective. Memory weak. Mild. Time** seems to pass too fast.
Uncommunicative.

The emotional state of people requiring *Cocculus* will result from a lot of stress, especially if that stress is sleep deprivation. Grief (the loss of a loved one, for example) or anger may also be part of this picture. The stress will make them tired, anxious and confused and they begin to forget things. Though they are easy-going characters they become introspective, uncommunicative and closed off from the world – appearing dazed to outsiders. They may become trembly if they have difficult emotional situations to deal with. They will say that time passes quickly, especially at night when they try to sleep but can't.

PHYSICAL COMPLAINTS

Exhaustion

Symptoms EXHAUSTION paralytic. With DIZZINESS; NERVOUSNESS; NUMBNESS; STIFFNESS; TREMBLING; VERTIGO.
Worse for walking in the fresh air.
Causes loss of sleep; irregular sleep; nursing the sick; nervous exhaustion.
People who have to nurse or work through the night may need this remedy to help them through difficult times when they feel worn out from exhaustion and lack of sleep. Their legs tremble whilst walking and

NB   SEE ALSO PAGES 203–26 FOR GENERAL ADVICE, DOS AND DON'TS.

their hands tremble whilst eating and when lifting them up high. Various parts of the body, hands and feet especially, go to sleep easily. The back and neck feel weak and stiff. They have to lie down and feel worse for sitting up.

Headache

Symptoms PAINS: in back of head; in forehead; at nape of neck. With NAUSEA (see below).
Causes irregular sleep; loss of sleep.
These headaches come on after disturbed sleep or from a lack of sleep, and the head can feel empty, sore and bruised. Headaches from nervous strain, overwork and from travel sickness can also benefit from this remedy if the other symptoms fit the general picture.

Insomnia

Symptoms DREAMS anxious; nightmares. Restless SLEEP.
Causes anxiety.
This remedy is useful for people whose sleep pattern has been disturbed by working night shifts or by nursing sick people through nights, and who become weak, tired and dizzy as a result (see Exhaustion above).

Nausea

Symptoms APPETITE lost. BELLY/STOMACH feels empty. BELCHES. TASTE: metallic taste in mouth. With FAINTNESS.
Worse during the afternoon; after eating; after drinking; for movement; for sitting up in bed; for smell and thought of food.

Period problems

Symptoms PERIOD painful. BELLY bloated. PAINS: cramping; gripping; severe.
Worse for movement; for breathing.
The tummy is blown right up, and passing wind does not relieve the pains. The person feels extremely weak before as well as during the period itself.

Travel sickness

Symptoms With DIARRHOEA; DIZZINESS; FAINT-LIKE FEELING; HEADACHE (see above); NAUSEA (see above); VOMITING.
Better for lying down.
Worse for fresh air; after eating; after drinking; for movement; for sitting up.
Getting up causes dizziness and nausea; the person has to lie down to prevent vomiting.

COCCUS CACTI (Cocc-c.)

Family name: Hemiptera
Other name: cochineal

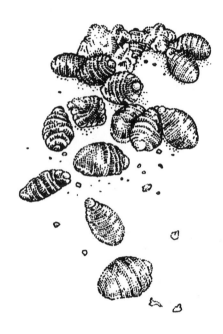

Coccus cacti are insects that live and feed on the prickly pear cactus of Mexico and Central America. They increase rapidly in size and lose their original shape until at last they look like protuberances of the plant itself. The dried, pulverised bodies of these insects yield the red dyestuff cochineal, which the Aztec Indians used as a body paint and for dyeing their fabrics a brilliant crimson. They also used cochineal for medicinal purposes.

It has been used as a pigment and as a colouring agent in cosmetics, paints and beverages, but the cost of producing cochineal is high – it takes 70,000 insects to make one pound of dye – and it has now largely been replaced by synthetic dyes.

The homeopathic tincture is prepared from the dried bodies of the female insects, which are larger than the males and have no wings.

GENERAL SYMPTOMS

This is a very small remedy that I have included because it is one of the main whooping cough remedies.

There are no marked general or emotional/mental symptoms.

PHYSICAL COMPLAINTS

Cough

Symptoms COUGH: choking; in fits; irritating; violent; whooping; racking. Tickling in LARYNX. MUCUS: copious after each coughing fit; sticky. THROAT dry.
Better for fresh air.
Worse in a stuffy room; around 11.30 p.m.
The mucus drips down the back of the throat and irritates the larynx, causing the person to hawk up which in turn causes coughing fits that end in retching and vomiting of mucus. The mucus hangs in strings from the mouth.

COFFEA CRUDA (Coff.)

Family name: Rubiaciae
Common names: coffee; coffea arabica; mocha bean

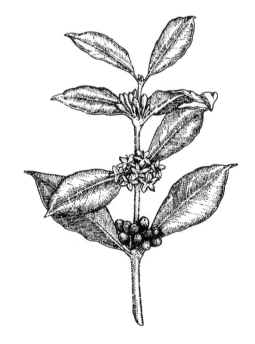

This evergreen shrub is grown in tropical regions throughout the world. It grows to about 30 feet in the wild but is kept to about 16 feet in cultivation. Its fragrant white flowers bloom for only two days, and the cherry-like berries are picked and dried in the sun; each plant yields between one and two pounds of coffee.

Coffee has been drunk in Ethiopia from time immemorial, where tradition has it that its power to cause wakefulness was first noticed by a shepherd who saw the effect it had on his goats. It was introduced to Mecca by the dervishes for religious purposes – so that followers could pass the night in prayer with greater zeal and attention. As coffee became a social drink and coffee houses spread rapidly throughout Arabia it became associated more with singing and dancing than with prayer. Efforts to forbid its usage failed and for hundreds of years Arabia supplied the world's coffee. By the mid-seventeenth century it had made its way to Europe. In England the religious order of the day came down heavily on coffee, calling it 'a poison which God made black that it might bear the devil's colour'.

Its medicinal virtues are few: it was used as a diuretic and was said to relieve headaches, enliven the spirits and prevent sleepiness, although it was found that its effects were lost with continued usage. It is used as an antidote to morphine poisoning and certain snake venoms.

Interestingly, coffee and wine counteract the ill effects of each other so that someone who has had a quantity of coffee to drink will find that a glass of wine will allow a night's sleep. Tea and beer act in a similar way, antidoting each other's bad effects.

The homeopathic preparation is made from the unroasted bean which is ground to a powder, mixed with alcohol and left to stand for eight days. The sediment is then boiled with water until greatly reduced, then strained and mixed with alcohol again before succussion.

GENERAL SYMPTOMS

Senses acute. Sensitive: to pain; to noise.
Worse for fresh air; at night; for touch; for wine.

Coffea affects the nerves, so that someone needing the remedy will be over-excited and over-sensitive. All the senses become acute; everything is felt, seen, heard, smelt, tasted. Pain and noise become intolerable. Fresh air likewise. The person will be sensitive to alcohol, especially wine – it will make his symptoms worse.
NB Both coffee as a drink and *Coffea* the remedy can counteract the effect of some homeopathic remedies. See page 28 for guidance on drinking coffee while taking a homeopathic remedy.

EMOTIONAL/MENTAL SYMPTOMS

Complaints from: excitement; joy. **Cheerful. Despair. Exhilarated. Excitable. Fearful** of painful death. **Lively. Screaming** with pain.

This is a remedy for someone who is very excitable and lively or who has received some news that has induced a state of exitement and joy to the extent that she has become 'wired up' and cannot calm down. This is typical of a child who has had a series of exciting events in his life, for example a birthday party followed by Christmas followed by a school outing. She becomes so excited that she cannot sleep at night and may suffer from headaches. This state – of merriness and excitement, with an active mind full of ideas and plans – can turn to fear in the face of pain. The slightest pain drives the person to despair and she will weep and make a fuss with her toothache or headache.

PHYSICAL COMPLAINTS

Headache

Symptoms HEADACHE nervous. PAIN: one-sided.
Worse for noise.
The headache may be worse out in the fresh air and it may feel as if a nail is being driven into the brain.

Insomnia

Causes over-active mind; over-excitement.
This is for people who sleep lightly and wake at every sound, who are unable to sleep because they literally may be so happy that their minds are full of excitement and ideas and plans. This is sleeplessness from *good* news!

Toothache

Symptoms IN CHILDREN. IN NERVOUS PEOPLE. PAINS: shooting/spasmodic.
Better for cold water.
Worse for hot food and drinks; heat.
The pains in the tooth are eased by holding cold water (especially ice-cold water) in the mouth, but they return again as soon as the water warms up.

COLCHICUM AUTUMNALE (Colch.)

Family name: Liliaceae
Common names: meadow saffron; naked lady; tuber root; upstart

This perennial plant grows wild in meadows throughout Europe, Asia Minor and North America. Its purple flowers are similar to crocus flowers and, as the name implies, appear in the autumn. The leaves grow up to a foot long and between one and two inches broad, and they contain an active poison; overdoses cause vomiting, violent purging, serious inflammation of the stomach and bowels, and death.
　　Colchicum has been used since before the thirteenth

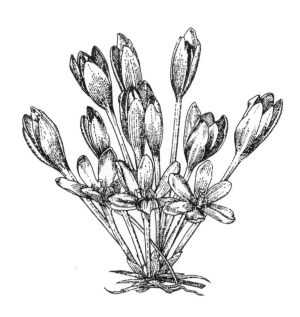

century to treat gout and rheumatism. It was the principle ingredient in all proprietary gout specifics although one sixteenth-century medic noted that the habitual use of the medicine encouraged more frequent attacks of these troubles (see sections on provings pages 4 and 11). It was nicknamed *Anima articulorum* or 'the soul of the joints'.
　　The homeopathic preparation is made from the fresh bulb, which is gathered just before flowering. It is chopped and pounded to a fine pulp, and the expressed juice is mixed with alcohol and succussed.

GENERAL SYMPTOMS

Exhaustion. Sense of smell acute. **Sweat** sour.
Thirstless.
Better for sitting.
Worse in the autumn; for cold; for damp; for movement; at night; for the sight of food; for touch.

This plant flowers in the autumn and its symptoms, such as the diarrhoea and the rheumatism are worse at that time of year, especially when the weather is damp. People needing *Colchicum* are usually sensitive to cold, are always sensitive to damp and their symptoms are worse at night. Movement of any sort, including walking, will aggravate their pains and the only position they feel better in is sitting down. A keynote of this particular remedy is that the sense of smell is extremely acute; if they are unwell the smell of food cooking will quickly exacerbate their symptoms and/or make them feel faint. This sensitivity to food smells is at its worst with eggs, which really do make them want to vomit.

EMOTIONAL/MENTAL SYMPTOMS

Complaints from anger. **Memory weak.**

This is a small remedy and does not have many strongly marked emotional characteristics. People needing this remedy may be absent-minded and forgetful. They are very sensitive to anger and conflict and symptoms – diarrhoea or nausea or painful joints – will be worse after, say, an argument.

PHYSICAL COMPLAINTS

Diarrhoea

Symptoms STOOLS: jelly-like; with mucus; watery. PAIN on passing stools.
Causes autumn.
This diarrhoea may well accompany the joint complaints that are worse in the damp weather of autumn.

Flatulence

Symptoms BELLY/STOMACH bloated. WIND obstructed (difficult to expel).

Joint pain

Symptoms PAINS: in hands and feet; acute; tearing. With SWELLING.
Better for warmth.
Worse for cold, wet weather; for movement; for warm weather.
This 'rheumatism' affects the small joints of the hands and the feet, which may be better for being wrapped up and kept warm and are worse for touch. The toes especially are so sensitive that stubbing them accidentally is agonisingly painful. The severe, tearing pains in the joints may also be accompanied by a great general weakness.

Nausea

Symptoms APPETITE lost. BELLY/STOMACH bloated. With FAINTNESS; VOMITING (see below).
Worse after eating; for smell and sight of food.
There is an intense loathing at the sight, smell or thought of food, and the nausea is exacerbated particularly by the smell of eggs and fish.

Vomiting

Symptoms PAINS: burning; sore, bruised. With RETCHING after vomiting.
Worse for smell of eggs.
The stomach is distended and may feel icy cold.

COLOCYNTHIS (Coloc.)

Family name: Cucurbitaceae
Other names: cucumis colocynthis; bitter cucumber; bitter apple; squirting cucumber

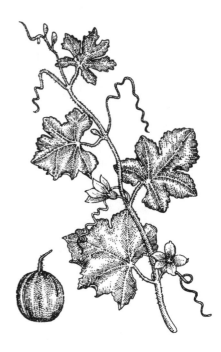

Colocynthis is a trailing plant that grows in sandy places in hot, dry regions throughout the world. It has a hairy stem that looks very like the common cucumber, yellow flowers and yellow fruit the size of oranges. The seeds are said to be highly nutritious but the pulp of the fruit is a strong poison which causes severe gastro-intestinal inflammation.

Because of its drastic purgative effects it has been in general medicinal use from earliest times for such complaints as lethargy and 'mania'. It is mentioned in the Old Testament when the prophet Elisha showed his divine mission by making this poisonous gourd into a wholesome vegetable during a time of famine.

For the homeopathic preparation the dried fruit is powdered, mixed with alcohol and left to macerate; it is shaken twice daily for a week and then strained and succussed as usual.

GENERAL SYMPTOMS

Colocynthis is one of the main colic remedies (see below). Other major colic remedies are *Staphysagria* and *Dioscorea*. *Staphysagria* children develop colic from anger (like *Colocynthis*) but will also have teeth which

NB   SEE ALSO PAGES 203–26 FOR GENERAL ADVICE, DOS AND DON'TS.

decay early, and *Dioscorea* bend right back with the pains.

EMOTIONAL/MENTAL SYMPTOMS

Complaints from: anger; humiliation; indignation. **Restless.**

The physical symptoms may develop as a result of feeling angry or humiliated, and the pains cause the sufferers intense anguish, as a result of which they become very restless and possibly irritable. The pains are so bad as to make them cry or scream out.

PHYSICAL COMPLAINTS

Colic

Symptoms In babies. Belly bloated. Pains: cutting; griping; tearing; violent; in waves. With diarrhoea (see below); nausea; vomiting.
Better for bending double; for pressure; for passing a stool.
Worse after drinking; for cold drinks when over-heated; before a stool; after eating fruit.
Causes anger; eating fruit; excitement; vexation.
The pains may be either in the stomach or in the belly and may be so severe as to cause vomiting. Young babies commonly pull their legs up to their bellies and scream if they are moved. Older sufferers will also double up with the pain and will press hard on the affected area (they may dig their fists into their bellies or bend over the back of a chair, twisting and turning to get some relief). Eating, especially fruit, will aggravate the pains.

Cramp

Symptoms Cramp: in thighs; legs; calves.

Diarrhoea

Symptoms Stools: green; pasty. With colic (see above).
Worse after eating fruit; after eating.
Causes anger; fruit.

Headache

Symptoms Pains: on left side of face; spread up to ear; tearing.
Worse for touch.
Causes excitement; vexation.

Sciatica

Symptoms Pains tearing.
Worse on right side of body.

The awful tearing pains are usually worse for movement, pressure and touch and although they may be better for warmth are often worse for the warmth of bed at night.

CONIUM MACULATUM (Con.)

Family name: Umbelliferae
Other names: common hemlock; spotted hemlock; poison hemlock; herb bennett; poison parsley

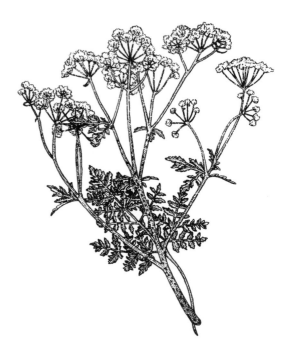

Common in this country as well as throughout most of Europe and in parts of Asia, North Africa and America, hemlock is found in hedges, meadows, by streams and on waste ground. It belongs to the same family as parsley and in fact its leaves have been mistakenly taken for parsley, but unlike the rest of its family every single part of this plant is extremely poisonous. The name *Conium* comes from the Greek 'konas', to whirl about, because when eaten the plant causes great vertigo before death.

Medicinally it has been used from as early as the tenth century for a wide range of illnesses including tumours, epilepsy, whooping cough and many others, to cure the bite of rabid dogs and as an antidote to strychnine poisoning. However, these treatments were fraught with danger because of the toxic nature of the herb and it eventually fell into disuse.

It was commonly used by the Romans and the

Greeks as a poison both legally (for criminals) and illegally. Hemlock was the poison that the condemned Socrates was made to drink. Poisonous doses produce complete paralysis which starts at the feet and moves up the body, the legs becoming cold at first and then the rest of the body following. There are no convulsions and no pain. The ability to think clearly remains right up until death, which is caused by asphyxia.

The homeopathic remedy is prepared from a tincture made from the fresh plant when in flower.

GENERAL SYMPTOMS

Complaints from accident/injury. **Dizzy. Sweating:** during sleep; hot; at night; on closing eyes.
Worse on lying down.
Better for sitting down.

The complaints are worse for lying down, from the cough, the sweating and the dizziness. A slightly strange symptom is that the person (and the complaints) are better for sitting down and letting the limbs hang down (not sitting cross legged). The sweating may be profuse and occurs on closing the eyes (another strange symptom) as well as during sleep.

EMOTIONAL/MENTAL SYMPTOMS

Anxious. Depressed. Memory weak. **Sensitive** to noise. **Slow.**

These are melancholic people whose brains seize up after a period of mental strain. They can't read, and they may sit looking vacant, feeling anxious and not wanting to work. They are easily startled by noise, and their eyes are sensitive to light (although not inflamed). Women feel worse, physically and emotionally, before their periods, when they find it more difficult to concentrate and when they feel generally miserable.

PHYSICAL COMPLAINTS
Breastfeeding problems

Symptoms BREAST LUMPS worse in right breast.
These breast lumps are not necessarily painful.

Cough

Symptoms COUGH: dry; irritating; tickling; violent; must sit up as soon as cough starts. EXPECTORATION: difficult; must swallow what comes up.
Worse lying down in bed; in the evenings; for deep breathing; during fever.
The cough is caused by a dry, tickling spot in the larynx; it starts on first lying down (day or night) and the person has to sit up to cough. He or she is unable to cough out the mucus; it is swallowed, and then the person has to lie down to rest. The cough is exhausting and is often accompanied by a fever.

Dizzy

Symptoms With TURNING SENSATION.
Worse for moving or turning the head quickly; for lying down.
The person feels as if he or she is turning in a circle, and cannot watch moving objects. Better when quite still with eyes closed.

Exhaustion

With TREMBLING; NUMBNESS.
Better for fresh air.
Worse for slightest exertion; after stool; for walking.

Injuries

Symptoms INJURIES: of breasts; of testicles; stony hard lumps, sensitive, swollen, cold, inflamed.
Injured parts become lumpy and painful and feel stony hard. After a bang or a bruise there is tingling with stitching pains.

Insomnia

Symptoms SLEEPLESS before midnight. With NIGHTMARES.

Period problems

Symptoms BREASTS: lumpy; stitching pains. With EXHAUSTION (see above).
Worse before menstrual period.
The breasts feel heavy, and swell before a period. The typical emotional/mental symptoms will also be present.

CUPRUM METALLICUM (Cupr.)

Common name: copper

Copper is a reddish-brown metallic element that is mined in many countries throughout the world. It is a malleable metal, and was the first metal used to make tools and weapons. Though it is very soft on its own, it can be hardened by being mixed with other metals (with tin to make bronze and with zinc to make brass, for example). Copper is a very good conductor of heat and electricity, and it is used to make electric wires and cables and water pipes. It is also used in a great variety of pigments for artists' powders, and was commonly used by doctors and vets at one time in ointments for wounds.

Copper's poisonous qualities were first noted in coppersmiths, when workers suffered from chronic poisoning, with colic, diarrhoea, cough, and difficulty with assimilation of food being the main symptoms. Acute poisoning is rare, with symptoms of violent stomach cramps, vomiting, pale face, icy-cold extremities, restlessness at night and violent headache. If the sufferer survives then liver disease always follows.

The homeopathic preparation is made from the triturated pure metal.

GENERAL SYMPTOMS

Extremities cold. Face: blue; pale. **Lips** blue. **Taste:** sweet. **Pains** cramping.
Better for cold drinks.
Worse for touch; for vomiting.

Cramps are an important part of the *Cuprum* picture; the muscles feel knotted up. The tiredness is from mental exhaustion or sometimes from loss of sleep, and the headaches and cramps may well follow a period of heavy work. *Cuprum* types look pale and drawn and have bluish lips.

EMOTIONAL/MENTAL SYMPTOMS

Restless at night in bed.

This remedy does not have a strong 'character'; its general symptoms and specific complaints will lead you to prescribe it.

PHYSICAL COMPLAINTS

Colic

Symptoms PAINS: cramping; violent. With NAUSEA; VOMITING.
The belly is sore, bruised, tender and hot.

Convulsions

Causes teething children; vexation.
These convulsions are accompanied by blue lips and cold hands and feet (see COUGH).
Seek professional advice immediately.

Cough

Symptoms BREATHING: difficult; fast. COUGH: in long fits at irregular intervals; uninterrupted; suffocative; violent; whooping.
Better for sips of cold water.
Although drinking cold water helps the cough (like

Causticum) cold air can aggravate it. There may be a metallic taste in the mouth. During a coughing fit the child loses his breath and then goes stiff, and then may go into a convulsion with fingers and toes twitching. Between the coughing fits the breathing is hurried and panting. This is a very serious cough and is frightening for parents – professional help should always be sought immediately. Meanwhile, *Cuprum* will give relief if prescribed at this time; the need for other medication may then be avoided.

Cramp

Symptoms CRAMP: in calves; feet; legs.
Causes childbirth.

Exhaustion

Symptoms HEADACHE between the eyes.
Causes loss of sleep; mental exhaustion.

DIOSCOREA (Dios.)

Family name: Dioscoreaceae
Other names: devil's bones; dioscorea villosa, wild yam, colic root

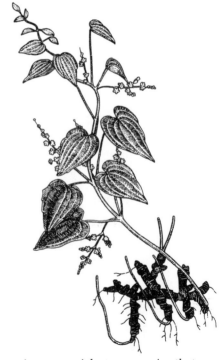

Dioscorea is a perennial creeper or vine that grows wild in hedges and entwined around trees and other objects in the southern States of North America. It has long been respected as an effective cure of certain types of bilious colic.

The homeopathic preparation is made from the plant's long, knotted root, which is gathered in September and chopped and pounded to a pulp. This is mixed with alcohol and left to stand for eight days in a dark, cool place before being strained and succussed.

GENERAL AND EMOTIONAL/ MENTAL SYMPTOMS

Dioscorea is a small remedy that has no great general or emotional/mental symptoms, but it is such an important colic remedy, especially in babies, that I have included it here.

PHYSICAL COMPLAINTS
Colic

Symptoms In babies. Belly: rumbling; windy. Pains: cramping; cutting; griping; around the navel; twisting.
Better for bending back; for stretching out.
Worse for bending forward; during the morning.
Infants arch back and scream (the opposite of the *Colocynthis* picture with its drawing up of legs). They have rumbly, windy tums and do not want to lie down but are better for being held upright.

DROSERA ROTUNDIFOLIA (Dros.)

Family name: Droseraceae
Other names: dew plant; round-leaved sundew, moor-grass; red rot; youth wort; rosée du soleil

Drosera rotundifolia is a small perennial carnivorous plant that grows close to the ground on mossy, turfy, marshy ground throughout Britain, northern Europe, northern Asia and North America. It flowers in July and August but the flowers themselves are open only in the mornings – they close when the sun is at its height. The leaves are interesting for their curious ability to trap insects; their upper surfaces are covered with long red hairs with glands that secrete a fluid to help trap the insect and then 'digest' it. These secretions shine in the sunlight and look like dewdrops, hence its nickname.

Drosera was used by physicians of the sixteenth century for treating tuberculosis but the herbalist Gerarde states that those who took it died sooner than those who were treated by other means. Herbalists used it as a cure for toothache, for madness (by hanging the plant around the neck), and to help during childbirth (by rubbing it on the abdomen).

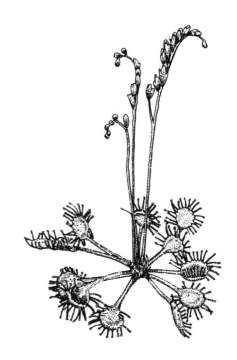

The homeopathic preparation is made from the entire fresh plant which is gathered when it is starting to flower (usually July) and the expressed juice is then succussed.

GENERAL AND EMOTIONAL/ MENTAL SYMPTOMS

Face blue during cough.
Worse at midnight; for lying down; for warmth of bed.

This is a small remedy whose usefulness in coughs, especially whooping cough, is such that I have included it here. It has no strongly marked general or emotional/mental symptoms, although children suffering from such a cough may be anxious. The chest complaints are usually worse for lying down in bed and especially around midnight.

PHYSICAL COMPLAINTS
Cough

Symptoms Cough: barking; deep; dry at night; in violent fits; hacking; irritating; suffocative; tormenting. Breathing: difficult; fast. Larynx tickling. Pain in chest: holds chest with hands to cough. With nosebleeds; blue face; hoarse voice; retching; vomiting of mucus.
Better for pressure.

NB   SEE ALSO PAGES 203–26 FOR GENERAL ADVICE, DOS AND DON'TS.

Worse after midnight; after drinking; for lying down; for talking.

Causes after measles.

The typical severe cough of whooping cough often starts with a tickling at the back of the throat and is usually accompanied in its acute phase by retching and vomiting and sometimes by nosebleeds. Breathing either speeds up during the coughing or is difficult (the coughing fit is so violent that it is often not possible to breathe and cough at the same time in which case the face goes a bluish colour). These coughing attacks follow each other rapidly, especially at night, and will often be set off as soon as the patient's head touches the pillow. The cough is painful and the chest becomes sore and bruised from coughing; patients are compelled to hold their chests with both hands when they cough as this pressure helps to ease the pain.

Sore throat

Symptoms IN BABIES. BELLY: rumblingl windy. PAINS: *Worse* for swallowing.

The larynx (voice-box) is sore and inflamed and there is an irritating feeling of dust in it. The voice becomes deep and husky.

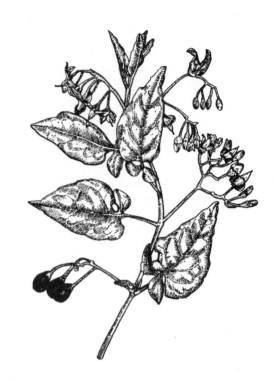

DULCAMARA (Dulc.)

Family name: Solanaceae
Common names: amaradulcis; bittersweet; felonwood; woody nightshade

Dulcamara is a perennial, shrubby plant common throughout Europe and the USA, where it is found in hedgerows and, more to its liking, moist banks around the edges of swamps. It has long, trailing branches and, from June to August, bluish-purple flowers. In the autumn it yields bright red poisonous berries.

Its common name *Amaradulcis* means bittersweet and refers to the fact that the root and stem, if chewed, taste first bitter and then sweet. The name felonwood refers to the country cure of the plant for felons or whitlows. Shepherds would hang the plant around their necks as a charm against the evil eye.

It has been used medicinally throughout history for most complaints known to man, from tuberculosis to leprosy, most skin conditions, diseases of the liver and for coughs and colds to name but a few. It was found to be reliable in its ability to cure rheumatism, fevers and many other inflammatory diseases. At one time it was also used as a tonic or restorative.

The homeopathic remedy is made from the fresh, green, still-pliant stems and leaves, which are gathered just as they are beginning to flower. The expressed juice is mixed with alcohol and succussed.

GENERAL SYMPTOMS

Catches colds easily. Complaints from change of weather to damp.

Better for movement; for walking.

Worse for change of weather to cold and wet; for cold; for damp; for lying down; at night; for sitting still.

These are people who lack 'vital heat'; they are extremely sensitive to the cold and to damp, and are greatly affected by a change of weather to cold and damp, when their complaints come on, especially if they get wet and cold themselves. In particular, they have a tendency to catch colds, especially in the winter, and they are then often better for keeping their heads warm; they may even sit with their heads under the blanket or with scarves pulled up over their noses. The winter colds clear once the warmth of summer is established and return with the cold weather the following autumn.

The symptoms are usually worse at night, especially the rheumatic ones and these are also generally worse for sitting and better for moving about. An unusual symptom is their very strong need to urinate (or pass a stool) after they have become chilled or spent some time in a cold place.

EMOTIONAL/MENTAL SYMPTOMS

There are not many strong emotional/mental symptoms for this remedy; the physical and general symptoms are much more important. However, there may be some depression, irritability, restlessness and/or confusion. These people may also be quarrelsome and impatient.

PHYSICAL COMPLAINTS

Backache

Symptoms PAINS: in lower back; aching; sore, bruised. With LAMENESS.
Better for movement; for walking.
Worse for wet weather.
Causes change of weather; damp weather; getting cold; getting wet.
The lower back aches as if from long stooping.

Breastfeeding problems

Symptoms MILK SUPPLY low. IN CHILLY WOMEN.

Cough

Symptoms COUGH rattling.
Causes damp weather.
The cough may develop from a sore throat. The person has to cough for a long time before expelling mucus.

Cystitis

Symptoms URINATION involuntary.
Causes getting cold and wet.
This is the remedy to give after *Aconite* (if you have given six doses and it has had no effect), where the cystitis has come on after getting cold *and* wet, and where there are as yet no remarkable symptoms apart from an inability to hold on.

Diarrhoea

Symptoms IN TEETHING CHILDREN. PAINFUL. STOOLS: yellow; watery.
Worse after eating cold food; at night.
Causes getting cold; getting damp; teething.
The pains will generally be worse before the stool and may be accompanied by nausea.

Eye inflammation

Symptoms With symptoms of COMMON COLD.
Causes wet weather.
This eye inflammation accompanies a common cold and is often seen in teething babies.

Flu

Causes cold, damp weather.

Hives

Symptoms SKIN RASH lumpy.
Worse for heat; after scratching.
Causes getting cold.
The rash burns after scratching and, although it is brought on by getting cold, it is worse for warmth, for example when heated after exercise.

Joint pain

Better for movement.
Worse for sitting; at night.
Causes damp; getting cold.
Pains in the joints that come on after staying in a damp house, or sleeping in a damp bed often need *Dulcamara*.

EUPATORIUM PERFOLIATUM (Eup-p.)

Family name: Compositae
Other names: agueweed; boneset; thoroughwort; vegetable antimony

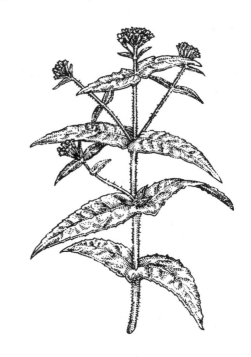

This is a perennial herb that grows in damp pastures and wet ground throughout the eastern States of America. It grows up to four feet high.

It was a favourite herb with the North American Indians, and it was probably the most widely used plant in American domestic medicine: every attic, woodshed and country farmhouse would have had bunches of dried boneset hanging tops downward from the rafters in case any member of the family or a neighbour should come down with a cold or 'break-bone' fever (a type of flu attended by pains which felt as if the bones were breaking). Boneset helps to promote perspiration, thereby giving relief from flus and fevers. It was also used as a tonic for general debility with indigestion, especially in the elderly.

The homeopathic preparation is made from the fresh herb when first in bloom, which is chopped and pounded to a fine pulp. It is mixed with alcohol and left to stand for eight days before being succussed.

GENERAL SYMPTOMS

Pains: sore, bruised; in bones. **Sweat** scanty. **Thirst:** for cold drinks; unquenchable.

Eupatorium is like *Bryonia* in that they have similar flu symptoms, but the pains in the bones are more marked with *Eupatorium*, and the *Eupatorium* patient is also more restless than the *Bryonia* patient, who likes to be completely still. The *Eupatorium* symptoms may be better whilst sweating, except the headache which is worse for it.

EMOTIONAL/MENTAL SYMPTOMS

Depressed.

These patients are sad and depressed during their flu, and lie about moaning during a fever.

PHYSICAL COMPLAINTS

Fever

The patient is sleepy with the fever and yawns and falls asleep all the time. With characteristic thirst and sweat (see General Symptoms).

Flu

Symptoms EYEBALLS aching. EYELIDS red. PAINS: in bones; bones feel broken. SKIN sore. With SHIVERING; CHILLS in back; HEADACHE (see below); NASAL CATARRH; SNEEZING.
Better for sweating.
This is an awful flu with intense aching pains in the bones of the arms, legs and lower back (and sometimes the hips as well). The bones feel as if they are broken and the skin all over the body feels dry and sore. Even the eyeballs and the scalp feel aching and sore.

Gastric flu

Symptoms With FEVER; NAUSEA; RETCHING; VOMITING: of bile; of food.
Better after chills; during fever.
The patient is very thirsty before vomiting.

Headache

Symptoms PAINS: in back of head; sore, bruised; throbbing. With FEVER (see above).
Worse for sweating.

EUPHRASIA (Euphr.)

Family name: Scrophulariaceae
Other name: eyebright

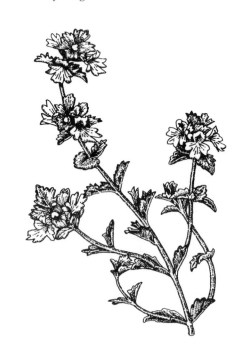

This annual plant grows in alpine meadows and other grassy places all over Europe. It is a small plant, two to eight inches high, which flowers from May to October. Its flowers look like hooded foxgloves in miniature and are white or purplish-white with a patch of yellow at the centre, pointing the way to the nectar. The plant will only grow in the wild as it leads a semi-parasitical existence with grass from whose roots it sucks its nourishment.

The name *Euphrasia* is derived from the Greek *euphrosyne*, meaning gladness. Euphrosyne was one of the three Graces, renowned for her joy, and it is believed that the plant was named after her because of its properties of preserving eyesight and the gladness that that brought into the life of the sufferer.

In the sixteenth century it was regarded by the great herbalists as a specific in diseases of the eyes, and was used by them to strengthen the head, eyes, memory and to clear the sight. It was taken internally either in soup, milk, wine or water; or the diluted juice was dropped into the eyes. Nowadays the dried herb is an ingredient in some herbal tobaccos that are said to be good for clearing the chest.

Euphrasia was first proved by Hahnemann, who found it had a definite irritating action on the eyes, indicating its most prominent symptom. The preparation uses the expressed juice of the plant, mixed with equal parts of alcohol.

GENERAL AND EMOTIONAL/ MENTAL SYMPTOMS

Worse during the evening.

This is a small remedy that has a tremendously useful place in the homeopathic first-aid kit but it has no notable general or emotional/mental symptoms apart from a general worsening in the evenings. As with many of the small remedies it is very important that the physical symptoms fit well.

PHYSICAL COMPLAINTS

Common cold

Symptoms NASAL CATARRH: bland; watery. With COUGH (see below); EYE INFLAMMATION.
The nasal discharge does not burn like the burning, watery discharge from the eyes. This is the opposite of *Allium cepa*, where the nasal catarrh irritates and the watering eyes do not feel irritated. The throat may also be sore; if it is, it will burn.

Cough

Symptoms COUGH during the day only. MUCUS copious.
Better for lying down.
Worse during the morning.
The person hawks up a mouthful of mucus at a time and clears the throat frequently.

Eye inflammation

Symptoms DISCHARGE: burning; watery. EYES: sensitive to light; watery. EYELIDS: burning; red; swollen. With COMMON COLD.
Worse for coughing; for light; for wind.
Causes with common cold.

The eyes stream on coughing and are very sensitive to light.

Eye injuries

Symptoms With EYE INFLAMMATION (see above).

Hayfever

Symptoms With COMMON COLD symptoms (see above); EYE INFLAMMATION (see above).

Measles

Symptoms With symptoms of COMMON COLD (see above); COUGH (see above); EYE INFLAMMATION (see above).
The fever is not usually very high and the patient does not necessarily feel very ill.

FERRUM METALLICUM (Ferr-m.)

Other name: iron

Iron is the most common metal in the Earth's crust, after aluminium. It has been mined for thousands of years, and it is still one of our most useful metals. The Iron Age was the third great stage, after the Stone and Bronze Ages, in the history of humans as tool and weapon makers.

Ferrum is one of the main constituents of the body, being present in considerable quantity in the blood. It is also present in many foodstuffs and, when given in excess to humans or animals, increases the amount of iron in the blood and stimulates the appetite as well as the energy. However, if the administration of iron is continued, secondary effects will ensue sooner or later and it is these that give the indications for homeopathic prescribing (in other words, which constitute a proving). Hahnemann said of people who live in areas with iron-rich waters, 'There we find more than anywhere else . . . weakness, almost amounting to paralysis of the whole body and of single parts, some kinds of violent limb pains, abdominal affections of various sorts, vomiting of food by day or by night, pulmonary ailments, often with blood spitting, deficient vital warmth, suppression of the menses, miscarriages, impotence in both sexes, sterility, jaundice and many other rare cachexias [weaknesses] are common occurrences.'

The value of iron has in fact been appreciated since the beginning of medical history for haemorrhages of all kinds, diarrhoeas and menstrual problems as well as for dropsies and intermittent fevers, especially if accompanied with great debility.

The homeopathic remedy is prepared from the pure metal by trituration.

NB   SEE ALSO PAGES 203–26 FOR GENERAL ADVICE, DOS AND DON'TS.

GENERAL SYMPTOMS

Appetite: lost, alternating with hunger. **Face:** pale; pasty; flushes easily; red with the pains. **Sweat:** clammy; cold; profuse; worse for lying down and for slightest physical exertion.
Better for walking slowly.
Worse on beginning to move; at night; for lying down.

These patients become exhausted and breathless very easily, and their pale faces become flushed, not only with exertion but when excited, and when in pain or with a fever. They in fact benefit from gentle exercise, which helps them generally and relieves many of their symptoms.

They are not actively hungry people and their appetite for eating will come in bursts; they also experience a sense of fullness after eating very little. The digestive disorders are marked and peculiar. People needing *Ferrum* have an intolerance of eggs. They suffer from diarrhoea while eating (the diarrhoea actually comes on when they begin to eat). This symptom is peculiar to *Ferrum*. They also experience periodic vomiting around midnight.

EMOTIONAL/MENTAL SYMPTOMS

Depressed. Irritable. Moody. Restless in bed.

These are anaemic, nervous, irritable and worn-out patients who are moody and physically restless, and who toss and turn in bed. If they are stuck in bed feeling ill they will be forever getting out of bed to wander around for a while.

PHYSICAL COMPLAINTS

Anaemia

Symptoms Lips pale. With EXHAUSTION (see below).
Causes loss of blood (heavy menstrual periods, pregnancy, bleeding).
People with anaemia who need *Ferrum* will have the characteristic pale face that flushes easily.

Backache

Symptoms In LOWER BACK.
Better for walking slowly.
Worse on beginning to move.

Cough

Symptoms COUGH in fits.
Better for walking slowly.
Worse after getting up; for movement.

Diarrhoea

Symptoms In TEETHING CHILDREN. PAINLESS. STOOLS: containing undigested food; passed with wind. With BELCHING; FLATULENCE.
Worse after drinking water; for movement; at night; while eating.
Causes teething.
The person burps after eating and it tastes of food recently eaten. He will pass wind with the diarrhoea – that is, at the same time.

Exhaustion

Symptoms With DESIRE to lie down.
Better for walking slowly in the fresh air.
Worse for exercise.
Causes anaemia; sweating.
This is a great tiredness that is actually better for a gentle stroll. The exhaustion is mental as well as physical, and the person doesn't want to work.

Fever

Better for being uncovered.
The patient will have the typical pale face which flushes easily.

Headache

Symptoms PAINS: in forehead; hammering; throbbing. With THIRSTLESSNESS.
Better for firm pressure; for lying down.
Worse for moving head.
These headaches last for two to three days at a time and are very draining. The patient feels she must lie down, and refuses drinks; her face is alternately hot and flushed or pale and drained.

Joint pain

Symptoms PAINS: in shoulder; in upper arm; stitching; tearing.
Better for gentle movement.
Worse on beginning to move; for lifting arm up; for bending arm backwards.

Nosebleeds

Symptoms In CHILDREN.

Sciatica

Better for gentle movement; for walking.

Varicose veins

Symptoms VARICOSE VEINS: painful; swollen.
Worse During pregnancy.
These are often accompanied by anaemia and tiredness.

Vomiting

Symptoms VOMITING sudden; of food.
Worse after eating eggs; after midnight; at night.
Food either comes up suddenly whilst eating or it lies in the stomach all day and then comes up around midnight.

GELSEMIUM SEMPERVIRENS (Gels.)

Family name: Loganiaceae
Other names: yellow jasmine; false jasmine; wild woodbine; Carolina jasmine

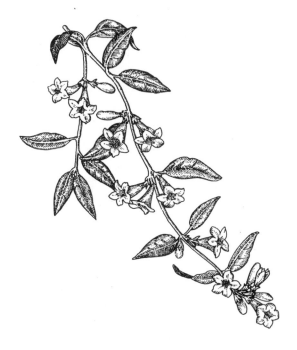

Gelsemium is a beautiful climbing plant found in moist woodlands and along sea coasts in the southern States of the USA. It belongs to the same family as *Nux vomica* and *Ignatia* and should not be confused with the true jasmine which belongs to a different botanical family. It can grow to a great height and bears fragrant yellow flowers in the early spring. All attempts to grow it in this country have failed.

Gelsemium is poisonous in large doses, causing paralysis of the motor nerves – its poisonous effects include mental and physical sluggishness, double vision, lack of balance, drooping of the eyelids, convulsions and, ultimately, death. The medical history of this plant is quite modern and began when it was used in error for another root by a Mississippi farmer who, after recovering from the poisonous effects of

Gelsemium, was cured of the bilious fever from which he had been suffering. This accidental poisoning and cure led to *Gelsemium* being marketed as a cure for fevers and finally to its homeopathic provings.

For the homeopathic preparation the fresh root is chopped and mixed with alcohol and left to stand for eight days before being succussed.

GENERAL SYMPTOMS

Exhaustion paralytic. **Eyelids** heavy. Feeling of **heaviness**. **Onset of complaint** slow. **Sweat** absent during fever. **Thirstless. Trembling.**
Better for sweating; for urinating.
Worse for physical exertion.

These are intensely weary individuals whose bodies feel heavy (their arms and legs feel as if they are weighted down with lead); they become trembly with exhaustion and consequently worse for any additional physical exertion. This heaviness and trembling and exhaustion is usually present in the anxiety or fear that precedes an exam or a public talk. The acute *Gelsemium* complaints (for example flu) come on gradually, taking days to develop (unlike *Aconite/Belladonna*). It is a remedy that is more often needed when the weather changes to warm after the cold of winter, and for people who spend their lives in overheated houses. *Bryonia* is similar, but people needing it keep still because of the terrible pain of moving, whereas *Gelsemium* people cannot move for heaviness and weariness. *Gelsemium* is thirstless whereas *Bryonia* is thirsty (at infrequent intervals). They have an unusual symptom in that they actually feel brighter after urinating.

EMOTIONAL/MENTAL SYMPTOMS

Complaints from: receiving bad news; excitement.
Depressed but cannot cry. **Desires** to be alone.
Dislikes company. **Exam nerves. Fearful:** of public speaking; in a crowd; of death. **Sluggish.**

These are dull, sluggish, depressed patients who just want to be left alone, who want to be quiet, and who do not want company. This is a common flu remedy and this sluggishness a familiar picture. *Gelsemium* is also one of the favourite remedies for people who become paralysed with fear prior to giving a talk or before an exam. This is not the active fear of *Argentum nitricum* or *Lycopodium*; it is an acute anxiety which causes a person to seize up both mentally and physically. These are people who may actually forget their lines (whereas *Lycopodiums* do very well on the extra adrenalin). People preparing for driving tests often need this remedy! They tremble and stutter and cannot collect their thoughts. They may even look, as well as feel, stupid. Like *Natrum muriaticum* and *Ignatia* they find it difficult to cry if depressed. The depression typically comes on after receiving a piece of bad news. Likewise over-excitement can make them ill – either emotionally or physically.

PHYSICAL COMPLAINTS

Diarrhoea

Causes anticipatory anxiety; bad/exciting news; fright/shock.

Fever

Symptoms HEAT: burning. With SHIVERING. Without sweating.
Better for sweating; for urinating.
Worse during the afternoon.
Waves of heat alternate with chills running up and down the back, and although the teeth may chatter the patient doesn't feel cold. The chills begin in hands and feet and move up the body. The patient may be breathing faster than normal.

Flu

Symptoms EYEBALLS aching. PAINS: in muscles. With EXHAUSTION (see General Symptoms); HEAVINESS; NUMBNESS; SHIVERING/CHILLS in back.
Better for sweating; for urinating.
Worse for exertion; for walking.
This is a flu that can come on in mild, damp weather or from getting chilled even though the person felt hot at the time. The tongue feels thick and heavy and the speech is slurred. The back aches all the way from the lower back up and over the head. The arms and legs ache and feel extremely heavy and tired. The patient is extremely chilly, and cannot get warm.

Headache

Symptoms FEET cold. HEAD: feels heavy. PAINS: in back of head; spreading to forehead; aching; sore, bruised. PUPILS dilated. Frequent URINATION. VISION blurred.
Better for urinating.
Worse for movement; for moving head.
The head feels so heavy that it needs support – of hands or a pillow. It also feels constricted as if a band or hoop were encircling it. The person has difficulty opening the eyes or keeping them open as the lids feel so heavy. The urine is copious and colourless. The person will have the characteristic lack of thirst and improvement from urinating.

Labour pains

Symptoms PAINS: distressing; in back; weak.

Measles

Symptoms ONSET slow. With FEVER (see above); HEADACHE (see above).
With typical *Gelsemium* heaviness, drowsiness and lack of thirst.

GLONOINE (Glon.)

Other names: nitro-glycerine; blasting oil; glyceryl trinitrate

Nitro-glycerine is a powerful explosive first made in 1846 by an Italian chemist called Sobrero, but early formulations were highly dangerous and the comparatively safe use of nitro-glycerine as a blasting explosive only became possible after Alfred B. Nobel developed a method for rendering it safe, and this became known as the first 'dynamite'. It is now an important ingredient of most dynamites and is used (with nitrocellulose) in some propellants for rockets and missiles.

The vapour produced in the manufacture of nitro-glycerine is absorbed through the skin and is mildly poisonous, causing violent headaches. Nitro-glycerine has been found to relax muscles of blood vessels when taken orally, and it is used medicinally to relieve heart pain in the treatment of angina.

The homeopathic preparation is made from nitro-glycerine diluted with alcohol.

GENERAL SYMPTOMS

Complaints from sunstroke. **Face** red.
Better for cold applications.
Worse for jarring movement; for heat; for exposure to sun.

The principal use of this remedy is for headaches that result from too much sun. Heat in any form aggravates, as does any jarring movement like walking.

EMOTIONAL/MENTAL SYMPTOMS

Confused. Forgetful. Time passes slowly.
Uncommunicative.

These patients are not willing to talk or answer your questions. They appear dull and confused. Their familiar surroundings feel strange and they have a sensation of time passing slowly.

PHYSICAL COMPLAINTS
Headache

Symptoms EYES red. FACE red. PAINS: bursting; hammering; throbbing; violent. With FAINTNESS; HOT FLUSHES.
Better for cold compresses; for pressure; at sunset.
Worse for heat; for jarring movement; during menstrual period; at sunrise; during the summer; for mental exertion; for walking.
Causes over-exposure to sun.
The headache increases when exposed to the sun and is better for being pressed firmly with the hands. The patient feels faint and flushed and as if the head will burst. An ice pack can ease the pains.

Sunstroke

Symptoms With HEADACHE (see above).

HAMAMELIS VIRGINICA (Ham.)

Family name: Hamamelidaceae
Other names: witch hazel; spotted alder; winterbloom; snapping hazelnut

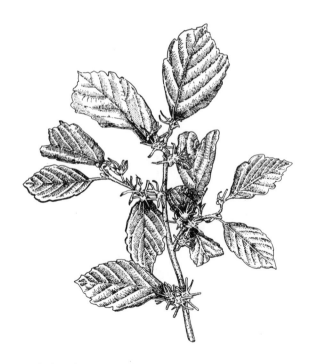

Witch hazel is a small deciduous tree that grows in damp woodlands throughout eastern and central North America. It grows to a height of twelve feet and produces clusters of yellow flowers in the autumn when the leaves have fallen. These are followed by edible seeds which are ejected violently from their shells when ripe, hence the name snapping hazelnut.

The leaves and bark are astringent and bitter. They were used by the North American Indians as a poultice for painful swellings and tumours. As a herbal remedy they were found to be a most effective treatment for piles, diarrhoea and wounds, both internally as a tea and externally. They have also been used as a general household remedy for burns, scalds and general inflammatory conditions of the skin including the calming of insect bites.

The homeopathic preparation is made from the fresh bark which is chopped and pounded to a pulp, mixed with alcohol and left to stand for eight days before being succussed.

GENERAL SYMPTOMS

Pains sore, bruised.
Worse for touch.

This is a small remedy whose use for acute complaints is limited to nosebleeds, varicose veins and piles, but because it is so useful (taken as a tonic) for these symptoms I have included it here. Symptoms cured by *Hamamelis* will be worse for touch.

There are no marked emotional/mental symptoms.

PHYSICAL COMPLAINTS
Nosebleed

Symptoms BLOOD: dark; thin.
Worse during the morning.

Piles

Symptoms PILES large; bleeding. PAINS sore, bruised.
Causes childbirth; pregnancy.
These are piles that occur towards the end of pregnancy, and also after childbirth (because of the pressure of the baby). If, once *Arnica* has been given as a routine prescription for the bleeding, a great deal of soreness persists and there are no indications for prescribing a bigger remedy, then *Hamamelis* will help. It is essential to seek professional help for both varicose veins and piles if the symptoms do not clear easily.

Varicose Veins

Symptoms VARICOSE VEINS: of legs and thighs; painful; swollen.
Worse for touch; after childbirth; during pregnancy.
These are hard, knotty varicose veins that feel sore and bruised and are sensitive to touch.

NB   SEE ALSO PAGES 203–26 FOR GENERAL ADVICE, DOS AND DON'TS.

HEPAR SULPHURIS CALCAREUM (Hep-s.)

Other names: calcium sulphide; sulphuret of lime

Hepar sulphuris calcareum is an impure calcium sulphide specially prepared by Hahnemann using oyster shells (*Calcarea carbonica*), instead of ordinary lime and flowers of sulphur. Being a chemical combination of *Calcarea carbonica* and *Sulphur*, it has some of the properties of both, but as a homeopathic remedy it is very different from either.

Before Hahnemann's time, ordinary calcium sulphide was used as an external remedy for itch, rheumatism, gout, goitre and tubercular swellings. Nowadays it is used in the manufacture of luminous paint, in medicine, for depilatories, and in veterinary medicine.

The homeopathic remedy is made by heating finely powdered oyster shell and flowers of sulphur in a hermetically sealed crucible. A white powder is produced which is dissolved in hot hydrochloric acid and then triturated.

GENERAL SYMPTOMS

Catches colds easily. Complaints from cold wind.
Likes sour foods. **Pains** needle-like. **Sweat:** cold; profuse; sour.
Better for warmth of bed; for heat; for wrapping up.
Worse for getting cold; for cold dry weather; for fresh air; for lying on painful side; at night; for pressure; for touch; for being uncovered; for cold wind.

This is one of the chilliest remedies in the Materia Medica. *Hepar* types hate the cold, especially dry cold and because they lack internal warmth they catch colds more easily than other more resilient people. When sick they are so sensitive to cold that if a part of the body escapes the bedclothes – a hand or a foot – they feel worse and start to cough or sneeze.

Their symptoms are usually worse at night and may develop when they are asleep – they may cough more in the night, for example. They are worse for pressure and consequently are worse for lying on the offending part of the body. They are only really better for lying in bed, well wrapped up, with the windows well shut and the heating on.

EMOTIONAL/MENTAL SYMPTOMS

Violently **angry. Impulsive. Irritable. Sensitive:** generally; to rudeness. **Speedy:** generally; eating; speaking.

Over-sensitivity is the special feature that runs throughout this remedy. *Hepar* types are extremely sensitive to pain and may weep or even faint in anticipation of or during their pains. Because they are sensitive to pressure they do not want to be touched when sick. They are as touchy mentally as they are physically. They are morose, difficult, irritable individuals who are easily offended and are prone to fits of anger. When sick they are extremely difficult, and will often be obstructive in giving information and at the same time demand (angrily) to be cured. They are also impulsive and speedy, like *Argentum nitricum*.

PHYSICAL COMPLAINTS

Abscesses

Symptoms Abscess: of glands; of roots of teeth.
Hepar is one of the major abscess remedies and is generally only useful before the abscess has opened and started to discharge. It is indicated at the swollen, painful stage, especially if this is accompanied by splinter-like pains and a great sensitivity to touch.

Boils

Symptoms Boils inflamed.
The boil is red around the edge, and very sore.

Common cold

Symptoms Nasal catarrh: drips down back of throat; smelly; yellow. With Sneezing on uncovering.
Worse for being uncovered.
The bones of the nose may feel sore and the sense of smell may be lost. The sneezing is brought on by draughts.

Constipation

Symptoms Stool soft.
This constipation may accompany any of the acute symptoms, such as the cough or the earache. The stool is passed with difficulty.

Cough

Symptoms Cough: barking; dry during the evening/night; loose during the morning; hacking; irritating; suffocative; violent. Mucus: copious; sticky; thick; tough; yellow. With hoarse voice; retching; sweating; vomiting.
Worse for cold dry air; for being uncovered; on single parts of the body; for uncovering hands; evening in bed; before midnight.
Causes exposure to cold dry wind.
This is a bad cough with irritation in the larynx, and the chest becomes sore from coughing. It is worse for being uncovered (an arm out of bed can cause a coughing fit). The simple act of going to bed can also

set the cough off (as soon as the patient closes his/her eyes to go to sleep the cough starts up again). Coughs up profuse, thick, yellow mucus.

Croup

Symptoms RECURRENT. With symptoms of COUGH (see above).

Many of the general symptoms and cough symptoms will be present in the croup. A *Hepar* croup is usually worse in the early morning (if it is worse in the evening it is more likely to be an *Aconite* croup), and the slightest breath of cold air causes coughing, as does uncovering. Patients choke and wheeze and rattle with the croup, but bringing up the mucus is difficult.

Diarrhoea

Symptoms DIARRHOEA painless.

There may be much rumbling in the abdomen accompanying this diarrhoea.

Earache

Symptoms DISCHARGE smelly. PAINS stitching.
Better for wrapping up warmly.
Worse for cold.

Fever

Symptoms HEAT alternating with chills.
Better for heat.
Worse for being uncovered.

The perspiration is cold, sour-smelling and profuse. The slightest exertion can bring on sweating and coughing; but the sweating will not provide any relief.

Injuries

Symptoms CUTS/WOUNDS: with inflammation; slow to heal; painful. PAINS: sore; splinter-like.

This is for cuts and injuries where the skin has been broken and healing is taking longer than expected. There is some redness (inflammation) around the site of the injury and it is generally sensitive, especially to touch.

Joint pain

Symptoms PAINS: in fingers; in hip; in shoulder; sore, bruised; pulling; tearing.
Better for heat.
Worse for cold.
Causes getting cold.

Sore throat

Symptoms PAINS: spreading up to ear; raw; splinter-like. TONSILS: swollen.
Better for hot drinks; for warm compresses.

Worse for breathing in cold air; for coughing; for swallowing; for turning the head; for cold drinks; in winter.
Causes getting cold; exposure to wind.

The throat feels as if there were a splinter or a fish bone stuck in it and the pains radiate up to the ear on swallowing, turning the head and sometimes even when yawning. The tonsils are swollen and ulcerated and the neck itself is sensitive to pressure/touch and better for being wrapped up warmly.

Toothache

Symptoms GUMS bleeding.
Worse for cold drinks; in winter.
Causes abscesses.

HYPERICUM PERFOLIATUM (Hyp.)

Family name: Hypericaceae
Other name: St John's wort

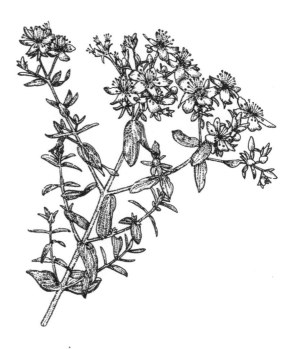

This herb grows wild in woods, along the borders of fields and meadows, and is also cultivated in many gardens throughout Britain, Europe, Asia and North America. It grows from one to three feet high and flowers from June to August with bright yellow flowers that exude a reddish-purple juice on bruising.

Its dark green leaves are full of tiny holes which are in fact oil glands; it was said that these holes resembled the pores of the skin and that the reddish juice of the flowers was like blood, so that it was therefore a plant which was useful for wounds to the flesh. Likewise, a plant with kidney-shaped leaves was thought to be capable of curing diseases of the kidneys and those with yellow sap were for diseases of the liver or bilious problems, and so on. This ancient way of looking at the healing potential of plants – of drawing similarities between the physical aspects of the plant and of the complaint – is called the 'doctrine of signatures', and it was for centuries the basis for many a herbal prescription.

Before the nineteenth century the great herbalist Gerard described *Hypericum*'s most important use as a 'most precious remedy for deep wounds . . . or any wound with a venomed weapon'. It was also used to reduce fevers, to expel worms and to stimulate the kidneys, amongst other symptoms, as well as a tonic or restorative to calm the nerves.

For the homeopathic preparation the fresh, whole flowering plant is chopped and pounded to a pulp, mixed with alcohol and left to stand for eight days before being succussed.

GENERAL SYMPTOMS

Complaints from accident/injuries to nerves/to coccyx. **Pains** shooting.
Worse for cold; for pressure.

Hypericum is the first remedy to think of when a nerve-rich part of the body is injured, that is, fingers, toes, spine (especially the coccyx), eyes, lips, and so on. Intense pains shoot along the course of wounded nerves towards the trunk or up the spine. They are usually tearing, severe pains and are sensitive to touch or pressure. It is often necessary to give *Arnica* first to prevent swelling and bruising and then to follow it with *Hypericum*, repeated every few minutes if the pain is excruciating. Use the external remedies to clean dirty wounds.

EMOTIONAL/MENTAL SYMPTOMS

Shock from injury.

This remedy has very few emotional symptoms but it is a marvellous first-aid remedy for certain types of injury and will also deal with the shock that accompanies such injuries.

PHYSICAL COMPLAINTS

Backache

Symptoms Pains: in coccyx; in lower back; sore, bruised; shooting; tearing.

Causes childbirth; forceps delivery; epidural; injury to coccyx; injury to spine.
Hypericum is useful for any trauma to spinal nerves. This might occur during childbirth, especially through the administration of an episiotomy or an epidural or after a forceps delivery; it might also result from a fall onto the coccyx (bottom), which can be unpleasant and can cause lasting pain and soreness, sometimes for years afterwards.

Bites/stings

Symptoms Bites inflamed. Pains: shooting; tearing.
Causes animal bites; insect bites.
Hypericum is for inflamed, exceptionally painful bites on nerve-rich parts; the pains are characteristically shooting or tearing up the nerve pathways.

Injuries

Symptoms Cuts/wounds: to nerve-rich parts; crushed; punctured; lacerated; slow to heal. Pains: shooting.
Causes accident; dentistry; splinter; surgery.
Hypericum wounds are inflamed and very painful. In fact the pain is often worse than it looks, because the nerves are injured (squashing a finger in a car door, stepping on a nail, tearing off a finger or toenail, and cutting the lips, or getting a splinter in the hand are all common injuries where a nerve-rich part is involved). If the pains are severe and shoot up the body then *Hypericum* is the correct first-aid remedy. It is also useful after any type of surgery where nerves are cut and painful or feel frayed or sore – for example teeth (root canals); gums (after dental work or an extraction); abdominal surgery (appendicectomy, Caesarean).

IGNATIA AMARA (Ign.)

Family name: Loganiaceae
Other name: St Ignatius' bean

This small shrub or tree grows in the Philippine Islands and China. It is a beautiful tree, with long, twining, smooth branches and fruit the size and shape of pears. The seeds (or beans) are one inch long and are very bitter, owing to the fact that they contain a large quantity of strychnine (more than in *Nux vomica*, and the provings show that in fact the two remedies have very different spheres of action).

The bean was named by the Spanish Jesuits who brought the seeds to Europe from the Philippines in the seventeenth century, where they were being worn by the natives as amulets, as a protection from all

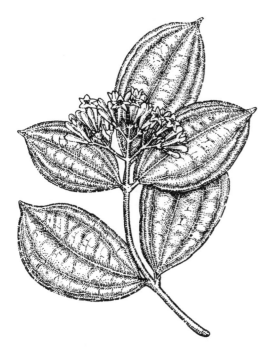

kinds of diseases. As an orthodox medicine it was then used for a variety of complaints such as gout, epilepsy, cholera and asthma.

In humans large doses are fatal, but small doses produce only unpleasant symptoms: a bitter taste, increased salivation, violent headache, loss of appetite, frightful dreams, trembling, twitching, cramps, giddiness, cold perspiration and nervous laughter. It is a fast-acting remedy that should be taken in the morning if possible as it has been known to cause insomnia when taken at night.

The homeopathic remedy is prepared from the powdered bean which is steeped in alcohol before being strained and succussed.

GENERAL SYMPTOMS

Symptoms contradictory. **Dislikes** fresh air. **Sweat**: hot; on single parts of the body.
Better after eating; for heat.
Worse after drinking coffee; for tobacco.

The *Ignatia* character is formed largely by the suppression of emotions, rather than by any general physical characteristics (see under Emotional/Mental Symptoms). *Ignatia* complaints often come on after extreme emotional upset, be it grief (from some sort of loss – a bereavement, perhaps), or shock, or anger where there is anxiety also present, or from being told off, punished or contradicted.

They experience contradictory symptoms, such as an empty feeling in the stomach that is not relieved by eating, or a sore throat that is worse when not swallowing. They are generally sensitive to coffee which makes them shaky, and tobacco which gives them headaches, amongst other things. People needing *Ignatia* feel worse for fresh air, where they quickly chill, and are better for warmth.

EMOTIONAL/MENTAL SYMPTOMS

Broody. Complaints from: anger; anger with anxiety; disappointed love; fright; grief; humiliation; reprimands; shock; suppression of emotions. **Conscientious. Depressed**: from suppressed grief. **Desires** to be alone. **Dislikes** consolation; contradiction. **Idealistic. Introspective.** Involuntary **weeping. Moody. Quarrelsome. Sensitive:** generally; to pain. **Sentimental. Sighing. Tearful:** cries on own.

Ignatia is valuable at all stages in life, for sensitive children who have developed sore throats or a tummy-ache or insomnia after being punished or severely frightened or if homesick; for teenagers who brood and pine after being ditched by a 'loved one' (they fall in love very easily); for men and women at all ages and in all walks of life who have suffered inwardly and become introspective and moody; and for older folks who, after losing a spouse or close friend or relative, grieve silently, without ceasing, struggling on and coping, and suffering from ill health as a result. They become anti-social, not wanting company or sympathy (although they will not be openly resentful of sympathy like *Natrum muriaticum* or *Sepia*), preferring to be alone to cry, but if they do break down and cry they cry convulsively and feel embarrassed so that they may laugh at the same time. They sit in company sighing and yawning, and because they are using so much tension in their chests to hold in their sadness the yawning becomes a reflex of the body to get oxygen.

They can experience great highs and lows. The highs are when everything is OK – only the sighing may give the game away then – and the lows are rarely seen because of *Ignatia* characters' secretiveness: they shut themselves away if they can. They are sensitive to being told off or humiliated and they torment themselves with recollections of offence or (emotional) injury they have received. *Ignatia* is the first remedy to think of when someone is overcome with grief, especially after a loss, for example when a woman miscarries, or loses a friend, or her boyfriend ditches her, or a child's pet dies. It is also for emotional shock, and someone needing *Ignatia* will have suppressed their feelings and developed 'hysterical' symptoms as a result. They are nervous, excitable types, gentle and refined idealists who have learned not to express their

NB   SEE ALSO PAGES 203–26 FOR GENERAL ADVICE, DOS AND DON'TS.

feelings. They become indecisive and scatty and are over-conscientious about doing everything correctly.

PHYSICAL COMPLAINTS

Cough

Symptoms COUGH: dry; irritating; racking; short; violent. PAIN IN CHEST: stitching. THROAT tickling.
Worse for coughing; during the evening in bed.
With this cough it feels as if a feather or dust were in the pit of the throat causing the cough. But suppressing the cough helps – the more the patient coughs, the worse it becomes (this contradictory symptom should guide you straight to this remedy). It may be useful in croup or whooping cough if the symptoms fit.

Fever

Symptoms THIRST with chills
Better for uncovering.
Worse during the afternoon; on front of body; for warm covers.
The patient is thirsty during the chilly stage rather than when hot and feverish, which is an *Ignatia* contradictory symptom. They want to be uncovered.

Headache

Symptoms PAINS: in forehead; stabbing; violent.
Worse in a smoky room.
These are nervous headaches that start gradually and stop suddenly, or start and stop suddenly. It feels as though a nail were being driven into the side(s) of the head. They are usually worse for being in a smoky room and are often set off by emotional upsets (see Emotional/Mental symptoms above).

Indigestion

Symptoms BELCHES sour. BELLY/STOMACH feels empty.
Better for belching.
Causes grief.

Shock

Causes emotional trauma.
Like *Phosphoric acid* the shock that needs *Ignatia* will have been sparked off by some emotional shock or loss.

Sore throat

Symptoms PAINS stitching. With LUMP SENSATION in throat; CHOKING SENSATION.
Better for swallowing.
Worse when not swallowing; evenings.

The sore throat is worse when not swallowing (a contradictory symptom) and liquids may be more difficult to swallow than solids. Along with the pain of the sore throat there is often a sensation of a lump in the throat which comes back up after swallowing. This is often associated with a suppressed desire to cry or express some upset.

IPECACUANHA (Ip.)

Family name: Rubiaceae
Other name: cephaelis ipecacuanha

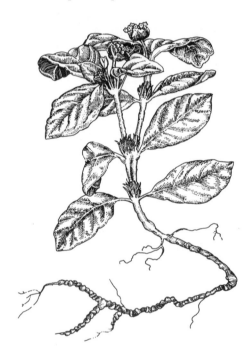

This small perennial shrub abounds in moist, shady woods in South and Central America. The roots of the plant have long been used medicinally. The name *Ipecacuanha* is from the Portuguese meaning 'road-side sick-making plant', and mention of it as a remedy for 'the bloody flux' or dysentery goes back as far as the late sixteenth century.

Large doses of the root cause gastro-enteritis (with vomiting), cardiac failure, severe bronchitis and inflammation of the lungs; in smaller doses it promotes sweating and expectoration (coughing up of phlegm from the lungs); and in still smaller doses it stimulates the appetite and digestion.

The powder of *Ipecacuanha* is irritating and causes redness, swelling and itching of the eyes and skin. If inhaled, it causes sneezing and breathing difficulties similar to asthma, all without relief until there is expectoration.

For the homeopathic preparation, the root is usually collected in January and February when the plant is flowering. It is dried, powdered coarsely and then either triturated or mixed with alcohol, left to stand and then succussed.

GENERAL SYMPTOMS

Face red, one-sided; blue during cough. **Nausea:** persistent; violent (see below). **Sweat** hot or cold. *Worse* at night.

Ipecacuanha is the first remedy to think of for violent and persistent nausea, which accompanies virtually all of its complaints (headache, diarrhoea, labour pains, whooping cough, haemorrhage, etc.). Patients look deathly, with a drawn, bluish face and dark-ringed eyes, and may be covered with a hot or cold sweat. They may feel chilly externally and hot inside. Their complaints recur periodically – at regular or intermittent intervals, and they feel generally worse at night.

EMOTIONAL/MENTAL SYMPTOMS

Anxious during a fever. **Capricious. Complaints from:** anger; vexation.

Ipecacuanha children are capricious. Nothing pleases them and they will scream or howl with frustration if they do not get what they want. When ill, these patients are anxious and are generally extremely unpleasant to look after. Complaints come on after getting angry or frustrated.

PHYSICAL COMPLAINTS

Colic

Symptoms PAINS: aching; cramping; griping.
Worse for movement.
These pains often accompany the *Ipecacuanha* nausea and vomiting.

Cough

Symptoms BREATHING: difficult; fast; wheezing. COUGH: choking; dry; in fits; irritating; rattling; tormenting; vomiting; whooping. EXPECTORATION: bloody; difficult to cough up. With NAUSEA (see below); NOSEBLEEDS; RETCHING; BLUE FACE.
Worse during a fever.
These coughs are nasty, and children have difficulty breathing during the coughing fits – they go stiff and blue in the face. They may complain of irritation in the larynx (voice-box), or air passages. The nosebleed that frequently accompanies the *Ipecacuanha* whooping cough produces bright red blood.

Diarrhoea

Symptoms IN CHILDREN. STOOLS grass green.
Ipecacuanha is useful for children with diarrhoea from over-eating.

Fever

Symptoms With ANXIETY. CHILLS: worse for heat; better for fresh air.
Better for fresh air (chills).
Worse for heat.

Flu

Symptoms CHILLS. PAINS: in bones; in back; in legs; aching; sore, bruised.
The patient feels weary, as if he has carried a heavy load, and the bones may feel torn to pieces. The chills are worse in a warm room and better for fresh air. Nausea may well be present.

Gastric flu

Symptoms of FLU (see above).

Headache

Symptoms PAINS sore, bruised. With VOMITING (see below).

Nausea

Symptoms Empty BELCHING. With PALLID FACE; RETCHING; copious SALIVA.
Worse after eating; for movement; for smell of food; for tobacco.
The person will feel nauseous but will be unable to vomit; even if he does vomit, the feeling of nausea will persist. The tongue is usually clean with an *Ipecac* picture.

Vomiting

Symptoms VOMIT: bile; food; green. With HEADACHE.
Worse after eating; after bending down; for coughing.

JABORANDI (Jab.)

Family name: Rutaceae
Other name: pilocarpus pinnatifolius

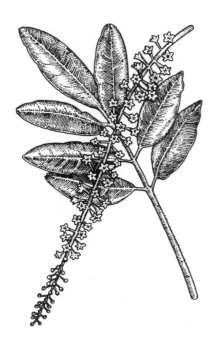

Jaborandi is a South American shrub, found mainly in Brazil. It grows to a height of four to six feet and has smooth grey bark, spotted with white dots.

The principal active ingredient is pilocarpine which is used to contract the pupils of the eyes, when, for example, they have been dilated with atropine for various eye tests. At one time it was used as a powerful and fast diaphoretic (sweat promoter); a single dose is said to bring out 9–15 ounces of sweat. It was used from the mid-nineteenth century onwards to promote salivation, a treatment for many ills.

The homeopathic preparation is made from the dried leaves and stems which are pounded and steeped in alcohol before being strained and the liquid succussed.

GENERAL AND EMOTIONAL/ MENTAL SYMPTOMS

This remedy does not have a strong picture, either generally or emotionally/mentally, but it is a very important mumps remedy and that is why I have included it in this book.

PHYSICAL COMPLAINTS
Mumps

Symptoms FACE red. GLANDS swollen. PAINS spread to breasts, ovaries or testicles. Copious SALIVA. Profuse SWEATING.

The sweat starts on the face and spreads all over the body. The saliva is like egg white, and although it runs freely the mouth is dry. The jaw is stiff and the tonsils are often swollen; given early enough, *Jaborandi* will prevent the involvement of other glands (breasts, ovaries, testicles). The sweaty stage, which is accompanied by an acute thirst, is followed by prostration and drowsiness and a general feeling of dryness.

Mercurius solubilis presents a very similar picture with its salivation and sweating but it will also have smelly breath and sweat which is not so marked with *Jaborandi*.

KALI BICHROMICUM (Kali-b.)

Other names: bichromate of potash; potassium bichromate

Kali bichromicum is prepared by adding neutral yellow potassium chromate in solution to a moderate quantity of one of the stronger acids; it is also obtained from chromium iron ore. It is a very caustic and corrosive poison.

As a chemical it is widely used in the dyeing of fabrics, staining of wood, photography and in electric batteries. It is a powerful oxidising substance.

The homeopathic remedy is prepared from pure potassium bichromate by trituration.

GENERAL SYMPTOMS

Discharges: stringy/sticky; thick. **Pains:** appear and disappear suddenly; in a spot; wandering. **Tongue** coated white.
Worse in the morning on waking; at night; for getting cold; after eating; in summer.

Kali bichromicum is a smallish remedy that is useful for colds and sinusitis if the indications fit. These are chilly individuals who are worse for cold, whose symptoms come on after getting cold. People needing *Kali bichromicum* become chilly when ill, yet feel worse in the summer's heat. The characteristic pains are 'in a spot' – the pain can usually be located with a fingertip. The pains may wander about from one part of the body to another and often come and go suddenly.

There are no strong emotional/mental symptoms.

PHYSICAL COMPLAINTS
Burns

Symptoms SLOW TO HEAL.
Deep burns that are not healing need this remedy.

Common cold

Symptoms NASAL CATARRH: crusty; dry; hard crusts; smelly; thick; green; yellow; yellow-green; sticky; stringy. PAINS: in sinuses. THROAT dry.

The catarrh forms sticky crusts in the nostrils which are hard to pick out; they leave raw, sore patches in the nostrils, and then re-form. The catarrh drips down the back of the throat, accumulates overnight, and is difficult to hawk out in the mornings; or it can block the nose entirely and be impossible to blow out.

Cough

Symptoms COUGH croupy. MUCUS: ropy; sticky; tough; thick; difficult to cough up. PAIN IN CHEST sore, bruised. With HOARSE VOICE.

Worse after eating; on waking in the morning.

The pains in the chest produced by the cough move from front to back, and the air passages are irritated and aggravate the cough. The ropy mucus tends to be coughed up in the morning only.

Croup

Symptoms With COUGH symptoms (see above).

Earache

Symptoms DISCHARGE: thick; yellow; smelly. PAINS stitching.

Worse on left side.

Headache ·

Symptoms PAINS recurring at regular intervals; in sinuses.

These headaches usually come on at the same time each day and although the pains will initially be in a small (localised) spot they may extend to the whole head, especially if the sinus congestion is severe.

Indigestion

Symptoms BELCHES: empty; sour.

Better for belching.

Worse after eating.

Causes beer.

This indigestion is usually caused by too much beer.

Joint pain

Symptoms PAINS: alternating with indigestion; alternating with cough; in a spot; sore, bruised; wandering.

The person is unlikely to suffer from joint pain and common cold symptoms at the same time.

KALI CARBONICUM (Kali-c.)

Other names: potassium carbonate; salt of tartar; potash, pearl ash

Potassium carbonate, a white crystalline substance, was obtained originally from wood, plant and seaweed ashes and was also known as potash or pearl ash. This was the major potassium compound in commerce before potassium chloride was obtained from salt mines in Germany in the 1860s. Potassium is now prepared commercially by various methods.

The Egyptians used potassium carbonate from the sixteenth century onwards for making glass, and it is still used commercially in the manufacture of glass and of soap, and in the production of other potassium compounds. It has also been used in dyeing processes.

As a medicine it has properties similar to those of potassium bicarbonate but because it is more caustic it is rarely administered internally. It has been used externally, though, as a lotion for eczema and urticaria.

The homeopathic remedy is prepared from potassium carbonate by trituration.

GENERAL SYMPTOMS

Anaemia. Catches cold easily. Exhaustion. Hot flushes. Pains stitching. **Sweat:** on single parts of the body; after eating; after the slightest physical exertion; profuse.

Better for warmth of bed.

Worse for becoming cold; for cold, dry weather; for draughts; for lying on side; around 2–4 a.m.; for getting overheated; at night; for touch; for being uncovered.

The *Kali carbonicum* picture can be hard to spot. People needing this remedy are extremely weak and weary and often anaemic. They sweat easily even with slight exertion, and, being chilly, they catch cold easily. They are sensitive to draughts and to cold air and dislike being overheated as this gives them hot flushes. But they feel generally better for warmth. Their pains are characteristically sharp, stitching, and their worst time is in the early morning between 2 and 4 a.m. Their faces are puffy, especially around the eyes and more especially the upper lids. They are touchy, both physically and mentally, and their symptoms are worse for lying on the affected part. It is a remedy that is more often needed for older people, although the coughs are seen in younger people or those prematurely worn out.

NB   SEE ALSO PAGES 203–26 FOR GENERAL ADVICE, DOS AND DON'TS.

EMOTIONAL/MENTAL SYMPTOMS

Angry. Anxious. Desires company. **Dislikes** being touched; being alone. **Expression:** haggard; suffering. **Fearful** of being alone. **Irritable. Jumpy. Sensitive** to noise. **Sluggish. Touchy.**

These are touchy individuals who are anxious, irritable and sluggish all at the same time. They do not want to be alone and yet they are not the welcoming type! They are highly strung, being easily startled both by noises and by unexpected touch, either while awake or asleep. They often talk and moan in their sleep.

PHYSICAL COMPLAINTS

Backache

Symptoms PAINS: in lower back; sore, bruised; stitching.
Better for pressure.
Worse around 3 a.m.; before menstrual period; after long sitting; for walking.
This backache may occur after injury, and the pains, which are much worse in the early hours of the morning, drive the person out of bed.

Cough

Symptoms BREATHING wheezing. COUGH: dry; hard; irritating; loose; racking; vomiting; violent; wakens person at night. PAIN IN CHEST: cutting; stitching. With NAUSEA; VOMITING.
Worse for deep breathing; for becoming cold; during fever; during the evening; for heat; for lying down; in the morning; at night; for talking; around 3 a.m.
Causes getting chilled.
The person has to sit up and lean forward to cough, and to get some relief. Chest pains with a cough (chest infection) are often right-sided and are cutting, knife-like or stitching, with a feeling of irritation in the whole respiratory tract.

Fever

Symptoms SWEATING: profuse; from slightest exertion.
Better in bed; for heat.
Worse after eating.

Headache

Symptoms PAINS: above eyes; in forehead; shooting; tearing.
Worse for cold; on left side of head.
Causes eye strain.

Indigestion

Symptoms BELLY/STOMACH: feels bloated; feels full. PAINS sore, bruised.
Better for belching.
Worse after eating.
Feels bloated and full after eating – everything turns to gas.

Insomnia

Symptoms DREAMS: anxious; nightmares.
Worse before midnight; around 1–2 a.m.
The person will be sleepy in the evening but will be unable to get to sleep, or alternatively will fall asleep easily, have awful and/or anxious dreams and wake in the early morning, unable to get back to sleep.

Joint pain

Symptoms ARMS feel weak. LEGS restless. PAIN: in arms/hip/legs/shoulder; sore, bruised; stitching; tearing.
Better for movement; for walking.
Worse around 2–3 a.m.; for lying on painful part.
There is jerking on going to sleep. Hands and feet feel cold and numb and legs fall asleep easily.

Labour pains

Symptoms PAINS: in back; distressing; ineffectual; weak; stop altogether.

Piles

Symptoms PILES large.
Causes childbirth.

Toothache

Symptoms PAINS stitching.
Worse while eating and drinking; cold drinks/food; hot drinks/food.

KALI MURIATICUM (Kali-m.)

Other names: chloride of potash; potassium chloride

Potassium chloride occurs naturally in the form of the mineral silvite. It is found in granular crystalline masses in salt deposits in Germany and Poland.

Potassium chloride is an important potassium compound and it accounts for most of the consumption of potassium salts because of its extensive use as a fertiliser. It also plays a major role in making chemicals. The homeopathic remedy is prepared from potassium chloride by trituration.

GENERAL SYMPTOMS

Discharges white. White-coated **tongue**.

This is a small remedy that does not have strong general symptoms but it is an important addition to any first-aid kit that deals with colds. Its keynote is whiteness – and this is found everywhere: on the tongue, in the mouth, and in all the discharges. It is worth considering for any cold that has moved beyond the first stage and settled in but has not as yet turned into a more serious infection, with yellow/green discharges.

There are no marked emotional/mental symptoms.

PHYSICAL COMPLAINTS

Common cold

Symptoms Nasal catarrh white.
This is for the second stage of a cold, when the nasal discharge has changed from clear and watery to white (before it turns yellow). It is for stuffy head colds with thick white mucus. The glands may be swollen.

Cough

Symptoms Cough: barking; hard; short.

Earache

Symptoms With noises in the ear. Deafness after a cold. Glands swollen.
Worse for swallowing.
The ears snap, crackle and pop on blowing the nose or on swallowing, and deafness remains after a cold because of catarrh in the Eustachian tubes.

Indigestion

Symptoms With: diarrhoea; stools pale.
Worse after eating starchy food.

Sore throat

Symptoms Tonsils: swollen; white.

Thrush

Symptoms In breastfeeding babies. Tongue/gums coated white.

KALI PHOSPHORICUM (Kali-p.)

Other names: potassium phosphate; phosphate of potash

Kali phosphoricum is a constituent of all animal fluids and tissues and especially of the brain, nerves, mus-cles and blood cells. It is produced by mixing aqueous phosphoric acid with potassium hydrate or carbonate.

The homeopathic remedy is prepared from potassium phosphate by trituration.

GENERAL SYMPTOMS

Anaemia. Exhaustion: caused by flu; nervous.
Sweating: when tired; profuse; after the slightest physical exertion.
Better for heat; for rest.
Worse for cold; for exercise; for excitement; for mental exertion; for worry.

Kali phosphoricum is a nerve nutrient found in the tissues and fluids of the brain and nerve cells. It is indicated in cases of nervous exhaustion where anaemia, nervous headaches and/or insomnia are present. It is especially useful for exhaustion that follows a bad case of flu and it is also useful in the convalescent stage of an acute illness where there is muscular weakness. This tiredness is often accompanied by sweating from even the gentlest exertion. The patients are very sensitive to cold air and cold in general, and all their complaints are worse for cold. They feel better for – and desperately need – warmth and rest.

EMOTIONAL/MENTAL SYMPTOMS

Anxious. Complaints from: mental strain; overwork.
Depressed. Forgetful. Jumpy.

This remedy is for those who are exhausted following a heavy work or study period and whose nerves are consequently frayed. They become sensitive, easily startled and depressed – a true sort of depression of the mind where the memory no longer works as well as it did, with resultant anxiety. The mind becomes exhausted and sluggish. Sensitivity to noise and light are often present.

PHYSICAL COMPLAINTS

Backache

Symptoms Pains: in spine; sore, bruised.
Better for movement.
The spine feels sore and bruised and the arms and legs heavy and cold.

Headache

Symptoms Headache nervous. Pains: one-sided.
Causes mental exertion; overwork.
These are the headaches of students who become worn out by over-study and are unable to think.

Indigestion

Symptoms INDIGESTION nervous. BELLY/STOMACH feels empty.
Causes nervous exhaustion; overwork.
There is a nervous, empty feeling in the stomach which is only temporarily relieved by eating. This indigestion accompanies the nervous exhaustion and depression.

Insomnia

Symptoms With EMPTY FEELING in pit of stomach.
Causes anxiety; excitement; mental strain; nervous exhaustion.
This is the sort of sleeplessness that follows a period of intense work or excitement. If you feel as if your nerves are worn out and have no other symptoms that would guide you to another remedy then take *Kali phosphoricum* at bedtime, every 5–10 minutes until sleep falls.

KALI SULPHURICUM (Kali-s.)

Other names: potassium sulphate; sulphate of potash; Vesuvian salt; glaserite

This salt occurs naturally in delicate needle-shaped crystals or crusting in many of the Vesuvian lavas. Various methods are used to separate the potassium sulphate from the ore.

Potassium sulphate is used commercially as a fertiliser for tobacco, citrus fruits and other crops that cannot tolerate much chloride; it is also used as an antiflash agent in smokeless powders and in the manufacture of potassium carbonate and glass.

Christopher Glaser, a sixteenth-century pharmacist and apothecary to Louis XIV of France, was one of the first independent discoverers and users of potassium sulphate as a medicine. Nowadays it is used in the manufacture of potassium alum which is used, because of its astringent properties, to treat certain skin conditions, to reduce excessive perspiration, and to stop bleeding from small cuts.

The homeopathic remedy is made from potassium sulphate by trituration.

GENERAL SYMPTOMS

Complaints from change of weather from cold to warm. **Discharges:** thick; yellow. **Pains** wandering. Yellow-coated **tongue.**
Better for fresh air.
Worse for heat; for change of temperature.

This remedy is very similar to *Pulsatilla* in that its symptoms are clearly aggravated by warmth in general (warmth of bed, stuffy rooms, and so on), and are greatly relieved by fresh air, especially a walk outside. Both remedies have thick yellow discharges and wandering pains, and most complaints are accompanied by a yellow, often slimy, coated tongue. The differences between the two remedies lie in the emotional/mental symptoms. A change of temperature from cold to warm in the spring/summer can set off a cold or cough which will be helped by *Kali sulphuricum* if the symptoms fit.

EMOTIONAL/MENTAL SYMPTOMS

Angry. Anxious when indoors; when overheated. **Irritable.**

There are very few emotional/mental symptoms with this remedy. These types feel ratty and anxious, especially when stuck inside the house; they are always improved by a walk in the fresh air.

PHYSICAL COMPLAINTS

Common cold

Symptoms NASAL CATARRH: profuse; thick; yellow.
Better for fresh air.
Worse in a stuffy room.
If *Pulsatilla* is well indicated for a cold but does not cure or only partly helps then *Kali sulphuricum* will finish the cure, as the symptoms are very similar. These cases are worse in a warm room, like *Pulsatilla*, and desire fresh air.

Cough

Symptoms COUGH: rattling; whooping. MUCUS: difficult to cough up; has to swallow what comes up.
Worse at night; in a warm room.
The person coughs up yellow phlegm into the throat but often has difficulty spitting it out so will swallow it.

Earache

Symptoms DISCHARGE: thin; yellow. With CRACKLING IN EARS when chewing.
This earache usually occurs in children. The child will be temporarily deaf because the Eustachian tubes are blocked with mucus, and there will be ringing noises in the ears when chewing. A course of *Kali sulphuricum* can help the mucus to disperse.

Headache

Symptoms PAINS: in forehead; in sides of head; stitching.

Better for fresh air.
Worse during the evening; in a warm room.

Joint pain

Symptoms FEET cold. PAINS: in hips; in legs; wandering.
Better for fresh air; for movement; for walking.
Worse for heat; in summer.
The feet will feel cold but the person and her symptoms are worse for heat.

LACHESIS (Lach.)

Family name: Ophidia
Other names: Surukuku snake; Churukuku snake; bushmaster snake

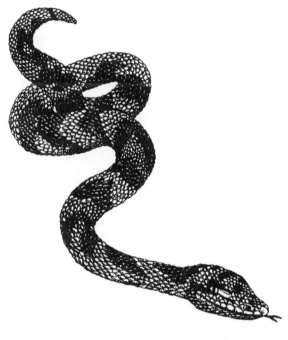

This remedy is derived from the venom of a South American snake supposed to be the *Trigonocephalus lachesis*, commonly known as the bushmaster or Surukuku. The snake is seven feet long and has one-inch fangs; it kills its prey both by constriction and by injecting its venom, and will hunt down a human being for prey.

The poisonous effect of snake venom on the nervous mechanisms of the heart causes death. If the dose is small and therefore not fatal, or if death is delayed, ensuing symptoms include a decreased ability of the blood to coagulate and the destruction of red blood corpuscles. *Lachesis* has both these symptoms strongly.

Constantine Hering was the first and principal prover of *Lachesis* during his zoological trip to Dutch Guyana in 1828. He offered a reward for a live specimen of the Surukuku snake; when this was found (after which the 'natives' accompanying him promptly fled) he stunned the snake with a blow and while expressing the poison in order to prove it accidentally handled some of it. His wife kept a record of everything he said and did during this accidental proving and these symptoms formed the basis for its use as a homeopathic remedy.

The homeopathic remedy is prepared from the venom by trituration.

GENERAL SYMPTOMS

Breath smells. **Lips** blue. **Palpitations. Sweat:** from mental exertion; from pain. **Symptoms** left-sided or start on the left and move to the right.
Better for fresh air; while eating.
Worse for alcohol; for humidity; before menstrual period; for heat; during the morning; for pressure; after sleep; for tight clothes; on waking.

Lachesis is a remedy that is often needed at the time of the menopause in women. They suffer from hot flushes and feelings of constriction, and headaches that throb or burst. Generally, *Lachesis* patients are worse for heat and feel better for cold compresses and fresh air. Their tiredness, which is often accompanied by trembling and a faint feeling, is not helped by sleeping. They and their symptoms are worse on waking and they may even begin to dread falling asleep because of this. Although these people enjoy a drink (too many at times), alcohol will aggravate their symptoms. They suffer from left-sided complaints, which may then move across to the right side of the body.

The *Lachesis* character is always worse for suppressing anything, be it emotions or natural bodily discharges so that, for example, the suppression of periods (by taking the pill or the cessation at the menopause) can create problems with headaches, sleeplessness, and so on. Similarly, they will often feel worse before a period and much better as soon as the period starts.

EMOTIONAL/MENTAL SYMPTOMS

Anxious on waking. **Cheerful. Complaints from:** grief; mental strain. **Confused. Depressed:** generally; on waking. **Excitable. Exhilarated. Expression** sickly. **Jealous. Lively. Sluggish** on waking. **Sensitive** to pain; to touch. **Shock** from injury. **Talkative.**

NB SEE ALSO PAGES 203–26 FOR GENERAL ADVICE, DOS AND DON'TS.

These are lively, excitable characters who enter fully into life's rich tapestry. They are terrible talkers, jumping from one subject to another so that it is hard to get a word in edgeways. These mental symptoms are not often seen in a minor acute complaint like a sore throat, but if you know your patient fits the *Lachesis* picture on a day-to-day, healthy basis, when she falls ill this remedy will be the one to help. Ill health often follows a period of overwork or a personal loss and this will cause depression, anxiety (which is worse on waking) and mental exhaustion. They do not want to work in this state and their talkativeness will degenerate into muttering. They are acutely sensitive to touch and cannot tolerate the slightest pressure especially around their necks (this corresponds to the snake's weak spot, for it is by gripping the snake firmly around the neck that the venom may be 'milked' without any harm coming to the person holding the snake).

PHYSICAL COMPLAINTS

Bites/stings

Better for cold.
Worse for heat.
Causes insects/animals.
The area around the bite looks bluish.

Cough

Symptoms COUGH: choking as soon as person falls into a deep sleep; dry; hacking; suffocative; violent; from tickling in larynx.
Worse for touch; at night.
The larynx is irritated and feels as if a crumb were lodged in it. This sets off a desire to cough, as does touching the neck. Patients may wake with a choking cough as soon as they have fallen into a deep sleep.

Croup

Symptoms With symptoms of COUGH (see above); LUMP SENSATION in throat.
Worse after a sleep; on waking.
The voice is hoarse and the air passages feel irritated, which aggravates the cough.

Earache

Symptoms PAINS on left side. With SORE THROAT (see below).
Worse for swallowing; for exposure to wind.

Exhaustion

Worse during the morning after getting up; for heat of sun; for slightest exertion; for walking; for mental exertion.
Causes mental exertion.

Food poisoning

Causes rotten meat.

Gums bleeding

Causes tooth extraction.

Hair loss

Causes pregnancy.

Headache

Symptoms HEAD: feels heavy; hot. PAINS: in forehead spreading to back of head; in temples and top of head; bursting; pressing; throbbing; violent.
Better after eating.
Worse on left side of head; for lying down; on waking; for pressure; for walking.
Causes alcohol; menopause; exposure to sun.
These headaches begin on the left side of the head and may move to the right. The pains are bursting and are worse for lying down and better for eating. The patient dreads going to sleep, knowing that the pain will be awful on waking.

Hot flushes

Symptoms With HEADACHE (see above); PALPITATIONS; HOT SWEATS.
Causes menopause.
These hot flushes are sparked off by the menopause; they may be accompanied by palpitations as well as hot sweats and headaches.

Injuries

Symptoms CUTS/WOUNDS: bleed freely; slow to heal. SCARS become red.
The skin around the wound looks dark or bluish and the blood is dark.

Mumps

Symptoms GLANDS: swollen/painful. With SORE THROAT.
Worse on the left side.
Patients are very sensitive to touch, especially the neck and glands, which are so painful that swallowing is extremely difficult.

Nosebleeds

Symptoms BLOOD dark.
Worse during the morning; before a menstrual period.
Causes blowing nose; menopause.

Sore throat

Symptoms PAINS: spreading up to ears; splinter-like. With CHOKING SENSATION; LUMP SENSATION in throat.

Better for swallowing solids.
Worse for heat; on the left side; for pressure; for touch; for swallowing liquids or saliva.

This sore throat is very painful and has the unusual symptom of being better for swallowing hard foods, such as toast, because this hard pressure helps, and light pressure or touch aggravates. Empty swallowing (of saliva) and swallowing drinks, especially warm ones, is very sore. The patient has a constant desire to swallow because it feels as if there is a lump in the throat, and swallowing helps this feeling, but only temporarily. It may feel as if there were breadcrumbs in the throat and this is relieved by hawking. The patient feels a sense of constriction around the neck and cannot bear to be touched there.

Toothache

Symptoms CHEEKS swollen. PAINS throbbing.
Worse for brushing teeth; for cold drinks; hot drinks/food; during menstrual period; in the spring.
Causes getting wet.

The teeth are sensitive to cold water, to being touched and to warmth in general.

LEDUM PALUSTRE (Led.)

Family name: Ericaceae
Other names: marsh tea; wild rosemary

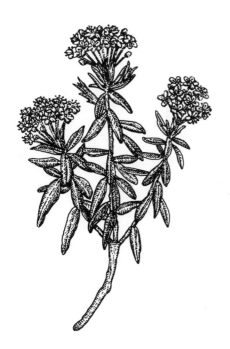

This evergreen shrub grows in marshes and bogs in the north of Europe, North America and Canada. It flowers from April to July and smells strongly of hops when crushed. The leaves resemble those of the herb rosemary, and rust-coloured down covers the soft, green upper branches. These woolly hairs probably gave the name *Ledum* to this plant, for *ledos* is the Greek for 'woolly robe'.

The flowers contain an oil that smells strongly of antiseptic; this, and the plant's bitter taste, protect it from being eaten by animals. *Ledum* has in fact served well as an 'antiseptic': the Swedes used it to wash their oxen in order to kill lice, and the Lapps and Finns used it to protect their grain from vermin. It has also been used as a tea substitute, and to replace hops in the manufacture of beer, though this causes an unpleasant sort of drunkenness accompanied by an obstinate headache and dizziness.

The homeopathic remedy is made from the whole plant which is dried and powdered then mixed with alcohol and left for eight days; the clear liquor is then decanted and succussed.

GENERAL SYMPTOMS

Pains wandering.
Better for cold bathing.
Worse for heat; for movement; for touch; for walking; for wine.

Ledum is effective in treating acute rheumatic and gouty afflictions of the joints, as well as preventing sepsis developing in a particular type of injury. The injured or painful part puffs up, becomes numb and is sensitive to being touched. It may look mottled or bluish, or can become pale. Although *Ledum* types are chilly, and although the painful part may feel cold (both internally and externally), the pains are actually relieved by cold compresses or by being bathed in cold (and even icy-cold) water. The pains are generally worse for movement and warmth and there will be a general aggravation after drinking wine.

There are no marked emotional/mental symptoms.

PHYSICAL COMPLAINTS

Bites/stings

Better for cold.
Worse for heat.
Causes insects/animals.

Ledum prevents a septic state setting in and should always be routinely administered after a person has been bitten by any animal, poisonous or not. Give also for any insect bite or sting unless another remedy is strongly indicated, and use the appropriate external remedy at the same time.

Bruises/black eye

Symptoms BLACK EYE. With DISCOLOURATION.
Causes injury.
If *Arnica* has been given but the bruising comes out, then give *Ledum*.

Eye injury

Symptoms With BRUISING; DISCOLOURATION.
Better for cold.

Injuries

Symptoms CUTS/WOUNDS: lacerated; punctured; to palm of hand/sole of foot.
Better for cold compresses.
Worse for heat.
Causes splinter; nails.
If prescribed early, *Ledum* will prevent sepsis from developing in wounds where the skin is punctured by a sharp, pointed instrument such as a knife, nail, splinter or needle, or by an insect sting or animal bite. The foreign object may have penetrated deeply into the flesh, so press gently around the wound to encourage bleeding and to expel it. '*Ledum* wounds' feel cold internally but are made worse by warmth – they are actually improved by cold compresses.

Hypericum is a better choice of remedy if the wound is in a nerve-rich area; if the wound is in an area around a joint, then *Ruta* may be better indicated.

Joint pain

Symptoms JOINTS: hot; icy cold; stiff. PAINS: in hands and feet; in right hip; in left shoulder.
Better after a common cold; for being uncovered; cold compresses; cold bathing.
Worse for movement; for heat; for warmth of bed; at night; for wine.
Pains may start in the lower limbs, especially in the small joints, and move upwards, for example from the feet to the hands. Although the patients feel cold, the warmth of bed is unendurable.

LYCOPODIUM (Lyc.)

Family name: Lycopodiaceae
Other names: wolf's claw; club moss; stag horn; witch meal; vegetable sulphur; muscus terrestris repens

Lycopodium is an evergreen trailing plant found on heaths, moors, pastures and in woods throughout Great Britain, northern Europe and North America. The plant's roots resemble a wolf's foot – hence its name.

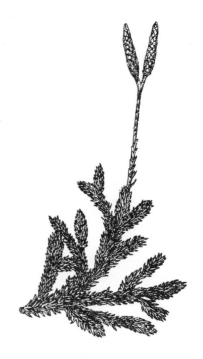

The useful part of the plant is the spores, or, more specifically, the pollen collected from the spores. This fine, odourless and tasteless, pale yellow powder has been used internally since the seventeenth century in treating diarrhoea, dysentery, rheumatism, and externally for wounds and diseases of the skin such as eczema. Before that time the whole plant was used mainly as a herbal remedy for kidney complaints. The powder's power to repulse water is so strong that if the hand is covered with the powder it can be dipped in water without becoming wet; it has been used as a covering for pills in order to prevent them sticking to one another in the box. The pollen is highly inflammable, and it was at one time used to produce false lightning in theatres as well as in the manufacture of fireworks.

The powder or spores are gathered towards the end of summer and are potentised by trituration.

GENERAL SYMPTOMS

Discharges yellow. **Face** pale; sickly. **Expression** confused. **Likes:** sweets; chocolate. **Pains** in glands.
Sweat: cold; profuse; clammy; smelly; sour; from slightest physical exertion; better for uncovering.
Taste: mouth tastes sour. **Symptoms:** right-sided; starts right side and moves to left.
Better for fresh air; for warmth of bed.
Worse around 4–8 p.m.; during the afternoon; during the evening; for pressure; in stuffy rooms; for tight

clothes; wind; for onions; for flatulent food (beans; cabbage, etc.).

Adult *Lycopodium* types are bright intellectually but tired and weak physically: the classic professor who lives a sedentary life. Their hair greys early and they may look older than their years, with a deeply furrowed forehead and a pale, sickly complexion with dark rings around their eyes. These types have a lot of trouble with food; they either feel full up and distended after eating very little or they have no appetite at all until they start eating, and then they become ravenous (and in this case the feeling of emptiness will not be helped by eating). These are big sweet cravers, often eating several bars of chocolate a day. They may feel sleepy after eating. They are bloated with gas, with acidity and sourness and feel worse for the pressure of clothes especially around the waist. They are often called 'thin, brainy and windy'!

Lycopodium symptoms are predominantly right-sided, or they may start on the right and move to the left. The symptoms are always worse between 4 and 8 p.m. Despite being chilly and worse for extremes of heat and cold, these people feel generally better for fresh air. Babies may sleep well at night but cry all day.

EMOTIONAL/MENTAL SYMPTOMS

Angry from contradiction. **Anxious:** generally; indoors; anticipatory. **Complaints from:** humiliation; mental strain. **Concentration** poor. **Depressed** on waking. **Desires** company. **Dislikes** being contradicted; being alone; company. **Exam nerves.** **Fearful** of public speaking. **Forgetful. Indecisive. Irritable** on waking. **Moody** (changeable). **Restless.** Lack of **self-confidence. Screaming:** during sleep; on waking. **Sensitive. Sluggish:** better for fresh air. **Shy. Tearful.**

EMOTIONAL/MENTAL SYMPTOMS

Lycopodium characters are generally anxious and will worry about most things because of an essential lack of self-confidence. Their biggest worries are in anticipation of an event where they either appear in public (acting or public speaking) or are tested (exams, driving test) – they dread taking on new things. Exams, interviews, new jobs and public-speaking engagements make them extremely nervous and they prepare for them meticulously. When the time comes, in spite of creating a scene about not being able to do it, they actually shine, and succeed in their exams well and easily. They are extremely sensitive, shy individuals whose rude, difficult behaviour is a front for their low self-confidence. They hate to be alone, but are not keen to have company, either; their ideal is to know that there is someone else in the house – in another room!

When sick they become dull and sluggish mentally and unable to concentrate. These mental symptoms are always worse in a stuffy room and better for some fresh air. After a big effort like an exam or the first night of a new play, or having to make a decision, which is also hard for *Lycopodiums*, they can become exhausted and go down with a minor acute illness.

Lycopodium children are irritable and dictatorial and will have a tantrum if contradicted. They kick and scream after a nap or on waking in the mornings and are generally difficult to live with.

PHYSICAL COMPLAINTS

Backache

Symptoms PAINS: in lower back. With STIFFNESS.
Better for movement; for passing wind; for urinating.
Worse on beginning to move; while passing a stool; on getting up from sitting.
Causes lifting.
The lower back feels sore, often because of wind that cannot escape.

Blisters

Symptoms BLISTERS: burning; on tip of tongue.

Common cold

Symptoms NASAL CATARRH yellow. NOSE: blocked; dry. SINUSES: blocked. With HEADACHE (see below).
Worse on the right side.
The nose and sinuses become quite blocked so that the person has to sleep with his mouth open. Nursing infants cannot breathe; this is one of the main remedies to consider for new babies with the snuffles.

Constipation

Symptoms DESIRE TO PASS STOOL ineffectual. STOOLS: hard; knotty.

Corns

Symptoms CORNS inflamed. PAINS: pressing; sore; tearing.

Cough

Symptoms COUGH: constant; dry, irritating; painful; disturbs sleep. BREATHING: difficult; fast. MUCUS: yellow; copious; white; green; tastes salty.
Better for hot drinks.
Worse on going to sleep; at night; in the evening in bed.

NB   SEE ALSO PAGES 203–26 FOR GENERAL ADVICE, DOS AND DON'TS.

This cough is aggravated by an overpowering tickling in the larynx, as if the larynx were being tickled by a feather. It is worse in the evening on going to bed and can prevent the patient from falling asleep. The chest infection is accompanied by a feeling of constriction or tightness in the chest. The sputum is yellow or white.

Cramp

Symptoms CRAMP in calf.
Worse at night.

Cystitis

Symptoms DESIRE TO URINATE: frequent; ineffectual. PAINS: aching; cutting; pressing; stitching. URINATION: frequent; slow (waits a long time for it to start).
Better after urination.
The person can pass only a few drops or a dribble of urine at a time. A child will scream before urinating because she cannot urinate and because of the pain.

Earache

Symptoms EARS feel blocked up. PAINS tearing. With NOISES IN THE EAR.

Eye inflammation

Symptoms DISCHARGE purulent. EYES: sensitive to light; watering. EYELIDS glued together.

Fever

Symptoms FEVER: one-sided; on the left side.
Worse in the evening.
One-sided sweating, or feeling hot on one side of the body and cold on the other, is a common symptom.

Flatulence

Symptoms BELLY/STOMACH: bloated; intolerant of tight clothing; rumbling.
Better for passing wind.
Worse after eating; before and after passing a stool.
The belly (below the navel) is bloated and uncomfortable; and the person has to loosen clothing around the waist.

Food poisoning

Causes shellfish (especially oysters).

Hair loss

Symptoms HAIR falls out.
Causes childbirth.

Headache

Symptoms PAINS: in forehead; in temples; pressing; throbbing.
Better for fresh air.
Worse for coughing; during menstrual period; for overheating; for warmth of bed; for wrapping up head.
Causes eye strain; mental strain.

Indigestion

Symptoms BELCHES: acrid; empty; sour. BELLY/ STOMACH: feels empty; feels full very quickly. PAINS: in stomach; pressing; cramping. With HEARTBURN.
Better for belching.
Worse after eating; for onions; for wearing tight clothing.

Joint pain

Symptoms PAINS: tearing.
Better for movement; for walking; for warmth of bed.
Worse on beginning to move; during a fever; for sitting.
The rheumatic pains may occur in any of the joints of the body, but the knee and finger joints are especially sore and stiff. The pains will often have started on the right side of the body and moved over to the left.

Mouth ulcers

Symptoms ULCERS under the tongue.

Mumps

Symptoms GLANDS swollen/painful. With FEVER (see above); SORE THROAT (see below); typical *Lycopodium* general and emotional/mental symptoms.
The pains move from the right side to the left side.

Sore throat

Symptoms THROAT: dry; with lump sensation. PAINS: raw; sore. TONSILS swollen.
Better for warm drinks.
Worse at night; on right side.
The throat is sore and inflamed, and feels full of dust. The patient may choke while drinking even though warm drinks actually soothe the pains.

MAGNESIA CARBONICA (Mag-c.)

Other names: light carbonate of magnesia; magnesite

Magnesia carbonica is a white, grey, brown or yellow material that occurs as a crystal in sedimentary beds or as veins in other rocks, mainly in southern California, Mexico and Venezuela. It is also made commercially. Its name comes from 'Magnesia', the name of the city in Thessaly near which the deposits of native magnesium carbonate occur.

It is used in the production of refractory bricks, in the manufacture of chemicals, cement, fertilisers and artificial stone flooring, rubber pigments, inks, glass, pharmaceuticals, toothpastes, cosmetics, mineral waters, free-running table salts, and in other magnesium salts.

It was known medicinally from the eighteenth century onwards and it became renowned as the 'terror of the nursery' as it was used extensively as a laxative. It has been widely used as an antacid and an anticithii (a medicine to aid the dissolving of kidney stones).

The homeopathic remedy is prepared by mixing a solution of epsom salts with sodium carbonate; this is then succussed.

GENERAL SYMPTOMS

Insomnia after 3 a.m.; sleep unrefreshing. **Sweat:** oily; sour. **Taste:** mouth tastes sour.
Better for fresh air.
Worse during the evening; at night.

These are often puny, sickly children, or worn-out individuals of any age who are debilitated from too many cares and not enough good food. They snack for comfort on junk food and so compound this situation. They have an 'unloved' look about them. They are generally worse at night, when they cannot sleep; they wake more tired in the morning than when they went to sleep. A walk in the fresh air helps a little. Children who need this remedy may have an aversion to vegetables and a craving for meat; they stay thin, have delicate digestive systems, and will have sour perspiration. Nursing children may refuse the breast. Milk passes through undigested.

EMOTIONAL/MENTAL SYMPTOMS

Anxious in bed. **Irritable** children.

Magnesia carbonica children are irritable, and are anxious in bed, particularly during a fever. They sleep restlessly and have disturbed dreams (about fires and dead people).

PHYSICAL COMPLAINTS

Diarrhoea

Symptoms PAINS: colicky; cramping. STOOLS: frothy; green; slimy; sour smelling.
Worse in the morning; before passing a stool.

Milk is poorly tolerated, and passes through the body undigested; nursing babies may even refuse the breast. Stools are like the scum of a frog pond.

Flatulence

Symptoms BELLY/STOMACH bloated. With RUMBLING before passing a stool.

Headache

Symptoms PAINS: recurring at regular intervals; spasmodic; shooting; tearing.
Better for pressure; for walking.
Worse for lying down.
The pains of this headache are better for walking; and the person may be obliged to walk about all night because the pains return in force as soon as he stops to rest.

Indigestion

Symptoms BELCHING: greasy; sour. BELLY: bloated; rumbling. With HEARTBURN; NAUSEA.
Worse after eating cabbage; after drinking milk.

Toothache

Worse for cold; at night in bed.
Causes occurs whilst travelling; during pregnancy.
The toothache comes on whilst travelling and forces the person to get up and walk about, as resting aggravates the pains.

MAGNESIA MURIATICUM (Mag-m.)

Common name: chloride of magnesium

Magnesia muriaticum occurs naturally in sea water and in carnallite, a combination of potassium chloride and magnesium chloride.

It is a by-product of the potash industry and its industrial uses are many – from its use as a catalyst in organic chemistry, for making other magnesium compounds; in the melting and welding of fluxes; as a cell food in metal production and as a dental cement.

The homeopathic remedy is made from hydrochloric acid which is neutralised with magnesia, mixed with ammonium carbonate and then heated.

GENERAL SYMPTOMS

Discharges: sour; of stools; of sweat.
Better for fresh air; for pressure.
Worse after drinking milk; at night; for swimming in the sea.

This is a small remedy that is useful for babies' colic or digestive upsets that are worse for milk or caused by drinking milk. These people are generally better for some fresh air, and the pains are better for pressure. The sweat and stools smell sour.

EMOTIONAL/MENTAL SYMPTOMS

Anxious. Restless in bed.

People feel rushed and hurried: they feel they must be doing something all the time. Though present during the day, the anxiety is always worse in bed at night, causing insomnia.

PHYSICAL COMPLAINTS
Colic

Symptoms Pains: cramping; sore, bruised. With CONSTIPATION (see below); DIARRHOEA (see below); INDIGESTION.
Worse after drinking milk.
Causes drinking milk; teething.

Common cold

Causes swimming in the sea.

Constipation

Symptoms STOOLS: passed with difficulty; crumbling; small balls; like sheep's dung/droppings; knotty. STRAINING ineffectual.
Causes drinking milk.

Diarrhoea

Symptoms IN CHILDREN. STOOLS green.
Causes drinking milk.

Headache

Symptoms PAINS: in temples; spreading to eyes. With BELCHING; THIRST.
Worse for pressure; for wrapping up head.

Insomnia

Symptoms SLEEP unrefreshing.
The person feels restless and anxious in bed, especially on closing his eyes, and he may be oversensitive to noise then, and unable to get to sleep.

Teething

Symptoms PAINFUL IN CHILDREN. With COLIC; GREEN STOOLS.

MAGNESIA PHOSPHORICA (Mag-p.)

Other name: magnesium phosphate

Magnesium phosphate is formed in hexagonal crystals which are sweet to the taste and are soluble in water. This salt is present in various body tissues and in the grain of certain cereals. It has an affinity with both the nervous and the muscular tissues, causing and curing neuralgic pains and cramps. If too much is taken, numbness and paralysis can ensue.

The homeopathic preparation is made from magnesium sulphate and sodium phosphate which is mixed in water and left to crystallise into prisms and needles. The remedy is then prepared by trituration.

GENERAL SYMPTOMS

Pains cramping.
Better for heat; for firm pressure.
Worse for cold; for swimming in cold water; for touch; for being uncovered; for walking in fresh air.

Magnesia phosphorica has been nicknamed 'the homeopathic aspirin' because of its success with curing minor aches and pains. These may be period pains, headaches, earaches, teething pains or even neuralgic pains of the face. For this remedy to be most effective, the general symptoms that characterise it must be present.

The pains are greatly relieved by heat, by the application of a hot water bottle or a hot compress, and are much worse for cold – for walking out in the cold, for swimming in cold water and/or for getting cold and wet. Firm pressure helps although light pressure may aggravate (like *Lachesis*).
NB. This remedy is best given dissolved in warm water. Add four pills to a glass of boiled and partially cooled water and stir vigorously. Sip frequently until the pains ease off. Repeat as and when needed. Scald the glass and spoon when you have finished with them, otherwise the next person to use them may get an inadvertent dose of the remedy.

There are no marked emotional/mental symptoms.

PHYSICAL COMPLAINTS
Colic

Symptoms PAINS: cramping; drawing.
Better for warmth; bending double.

Cramp

Symptoms CRAMP: in arms; in fingers; in hands; in wrists.

Better for heat.
Causes prolonged use of hands.
For writers, pianists and violinists, and other occupations that involve prolonged use of the fingers and hands.

Earache

Symptoms PAINS: spasmodic; shooting.
Better for heat; for firm pressure.
Worse for cold; for turning the head.
Causes cold wind.
This is an earache that can come on after a walk in a cold wind; the characteristic *Magnesia phosphorica* general symptoms will also be present.

Headache

Symptoms PAINS: on right side of head; spasmodic; shooting.
Better for heat; for firm pressure.
Worse for cold.
Causes getting chilled.
These headaches are often right-sided and may be accompanied by pains in the face that come and go throughout the day.

Period problems

Symptoms PERIOD painful. PAINS colicky; cramping.
Better for doubling up; for heat; for pressure.
Worse for cold.
The person will go to bed and curl up with a hot water bottle, with a fist kneading the abdomen or the back (for the firm pressure). This is a wonderful remedy for non-serious period pains but it is extremely important that you seek professional advice if it does not help.

Sciatica

Better for heat.
Worse for cold.
This can be sciatica or any cramping, neuralgic pains in the back. The pains are often caused by cold, and are much better for hot applications and firm massage.

Teething

Symptoms PAINFUL IN CHILDREN.
Better for external warmth.
A hot water bottle (wrapped in a towel) relieves the pains. *Magnesia phosphorica* in a bottle or cup will then also help.

Toothache

Better for heat; for warm compresses.
Causes teething.
Anything cold (air, drinks, water and food) aggravates the pains, and warmth in almost any shape or form helps them. This is for those teething babies whose gums are made worse by biting on cold things and are better for chewing on a warm finger! Teething babies bite hard on their fists – or on anything they can get in their mouths – and are actually worse for being out in the cold air.

MERCURIUS CORROSIVUS (Merc-c.)

Other names: corrosive sublimate; mercuric chloride

Mercurius corrosivus, a chloride of mercury, is a salt which occurs in the form of a heavy, colourless, transparent, glistening, rhombic prism. It has an acrid, disagreeable, metallic taste. It is soluble, and is extremely poisonous: when swallowed it produces a suffocating, constricting sensation as well as burning in the throat along with violent pains in the stomach.

During the seventeenth and eighteenth centuries it was used externally by orthodox doctors as a disinfectant or antiseptic. The treatments were fraught with danger as many deaths occurred before the correct dosage was ascertained.

Mercury's industrial uses are now carefully controlled but the poisonings from mercury were once common in some trades, including the preparation of felt: 'mad as a hatter' is a reminder of the effect of mercury on the nervous system.

The homeopathic remedy is prepared by succussing a solution of mercuric chloride in rectified spirit.

GENERAL SYMPTOMS

Exhaustion. Likes cold drinks. **Sweat** cold. **Thirst** extreme. **Tongue** coated yellow.
Worse for pressure.

This remedy has a similar sphere of action to *Mercurius solubilis* but its picture is stronger: it has *more* pains and *more* burning than *Mercurius solubilis* and is more violent, more active. There is an unquenchable thirst and increased saliva in the mouth.

EMOTIONAL/MENTAL SYMPTOMS

Mercurius corrosivus is different from its good friend *Mercurius solubilis* in that it does not have marked emotional symptoms. However, the physical symptoms are nearly always accompanied by a general feeling of nervous exhaustion, and, in view of the seriousness of the physical symptoms, you will see some anxiety, irritability and/or depression, and a general sluggishness.

NB   SEE ALSO PAGES 203–26 FOR GENERAL ADVICE, DOS AND DON'TS.

PHYSICAL COMPLAINTS

Cystitis

Symptoms Desire to urinate: constant; painful; frequent. Pains: burning; severe. Urine: burning; dark; green; red; scanty. Urination: dribbling; frequent; difficult.

Worse during urination.

This is for very severe cystitis where terrible pains are felt both in the bladder and in the rectum. Urine is passed in drops only or in a feeble stream in spite of a constant, extremely painful urge to urinate. The patient has to strain to pass urine and this is also excruciatingly painful. The urine itself burns and may have blood in it. Seek professional help immediately.

Diarrhoea

Symptoms Pains severe. Stools: bloody; frequent; green; slimy; smelly; yellow. Straining: frequent; painful.

Worse before/during/after passing a stool.

This is for an extremely severe diarrhoea (dysentery) where there is a constant, incessant, excruciatingly painful straining that is not relieved by passing a stool. It may be accompanied by vomiting, and if so the patient will vomit bile and end up with a bruised stomach.

Sore throat

Symptoms Gums: bleeding; swollen. Pains: burning; raw. Saliva increased. With ulcers in throat.

Better for eating.

Worse for pressure; for swallowing liquids.

The patient has a choking sensation in the throat and an increase of sticky saliva in the mouth, which create a constant desire to swallow. The breath is smelly and the gums may be swollen and may bleed easily.

MERCURIUS SOLUBILIS (Merc-s.)

Other name: ammonio-nitrate of mercury

Mercury is mined from the ore cinnabar. It is the only metal that is liquid at room temperature; if it is spilt on a flat surface it forms small, scattered droplets, and for this reason it is also known as quicksilver. *Mercurius solubilis* is a powdered impure oxide of mercury prepared according to Hahnemann's original formula.

Despite the fact that mercury in compound is extremely toxic, it has had a long history in medicine because of its ability to promote body secretions, including saliva and perspiration – two elements of 'heroic medicine' alongside bloodletting and purging.

It was long used as a specific in the treatment of syphilis and in Hahnemann's time the side effects from overdosing with mercury were well known. It is used in dental amalgam for fillings, where it is mixed with other metals, and is an ingredient of commercial herbicides, fungicides and water-based paints, and consequently accidental poisoning remains a problem.

The homeopathic remedy is prepared by trituration.

GENERAL SYMPTOMS

Breath smells. **Complaints from:** getting chilled. **Discharges:** burning; blood-streaked; smelly; yellow; watery. **Face** pasty. **Glands** swollen. **Likes:** bread and butter; cold drinks. **Mouth** dry. **Pains:** in bones; pressing in glands. **Saliva:** increased; during sleep. **Sweat:** cold; profuse; smelly; from pain. **Taste:** mouth tastes bad; bitter; metallic. **Thirst** extreme. **Tongue:** cracked; coated yellow.

Worse for cold; during the evening; for heat and cold; for lying down; at night; for light touch.

Mercurius patients are smelly! All their discharges – stools, urine, saliva, catarrh, etc. – smell strongly. When they are very sick with a fever their sweat can usually be smelled on entering the room. They sweat profusely, without relief, especially at night when they feel generally much worse.

They are sensitive to extremes of temperature so that they dislike both heat and cold. They may feel chilly and want a hot water bottle, then feel over-heated so open the window, which chills them quickly, whereupon the cycle begins again. A change of two degrees either way will make them feel worse. Resting in bed in a moderate temperature affords them the greatest relief.

They have a lot of trouble with their mouths – ulcers, abscesses, pain in the teeth and a burning, intense thirst, in spite of having a lot of saliva. In fact they are constantly swallowing and may dribble onto their pillows at night. They have a bitter, metallic taste in the mouth and their flabby tongues take the imprints of their teeth so that they are indented around the edges.

All their symptoms are worse at night generally and especially in bed if they become hot. They are prone to catching colds, to recurring abscesses (anywhere) and swollen glands. These are all extremely painful.

EMOTIONAL/MENTAL SYMPTOMS

Confused. Depressed. Discontented. Forgetful. Restless.

These are nervous, anxious, restless types who find it difficult to stay still. They do slow down, both mentally and physically, when they become sick, although they will always feel hurried inside. In this slowed-down state their memories weaken and they may then become confused and have trouble thinking.

They may feel depressed and weepy but their crying will alternate with laughter – they are restless even in their emotions!

Children who need *Mercurius* are mischievous and are always getting up to no good. They are restless and always rushing from one thing to another.

PHYSICAL COMPLAINTS

Abscesses

Symptoms ABSCESSES: of glands; of roots of teeth. Abscesses accompanied by *Mercurius solubilis* general symptoms – i.e. increased saliva, foul taste and smelly breath.

Backache

Symptoms PAINS: in lower back; burning; shooting. *Worse* for breathing; for coughing; on getting up from sitting; for sweating.

Breastfeeding problems

Symptoms BREAST ABSCESS painful.

Chicken pox

With typical *Merc-s.* general symptoms – i.e. worse at night, weak and smelly. The rash suppurates and is smelly.

Common cold

Symptoms NASAL CATARRH: bloody; burning; green; yellow; yellow-green; smelly; watery. With LOSS OF SMELL, FEVER (see below); HEADACHE (see below); frequent SNEEZING; SORE THROAT (see below); VOICE HOARSE. *Worse* for cold; at night; for heat.

The nasal discharge burns the upper lip, and the nostrils may become ulcerated. The nose may bleed during sleep.

Cough

Symptoms COUGH racking; MUCUS green. *Worse* during the evening in bed; at night; for lying on right side.

Cystitis

Symptoms DESIRE TO URINATE: constant; ineffectual. PAINS burning. URINE: dark; scanty. URINATION frequent. *Worse* at beginning of urinating; when not urinating.

The pains are terrible and urinating is very slow and difficult.

Diarrhoea

Symptoms IN CHILDREN. PAINS burning. STOOLS: bloody; green; slimy; smelly; yellow. SWEATING: before/during/after stool. *Worse* for cold; during the evening; at night after passing a stool.

The burning pains come on when passing a stool and remain for a time afterwards, when the person also feels faint and weak (see EXHAUSTION). There may be a frequent desire to pass a stool that is worse after the stool has been passed.

Earache

Symptoms EAR feels blocked. DISCHARGE from ears: blood-streaked; smelly. PAINS: boring; burning; pressing; tearing. *Worse* at night; for warmth of bed.

The eardrum may perforate and the discharge will then be smelly and blood-streaked.

Exhaustion

Symptoms HEAVINESS in limbs. *Worse* after sweating; after passing a stool. *Causes* sweating.

This exhaustion may well accompany a fever or an attack of diarrhoea, and a wave of tiredness with a feeling of heaviness will come on after passing a stool or after a heavy bout of sweating. The patient will tremble with exhaustion.

Eye inflammation

Symptoms DISCHARGE purulent. EYES: sensitive to light; watering. With symptoms of COMMON COLD (see above). *Worse* for heat of a fire; warmth of bed.

Fever

Symptoms HEAT alternating with chills. With SWEAT (see General Symptoms). *Worse* for fresh air; at night in bed.

The person feels chilled out in the fresh air, but can feel overheated in a stuffy room. The fever may precede a common cold.

Headache

Symptoms PAINS: in forehead; burning; pressing; sore, bruised. *Worse* at night; for bending down. *Causes* common cold; rheumatism.

The head feels as though there is a band around the

forehead or as though the head is in a vice. There will usually be an increased amount of saliva in the mouth as well as other *Mercurius* general symptoms.

Indigestion

Symptoms With HEARTBURN.
Causes pregnancy.
The stomach feels empty and out of sorts and the person will also hiccup and burp.

Joint pain

Symptoms PAINS: burning; tearing.
Worse in bed; at night; for wet weather.
The rheumatic pains are severe and always worse at night in bed, when they drive the sufferer out of bed.

Mouth ulcers

Symptoms ULCERS: on gums; in mouth; on tongue. PAINS: stinging; throbbing.
This is the major mouth ulcer remedy, but you should take the general symptoms into account as well as the ulcers themselves; the increase in saliva and the flabby, indented tongue usually point to *Mercurius* as the remedy that is needed.

Mumps

Symptoms GLANDS: hard; swollen/painful; worse on right side. With FEVER (see above); COPIOUS SALIVA; PROFUSE SWEATING.
Worse for blowing nose; at night; on right side of body.
The typical *Mercurius solubilis* tongue and smelly breath are also present. The bones in the face may ache.

Sore throat

Symptoms PAINS: spreading up to ears and neck; sore; stitching. TONSILS: swollen; ulcerated.
Worse at night; on right side of body; for swallowing.
These are very painful sore throats with ulcers on the tonsils and swollen glands. The pains shoot up into the ear or into the neck on swallowing.

Thrush (genital)

Symptoms DISCHARGE: burns; greenish; smelly.
Worse at night.

Thrush (oral)

Symptoms IN BABIES AND CHILDREN. With EXCESS SALIVA.
The characteristic smelly breath is usually present. There may be some ulceration.

Toothache

Symptoms CHEEKS swollen. PAINS: spreading up to ears and face; pressing; sore, bruised; tearing.
Better for warm compresses; for rubbing cheeks; heat.
Worse for cold air; for drawing in cold air between teeth; at night in bed; while eating; warmth of bed; winter.
Causes abscess; cold, damp weather.
These toothaches can indicate the presence of an abscess, and persistent toothache should always be taken to a dentist. *Mercurius* will provide relief in the meantime, however, if the symptoms fit.

NATRUM CARBONICUM (Nat-c.)

Other names: sodium carbonate; soda ash

Sodium carbonate is an important commercial chemical and is known variously as 'soda', 'sal soda' or 'washing soda'. It occurs naturally as a mineral deposit left behind by the evaporation of ancient saline lakes and seas as can be seen in the extensive deposits that occur in desert areas. It is also produced commercially.

The largest consumers of soda ash are the glass and chemical industries. It is also used in the manufacture of soap, paper, water-softening agents; and in the form of soda crystals it serves as a common cleanser.

Until Hahnemann proved it, it was used chiefly as an external application for burns, eczema and as a douche for nasal and vaginal catarrh.

The homeopathic preparation is made by dissolving purified common shop soda in two parts boiling distilled water, and filtering the solution through blotting paper to form crystals. One grain of these crystals dried on the blotting paper is taken for the trituration.

GENERAL SYMPTOMS

Ankles weak. **Complaints from** sunstroke. **Dislikes** milk. **Face** pale. **Sweat:** from slightest physical exertion; from pain. **Taste:** mouth tastes metallic.
Better after eating; for massage.
Worse before eating; during a storm; for fresh air; mid-morning; for physical exertion; for sun.

Natrum carbonicum types have pale faces with blue circles around the eyes, and their eyelids may be puffy. They are aggravated generally by excessive summer heat and exposure to the sun (especially the head), but there is also an aversion to fresh air. Once run down, any exercise will aggravate their general condition. They are extremely sensitive to thunderstorms and can sense them coming, often getting a headache then. These people are better after eating, when they feel warmer. They dislike milk – this can cause diarrhoea. Massage also helps.

This remedy is especially valuable for nervous children who cannot tolerate sunshine and who suffer from weak ankles. If they fall ill with, say, a severe headache or a cold, then *Natrum carbonicum* will not only help the acute symptom but will strengthen their whole body, including the emotional part!

EMOTIONAL/MENTAL SYMPTOMS

Anxious. Cheerful. Complaints from: mental strain. **Confused. Depressed. Fearful. Forgetful. Gloomy. Jumpy. Lively. Sensitive:** generally; to music. **Shy. Sluggish.**

These people put on a brave face when really they are feeling miserable. They are sensitive generally but especially to emotional hurts which they harbour quietly inside, though without the bitterness of *Natrum muriaticum*. They avoid conflict by appearing cheerful, but this masks a feeling of being cut off, depressed and anxious with persistent sad thoughts. Listening to music increases their sense of melancholy in a comforting but negative way. Their sensitivity is such that they are easily startled by noise.

They become mentally weakened from emotional pressure and find it difficult to think. Complaints come on in this weak state, and after mental strain (overwork), when a person has been feeling sad and depressed.

PHYSICAL COMPLAINTS

Common cold

Symptoms Nose blocked. Nasal catarrh: drips down back of throat; smelly; thick.
This is the sort of catarrh that runs down the back of the throat, constantly making the person want to hawk up. The nose also becomes blocked. There may be a sour or metallic taste in the mouth.

Exhaustion

Symptoms Legs: heavy; weak. Nervous exhaustion. With icy-cold extremities; heaviness in limbs.
Worse for heat of sun; for mental exertion; for slightest exertion; for sun.
Causes mental strain; sun.
This nervous exhaustion follows a period of overwork where the circulation grinds to a halt: the feet and hands become cold and the legs feel heavy and weak. It can also be caused by an overdose of sunshine (which is not a great deal for a *Natrum carbonicum* type); like *Pulsatilla* these types are more prone to becoming

tired in hot weather, and any thinking, sunshine or exertion will make this tiredness worse.

Headache

Symptoms Head feels heavy. Pains pressing. Sweating on forehead.
Worse after eating; for thinking.
Causes mental strain; mental exertion; summer; sunstroke.
Although the person feels generally better after eating, the headache itself may actually be worse. The headache may be a result of too much study or mental strain, and the person can't think any more because the brain is worn out. It may also be a hot-weather headache; these are people who are sensitive to too much sun. The person may feel dizzy with this headache, especially if the stress is mental.

Indigestion

Symptoms Belches sour. Pains: in stomach; sore, bruised. With nausea.
The person feels nauseous in a stuffy room and has trouble digesting food because the nervous system is run down.

Insomnia

Symptoms Anxious dreams. Waking early.
The person wakes early in the morning after a night of anxious dreams and cannot get back to sleep again.

NATRUM MURIATICUM (Nat-m.)

Common names: sodium chloride; table or common salt

Common salt is, next to water, the most widely distributed substance in nature. It occurs naturally in the form of rock salt, as crystals of the mineral halite, and it is also extracted from seawater. Huge deposits of solid salt are found throughout the world, some of them several thousand feet thick. These are formed by the evaporation of ancient lakes and seas, and are found both underground and exposed on the earth's surface through erosion.

Salt has been widely valued as a major item of trade throughout history. The word 'salary' is derived from the Latin word *Salarium* which referred to the money allotted to Roman soldiers for the purchase of salt. It is an essential element in the diet of all mammals and has been used widely to preserve and flavour food. Commercial salt is also important in the preservation of hides in the leather industry. At one time it was used in various refrigeration operations, and it still plays an

NB SEE ALSO PAGES 203–26 FOR GENERAL ADVICE, DOS AND DON'TS.

important part in keeping our streets ice-free in the winter.

Unfortunately, the excessive intake of salt in the modern diet is contributing to much ill health, and homeopaths frequently see patients who are conducting their own accidental proving by taking an excessive amount of salt daily, so that they become, for example, gloomy and depressed and suffer from headaches, cold sores of the lips and other *Natrum muriaticum* symptoms. Salt was used traditionally as a remedy in some diseases like malaria, but by and large it was thought to have little value medicinally until Hahnemann conducted his provings in the 1820s. Nowadays it is used in solution (often intravenously) in orthodox medicine to prevent dehydration of body fluids.

For the homeopathic preparation, pure sodium chloride is dissolved in boiling distilled water, then filtered and left to crystallise by evaporation at 122°F. It is then dissolved in water or triturated before succussion.

GENERAL SYMPTOMS

Anaemia. Catches colds easily. Discharges like egg white. **Dislikes** bread. **Dryness** generally. **Face** pasty. **Lips** cracked. **Mouth:** dry; with thirst. **Taste:** mouth tastes bitter. **Thirst:** extreme; for large quantities.
Better for lying down; after a rest; after sweating.
Worse 10 a.m.; after eating; for exposure to sun; before menstrual period; for heat; mid-morning; for physical exertion; for sun.

The water balance of people needing *Natrum muriaticum* is disturbed. They suffer from dryness and extreme thirst, especially with a fever. Their lips dry up and become chapped and cracked, and the lower lip often has a centre crack. Look also for hangnails as people who need this remedy often suffer from them.

Their discharges are profuse and watery (often like egg white) or thick and white. They will sweat a lot when ill and feel better for doing so.

People needing *Natrum muriaticum* may feel chilly in their bodies but they dislike hot weather and always feel worse for the heat of the sun or for being incarcerated in stuffy rooms. They may suffer from exhaustion and headaches if they sit in the sun without a hat. In the winter they may well have cold hands and feet, but they do not mind feeling cold.

Their symptoms and general condition are often worse in the morning around 10 or 11 a.m. They also feel worse for exercise and better for lying down.

Women with pre-menstrual tension may need *Natrum muriaticum* if the rest of the symptom picture agrees.

An uncommon symptom that will lead you to prescribe *Natrum muriaticum* is that these people are completely unable to pass urine in the presence of others. Children will want the toilet door closed. Adult *Natrum murs* find it difficult to urinate in a public toilet.

EMOTIONAL/MENTAL SYMPTOMS

Absent-minded. Angry. Complaints from: disappointed love; grief; humiliation; suppression of emotions. **Confused. Depressed:** but cannot cry; from suppressed grief. **Desires** to be alone. **Discontented. Dislikes** consolation. **Introverted. Irritable. Sensitive** generally. **Tearful:** with difficulty crying; cries on own.
Worse for consolation; before a menstrual period.

Despite being emotional types, *Natrum muriaticum* characters appear very cool as they find it difficult to express their emotions. They close themselves away to avoid being hurt, and suppress their grief, and so appear quite hard to the world. Their feelings can burst out uncontrollably under certain conditions, especially if they have a very sensitive, sympathetic ear, and then they may cry in spite of themselves. In that state they hate to be consoled and actually feel worse for any comforting. They find it very difficult to cry and would much prefer to cry alone, in fact it is rare to see a *Natrum muriaticum* crying in public and they will feel humiliated if that actually happens. They are prickly types.

Their depression and their irritability are worse pre-menstrually, when they become discontented with everything and everyone, and indifferent to having any fun or excitement. They prefer to be alone when depressed and will refuse all invitations. These types hate parties and small talk and would much rather stay at home on their own.

If hurt (which is very easy!) they do not show it; they harbour hurts inside and become bitter about people and life in general. They are haunted by persistent, unpleasant thoughts, of past wrong-doings, and their minds dwell on these past disagreeable circumstances and make them ill.

The children are serious and dislike too much physical contact. They hate to be teased, and it may be best to ignore them if they get upset, leaving them to come round in their own time. They are also often very slow to talk, not uttering words until their second or even third year, and, like *Calcarea phosphorica* children, they may be slow learning to walk.

PHYSICAL COMPLAINTS

Backache

Symptoms PAINS: in lower back; aching; back feels as if it were broken; sore, bruised.

Better for lying on a hard surface.
Causes manual labour.
The back feels weak and tired after exertion or after bending down for a long time (after gardening, for example).

Blisters

Symptoms BLISTERS on tip of tongue.

Cold sores

Symptoms SORES: on lips; around mouth.
Causes sun; suppressed grief.
This is our major cold sore remedy, but it would be a mistake to prescribe it on this symptom alone: the general symptoms and the emotional picture are both important. A *Natrum muriaticum* person will often produce cold sores after a disappointment or a grief that wasn't expressed. The sores are usually sited around the mouth on the lips and will often be found at the corners of the mouth.

Common cold

Symptoms DISCHARGE FROM EYES watery. NASAL CATARRH: drips down back of throat; profuse; white; watery alternating with blocked up nose; like egg white. With: LOSS OF SMELL; LOSS OF TASTE.
The discharge is profuse and resembles egg white; it may be post nasal (that is, it may drip down the back of the throat). There is a bitter, salty taste in the mouth which feels dry, and a big thirst. The person may sneeze a lot, and the lips will be dry and cracked.

Constipation

Symptoms STOOLS: crumbling; small balls; like sheep dung. STRAINING ineffectual; with unfinished feeling.
Worse during a menstrual period.

Cough

Symptoms COUGH: dry; hacking; irritating; tickling. MUCUS: like egg white; transparent; white.
Worse during fever; evening in bed; from tickling in larynx.
The cough is excited by a tickling in the larynx and air passages. The eyes water when coughing (or laughing).

Diarrhoea

Symptoms BELLY/STOMACH bloated. DIARRHOEA during the day only. STOOLS: gushing; painless; smelly; watery.
Worse after eating starchy food.
There may be pains before passing the stool.

Exhaustion

Symptoms With HEAVINESS.
Worse during the evening.
The person's energy may well increase for a short while after eating, but he or she feels tired and heavy, especially in the evenings.

Eye inflammation

Symptoms EYES: gritty; sensitive to light; watering.

Fever

Symptoms HEAT burning. With NAUSEA.
Better for being uncovered.
Worse mid morning; in the autumn.
The patient will look dazed and sleepy and will fall asleep when hot, although the feeling of burning heat may alternate with a great, intense chilliness. Sweating will help. There will be an extreme thirst for large quantities of liquids during the fever.

Hayfever

Symptoms With COLD SORES (see above); symptoms of COMMON COLD (see above).
The *Natrum muriaticum* general symptoms will also be present.

Headache

Symptoms EYES: sore; watering. PAINS: in forehead; in temples; hammering; pressing; splitting; throbbing.
Better for firm pressure.
Worse around 10 a.m.–3 p.m.; after eating; for coughing; during menstrual period; for emotions; for excitement; during a fever; on waking; for reading/writing; talking; thinking.
The patient may have trouble seeing, with flickering and zig-zags appearing before the eyes during the pains. This is in fact typical of migraines; these headaches should always be taken to a professional.

Indigestion

Symptoms BELCHES: incomplete, ineffectual; sour; tasting of food just eaten. MOUTH: tastes bitter; salty. PAINS: cramping; pressing; in stomach. With violent HICCUPS.
Worse after eating starchy food.
After suppressing emotions the stomach can become 'disordered', and stodgy foods are no longer easily digested. The patient will burp after eating but with difficulty and this does not relieve the indigestion. May also have violent hiccups.

Insomnia

Symptoms Dreams; anxious; vivid.
Causes grief.
The person may find it very difficult to get to sleep after a loss or disappointment and may then wake in the night and be unable to get back to sleep. May have anxious, vivid dreams.

Prickly heat

With *Natrum-mur.* general and emotional/mental symptoms.

Retention of urine

Causes presence of strangers.
Can only pass urine when on own.

Sore throat

Symptoms Pains burning. Throat dry; with lump sensation. Voice hoarse.
Can only swallow liquids; solids come up after they reach a certain point and the person may choke (may also choke when drinking). The voice is hoarse, and when swallowing there is a sensation of a lump in the throat which rises up. Hawks up egg-white mucus from the back of the throat.

Thrush (genital)

Symptoms Discharge: white; like egg white.

Thrush (oral)

Symptoms Gums/tongue: coated white.
With characteristic dry mouth and thirst.

NATRUM PHOSPHORICUM (Nat-p.)

Other names: phosphate of soda; sodium phosphate

Sodium phosphate is made commercially in various forms by combining phosphoric acid and sodium carbonate. It is used in the manufacture of ceramics, in fireproofing and as a detergent, in the making of baking powder, in photographic developers, as an emulsifying and cleansing agent and in boiler-scale treatment. It emulsifies fatty acids and regulates the production of bile and the absorption of water in the body.
    The homeopathic remedy is made from pure phosphate of soda by trituration.

GENERAL SYMPTOMS

Discharges sour. **Nervous exhaustion. Tongue** yellow at back.
Worse during the evening.

The *Natrum phosphoricum* picture is full of sourness. It has been called the acid neutraliser – these people have sour sweat, stools, urine, and so on. A yellow-coated tongue (usually the base only) accompanies nearly all the symptoms. Patients are weak; they have acidic digestions, and they may have weak ankles and cold extremities (like *Natrum carbonicum*).

EMOTIONAL/MENTAL SYMPTOMS

Apathetic. Indifferent.

These people are apathetic and dull, like *Phosphoric acid*.

PHYSICAL COMPLAINTS

Colic

Symptoms Vomit sour.
Babies suffer from colic with acidity, vomiting or curdled milk and sour-smelling, green, watery diarrhoea. This is a good remedy for simple colic with acidity (and sourness) where there are no other guiding symptoms that would lead you to prescribe another remedy.

Headache

Symptoms Face pale. Pains in forehead.
Causes mental exertion.

Indigestion

Symptoms Belches sour. Belly/stomach bloated. With heartburn.
Acidity, sour burps and pains will come on two hours after eating. *Natrum phosphoricum* will neutralise this acidity. The heartburn of pregnancy is often relieved by taking this remedy.

NATRUM SULPHURICUM (Nat-s.)

Other names: sodium sulphate; Glauber's salt

This mineral salt is found combined with calcium sulphate in the mineral glauberite, in sea water, in the waters of most saline springs (mineral spa waters) and in many salt lakes in Russia. It is also found in the minerals mirabilite and thenardite.

Sodium sulphate was first isolated by seventeenth-century German chemist Johann Glauber (hence the name Glauber's salt, and the mineral name glauberite). He called the salt 'sal mirabilis' and extolled its medicinal qualities as well as its potential for benefit to industry. Glauber was in advance of his time in foreseeing the likely benefits of the application of chemistry to industry and published many of his forty published works to that end.

Commercially, the salt is used in the manufacture of certain papers, paperboard, glass, in dyeing and tanning processes, in the manufacture of detergents and as a raw material for the production of various chemicals and medicines. Medically, it is used mainly as a laxative and externally for infected wounds.

The homeopathic preparation is made from sodium sulphate by trituration.

GENERAL SYMPTOMS

Complaints from accident/injury to the head. **Hot flushes. Likes** cold drinks. **Sweat** from pain. **Taste:** mouth tastes bad in the morning; bitter. **Tongue** green.
Better for fresh air.
Worse for damp; for humidity; for wet weather; for lying down; during the morning; after eating starchy food.

Those benefiting most from this remedy are extremely sensitive to damp, to cold and wet, or to hot and wet. Their complaints may result from living in a damp house for a long period of time. They dislike hot, stuffy atmospheres and always feel better for some fresh air. They are at their worst in the mornings.
Natrum sulphuricum is the remedy that is most often needed for complaints that arise after a head injury.

EMOTIONAL/MENTAL SYMPTOMS

Depressed. Jumpy. Weary of life.

These individuals feel confused and depressed, especially after a head injury. They become utterly sick and tired of life (having been quite happy before the injury) and may also become over-sensitive to noise in this state.

PHYSICAL COMPLAINTS

Backache

Symptoms PAINS sore, bruised.
Causes injury to spine.

Colic

Symptoms With INDIGESTION (see below).

Cough

Symptoms COUGH during the day only. MUCUS green.
Worse for damp, wet weather.

Diarrhoea

Symptoms BELLY/STOMACH: gurgling; rumbling. STOOLS: smelly; thin; watery. WIND: loud; smelly; spluttering.
Better for passing wind.
Worse after getting up; during the morning; after eating fruit/starchy food.
Causes eating fruit.
The diarrhoea may come on after eating starchy food like potatoes and bread or after fruit or vegetables. The person feels exhausted after the diarrhoea, and passes wind with it or wants to pass a stool but only manages to pass wind. It is worst in the morning after first getting up and moving about.

Flatulence

Symptoms WIND: loud; loud during stool; smelly. With DIARRHOEA (see above); RUMBLING.
Better for passing wind.
Worse after breakfast.
There is an urge for a stool but only spluttering wind is passed.

Headache

Symptoms EYES sensitive to light.
Causes head injury.
Give after *Arnica* if that remedy has not worked and the pains remain.

Head injuries

Symptoms of HEADACHE (see above).
If *Arnica* has been given for a head injury and the swelling has subsided but pain remains, or if there are any other symptoms after a bang or a fall, then a course of *Natrum sulphuricum* will clear these symptoms. Sometimes small children change character after a bad fall, from being cheerful and easy-going to obnoxious and screaming all the time, and it is possible to mistake this for teething and give *Chamomilla*, to no avail. Do be careful with head injuries, especially with small children, who are accident prone.

Indigestion

Symptoms BELCHING: bitter; sour. BELLY/STOMACH bloated. FLATULENCE: wind after breakfast.
Better after passing a stool.
Worse after eating starchy food.
The person cannot digest starchy food, such as potatoes, and the tongue may look greenish brown or dirty

NB   SEE ALSO PAGES 203–26 FOR GENERAL ADVICE, DOS AND DON'TS.

green. This colic or rumbling in the stomach is better for passing a stool.

NITRICUM ACIDUM (Nit-ac.)

Other names: aqua fortis; nitric acid

Nitric acid is an important mineral acid. It is one of the earliest nitrogen compounds to be prepared and used; in the thirteenth century it was known as *aqua fortis* or *eau forte*, and it was used as a tonic.

Pure nitric acid is a colourless, extremely corrosive liquid which fumes strongly on contact with moist air. (Free nitric acid is found in moist air in the discharge of atmospheric electricity, or lightning.) The fumes can cause nitrous gas poisoning, and spillage of the acid causes severe burns and stains the skin yellow. Poisonings produce gastro-enteritis with burning pains in the oesophagus and abdomen, bloody diarrhoea, collapse and death.

Commercially, it is used primarily in the manufacture of ammonium nitrate for fertilisers and explosives, although it is also used in dyes and drugs, plastics, lacquers and synthetic fibres. Medicinally, its powerfully corrosive action is used to remove warts, although much care needs to be taken in its application.

The homeopathic preparation is made from nitric acid prepared by mixing pure, pulverised nitre with an equal amount of phosphoric acid; this is then distilled and succussed.

GENERAL SYMPTOMS

Anaemia. Breath smelly. **Discharges** like ammonia. **Likes** fat/fatty foods. **Pains:** in bones; flying around; needle-like; splinter-like; appear and disappear suddenly. **Sweat:** on single parts of the body; smelly; sour; from slightest physical exertion. **Tongue** cracked.
Better for lying down.
Worse for cold; for fresh air; at night; on waking; for loss of sleep; for touch; for jarring movement; for walking.

Nitricum acidum is very similar to *Hepar sulph* with offensiveness on both physical and emotional levels. Their urine smells strongly (it is often compared to that of horses) and their sweat is also foul smelling. They will often have smelly breath and a cracked tongue. They love fatty, fried foods and will eat the fat on meat.

Nitricum types are weak and chilly and worse for cold and at night. This is one of the 'coldest' remedies in the Materia Medica.

Their pains come and go and are deep in the bones. These people are very sensitive to being touched or jarred, which aggravates their splinter-like pains. They always feel generally better for lying down.

They suffer from nervous exhaustion caused by insufficient sleep or from having broken nights.

EMOTIONAL/MENTAL SYMPTOMS

Violently angry. Anxious. Depressed. Fearful of death. **Irritable. Sensitive** to noise; to pain. **Sluggish. Tantrums. Unforgiving.**

These people feel anxious and depressed, especially in the evenings. They have a lot of anxiety about their health and may well consult doctor after doctor in order to find out what is wrong, not believing the diagnoses, particularly if they are told they are not seriously ill.

They often become sick in the first instance because they have a very unforgiving streak and feel an enormous amount of anger towards those who have offended them. They may use the word 'hate' when describing the object of their derision. Their anger can explode and cause them to swear and tremble. They are (in this unforgiving state) not moved by apologies and carry this hatred around with them. This eats away at them like an acid, and they then become sensitive.

They may throw themselves into their work and then become worn out mentally and swing to the opposite extreme of not wanting to work at all. In this state they become over-sensitive to noise, especially shrill noises, which will make them jump.

PHYSICAL COMPLAINTS

Common cold

Symptoms NASAL CATARRH: bloody; burning; dirty yellow; thin; watery in the fresh air.
Worse for fresh air; at night.
The nose is blocked and feels sore and bruised and sensitive to touch. There may be ulcers in the nostrils.

Earache

Symptoms Crackling in EARS when chewing. PAINS splinter-like; throbbing. With symptoms of SORE THROAT (see below).
Worse on right side, for swallowing.
The pains are usually splinter-like and the hearing becomes acute – more sensitive than normal.

Exhaustion

Symptoms Nervous.
Worse after passing a stool; for walking.
Causes diarrhoea; loss of sleep; nursing the sick.
This weakness results from loss of sleep and accompanies or follows an attack of diarrhoea. It is worse after passing a stool or for taking a walk.

Eye inflammation

Symptoms IN INFANTS. EYES watering. EYELIDS swollen.
It is important to take general symptoms – such as chilliness and smelly urine – into account, as well as the sore, watery eyes.

Flatulence

Symptoms WIND: smelly; obstructed (difficult to expel).

Headache

Symptoms HEAD feels constricted. PAINS: spreading to eyes; in bones; recurring at regular intervals; pressing.
Worse for jarring movement; for movement; at night; for noise; for pressure; on waking; for walking.
This is a severe headache that is worse at night. The bones of the face are sore, and the slightest pressure, even that of a hat, makes it worse (the head feels constricted, as if it were bandaged up tightly). The pressing pains in the head extend to the eyes which also feel sore. They may come and go suddenly (see General Symptoms); if they do, this may follow a pattern, for example the headache may return every evening or night.

Insomnia

Symptoms DREAMS anxious. SLEEP unrefreshing.
Worse after 2 a.m.
The person wakes around 2 a.m. and is unable to get back to sleep.

Joint pain

Symptoms PAINS: in bones; in legs; splinter-like; stitching; tearing.
Worse at night.

Mouth ulcers

Symptoms ULCERS: on edges of tongue; painful.
These are painful ulcers or pimples on the edge of the tongue. There is an increase of saliva in the mouth, and the gums may also bleed easily. The breath is very smelly.

Piles

Symptoms PAINS: burning; splinter-like. PILES: bleeding; large.
Worse after a stool.
The pains may last for one to two hours, even after a soft stool.

Sore throat

Symptoms PAINS: burning; pressing; raw; splinter-like; stitching; spreading to ear. TONSILS: swollen; ulcerated.
Worse for swallowing.
The pains are severe – it feels as if something sharp were stuck in the throat – and they extend to the ear on swallowing. Swallowing is extremely difficult; even tiny amounts of food seem to lodge in the throat.

Thrush (genital)

Symptoms DISCHARGE: burning; smelly; itching; thin.

NUX VOMICA (Nux-v.)

Family name: Loganiaceae
Common names: poison nut; Quaker buttons; semen strychnos

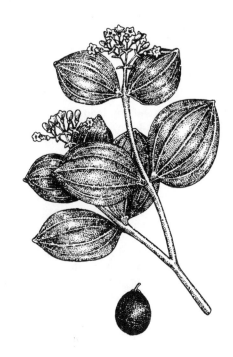

Nux vomica seeds are produced by a large evergreen tree native to certain parts of India, Burma, Thailand, China and Northern Australia. It produces small, unpleasant-smelling flowers, and beautiful orange-coloured fruit the size of large apples, which contain a soft white jelly-like pulp and five seeds covered in soft hairs; these seeds have no smell but taste extremely bitter owing to the strychnine contained in them.

The plant was known as the 'Vomiting nut' and was thought to have limited medicinal value on account of the seeds' poisonous nature, although in Germany it was used as an antidote to the plague, to treat worms, mania, rabies, hysteria, rheumatism and gout.

As a poison, small doses promote the appetite, aid digestion and increase the frequency of urination. Larger doses cause loss of appetite, an increased sensitivity generally, depression, anxiety, disordered muscular system with trembling, rigidity or stiffness of the limbs and staggering when walking. Still larger doses cause convulsions and death from asphyxia (suffocation).

The seeds are powdered finely in a heated mortar and triturated with sugar of milk.

GENERAL SYMPTOMS

Catches colds easily. Complaints from: getting chilled; cold, dry wind. **Likes** spicy food. **Pains** cramping. **Sense of smell** acute. **Sweat:** hot; one-sided; smelly. **Symptoms** right-sided. **Taste:** mouth tastes bitter; sour in the morning.
Better for heat; for lying down; for sitting down; for hot drinks.
Worse after drinking alcohol/coffee; after eating cold food; for tobacco; for cold; cold, dry weather; cold wind; fresh air; for loss of sleep; during the morning; in the winter; touch; for being uncovered; for walking.

These are extremely chilly individuals who hate the cold in any shape or form; they catch cold easily, especially if exposed to draughts or after becoming chilled, and they hate dry, windy weather. They are always better for warmth and if sick will not want any part of their bodies to be uncovered; they become so sensitive to cold that the slightest draught under the bedclothes will upset them. All they want to do when sick is to sit or lie down and keep warm – this is what helps.

Nux vomica is useful for all sorts of disturbances that follow over-indulgence in food, alcohol, coffee or tobacco. Once sick, any further indulgences will make them worse, but they find it hard to stop and will often carry on drinking and smoking in spite of feeling ghastly.

Mornings are their worst time of day, especially after a disturbed night, which is not unusual. They will be irritable and feel generally at their worst then.

Losing sleep always affects them. The *Nux vomica* mother with a new baby has an awful time.

EMOTIONAL/MENTAL SYMPTOMS

Angry: violently; when has to answer. **Complaints from** anger; anger with anxiety. **Concentration** poor. **Excitable. Impatient. Impulsive. Irritable. Quarrelsome. Sensitive:** generally; to rudeness; to light; to music; to noise. **Spiteful. Stubborn. Tidy.**

Nux vomica types are self-indulgent workaholics! They overdo everything: they work too hard, stay out too late, take no exercise, eat too much rich food, drink too much alcohol, become too wound up to sleep and then consume vast quantities of coffee in order to get going the next day. Then they find it difficult to concentrate and lose interest in their work. They become a bag of nerves. In this state they are extremely sensitive to both light and noise; even small noises will irritate them.

These are extremely impulsive, quarrelsome, stroppy individuals who know what they want and who 'want it now'! They are extremely impatient and do not like to be kept waiting. They are critical, fussy and exacting, easily frustrated by any limitations. They can be tidy but not fanatically so (like *Arsenicum*).

They hate to be contradicted, are irritable if questioned and then enraged if they are obliged to reply when they do not want to. Their irritability must have an outlet and it usually does – they tend not to keep their anger in and will always feel better for a good row. If they do suppress their anger they feel awful and often get sick.

Nux vomica children are mischievous and full of contradictions. They can be spiteful, stubborn and irritable on the one hand, and extremely sensitive and very easily offended on the other. As they grow up they become difficult and easily morose if things are not going their way.

Some homeopaths believe that *Nux vomica* works more effectively on meat eaters than on vegetarians, who have been observed to be less aggressive. Interestingly, the old homeopaths thought of *Nux vomica* mainly as a remedy for men. Anxious wives put it in the soup of those husbands who were getting out of hand with working all hours, drinking and smoking too much and becoming generally abusive. Since the advent of women asserting themselves more and more, this division is no longer true – *Nux vomica* is now needed as often for women as it is for men.

PHYSICAL COMPLAINTS
Backache

Symptoms PAINS: in lower back; aching; pressing; sore, bruised.

Worse in bed; during the morning; for movement.
Causes getting cold.
The person has to sit up in order to turn over in bed. The pain comes on after being chilled, and is often accompanied by a desire to pass a stool.

Colic

Symptoms PAINS: cramping; griping; pressing; sore, bruised.
Better for passing a stool; for hot drinks; for warmth of bed; for passing wind.
Worse after eating; for coughing; during the morning; during a fever; for wearing tight clothing.
These pains come on after over-indulging. They may accompany the nausea or the indigestion (see below) but the basic pattern is very similar. Children who have stomach-ache after a party where they have eaten a lot of junk food may well develop this sort of colic. The person feels full and bloated after eating, and the pressure of tight clothes around the waist is excruciating.

Common cold

Symptoms EYES watering. NASAL CATARRH: burning; watery. NOSE: runs during the day, blocked at night. With HEADACHE (see below); frequent SNEEZING; SORE THROAT (see below).
Better for fresh air.
Worse after eating; after getting up; during the morning.
Causes draughts.
The cold may start with an irritated spot high up at the back of the nose/nostril. Breastfeeding babies whose noses block up at night and who then find it difficult to feed will benefit from *Nux vomica*, particularly if they are also very sensitive to what their mothers eat.

Constipation

Symptoms Alternates with DIARRHOEA. DESIRE TO PASS STOOL ineffectual; constant. STOOLS: hard; large. With UNFINISHED FEELING.
Causes alcohol; over-eating; pregnancy; sedentary habits.
Wants to pass a stool but cannot, or just passes small amounts each time.

Cough

Symptoms BREATHING difficult. COUGH: distressing; dry; racking; suffocative; tickling; in violent fits. LARYNX raw. MUCUS tastes sour. With VOMITING when hawking up mucus.
Better for hot drinks.
Worse for getting cold; for cold air; during the early morning; on waking up; for slightest movement of chest; after eating; during a fever.

The person has difficulty breathing because of the cough. The cough is dry during the fever; it is also dry, and worse, after midnight until daybreak. The person may cough up sour-tasting mucus. Tickling in the larynx excites the cough.

Cystitis

Symptoms DESIRE TO URINATE: frequent; ineffectual; urgent. PAINS burning; pressing. URINATION: frequent; ineffectual. URINE: burning; scanty.
Worse during urination.
There is a constant urge to urinate, and slight incontinence; the patient wants to pee but can't.

Earache

Symptoms PAINS stitching. With ITCHING.
Worse for swallowing.
The Eustachian tubes itch and force the patient to swallow to relieve this, even though it may make the pain worse. Hearing is very acute.

Exhaustion

Symptoms EXHAUSTION nervous.
Worse on waking in the morning.

Fever

Symptoms HEAT: alternating with chills; dry; one-sided. With BACKACHE; extreme CHILLINESS; SHIVERING; SWEATING (see General Symptoms).
Worse for fresh air; for draughts; for movement; for being uncovered; for the slightest movement of the bedclothes.
The patient wants to be completely covered with warm bedding; he will become chilled if he turns over in bed or puts a hand out of bed. The fever may be on one side of the body only and the patient will feel dry heat externally, and chilly internally. Limbs feel heavy and tired. Is usually thirsty.

Flatulence

Symptoms BELLY/STOMACH: bloated; intolerant of tight clothing; rumbling.
Better for passing wind.
Worse for eating.

Flu

Symptoms PAINS in bones; in joints; sore, bruised. With symptoms of COMMON COLD (see above); CHILLINESS; FEVER (see above).
Better for warm compresses; for warmth of bed.
Worse in bed; for cold; during the morning.

NB   SEE ALSO PAGES 203–26 FOR GENERAL ADVICE, DOS AND DON'TS.

The *Nux vomica* flu is similar to the common cold. The person will be extremely chilly and unable to get warm. The typical *Nux vomica* general symptoms should be present.

Gastric flu

Symptoms of FLU (see above).

Hayfever

Symptoms With COMMON COLD symptoms (see above).
Nux vomica types suffering from hayfever with common cold symptoms will benefit from this remedy. This hayfever may last the entire year, with no relief in winter.

Headache

Symptoms HEAD feels heavy; PAINS: in back of head; in forehead; pressing; sore, bruised; stupefying; tearing. With BILIOUSNESS; DIZZINESS.
Better for excitement; on getting up in the morning; for pressure; for wrapping up head; during the evening in bed.
Worse after eating; for cold; for moving eyes; for shaking head.
Causes alcohol; cold wind; common cold; damp weather; loss of sleep; mental strain; over-eating.
This is the typical 'hangover' headache that comes on the morning after a night of excessive eating and drinking. The eyes often feel sore.

Indigestion

Symptoms BELCHES: bitter; sour. BELLY/STOMACH: bloated; empty. PAINS: in stomach; cramping; pressing; sore, bruised. With HEARTBURN.
Better for hot drinks; for warmth of bed.
Worse after eating; for wearing tight clothing.
Causes alcohol; coffee; mental strain; over-eating; rich food.
Food lies like a knot in the stomach for 1–2 hours after eating, and the stomach feels full, heavy and tender. See also Colic.

Insomnia

Symptoms WAKING: early; late; around 3 a.m.
Causes alcohol; excitement; mental strain; overwork; over-active mind.
The person is sleepy on going to bed but cannot sleep, or gets to sleep but wakes in the early hours of the morning, when anxious thoughts prevent her from getting back to sleep. May fall into a deep sleep just before the alarm goes off, and so wake tired and worn out.

Nausea

Symptoms NAUSEA constant.
Worse after eating; morning in bed; for sweating; for tobacco.
Causes pregnancy; travelling.
The nausea may make the person feel faint. It may occur with a painful period.

Period problems

Symptoms PERIODS: heavy; painful. PAINS: aching; cramping; in lower back.
Better for doubling up.
Worse during the period.

Piles

Causes pregnancy.

Sore throat

Symptoms PAINS: spreading up to ears; raw; stitching. With LUMP SENSATION in throat.
Worse for cold air; for swallowing; for uncovering throat.
Swallowing is difficult; the throat feels rough and the pains radiate to the ears on swallowing. The rawness may have been caused by coughing and the air passages may feel irritated.

Toothache

Better for external warmth; for wrapping up head; for heat; winter.
Causes after a filling/extraction.
The toothache is better for lying on a hot water bottle wrapped in a towel.

Travel sickness

Symptoms With FAINT-LIKE FEELING; NAUSEA.
Better for lying down.
Worse for tobacco.

Vomiting

Symptoms VOMIT: bile; mucus; bitter; sour; smelly.
Worse for expectorating (hawking up mucus).
Causes alcohol; anger; pregnancy.
This biliousness (with or without vomiting) occurs after over-eating or indulging in rich or unusual foods. It can feel like food poisoning and is common when travelling.

OPIUM (Op.)

Family name: Papaveraceae
Other names: white poppy; *Papaver somniferum*; mawseed

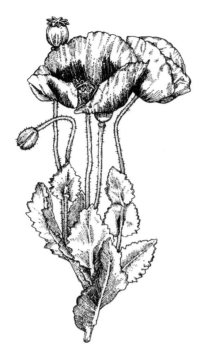

The opium poppy is a herbaceous annual native to Asia Minor. Its delicate flowers vary in colour from white to reddish purple, and in the wild they are pale lilac. They are easily bent and broken by wind and rain, and quick to drop their petals.

The plant is extensively cultivated in the East – in Turkey, Iran and India – for its narcotic properties (the red poppy more familiar in the West does not possess these properties). Opium is in fact the dried juice extracted from the green unripe seed capsules, hence the word 'opium' which derives from the Greek *opos* or 'juice'. The juice contains two acids and twenty-one different alkaloids, of which morphine, opium's 'active ingredient', is the most important. Morphine is named after Morpheus, the god of sleep, who is said to have discovered the sleep-bringing and pain-reducing power of the poppy.

The poppy was sacred to Ceres, the goddess of harvest and fertility, because of the abundance of seeds contained in the capsules. The seeds contain no morphia, only pale yellow oil which artists use as a drying oil. They are also used in the kitchen in pastry and bread making.

The plant and preparations from it were employed in medicine as early as the days of Hippocrates, though it was recognised as poisonous and great care was taken in its administration. It was used as a sedative and a pain reliever, externally for gout and earache and headaches, internally for dysentery and certain types of cough. In small doses opium acts as a stimulant; ideas flow, exhilaration is experienced, as well as a capability of greater exertion and a great ability to endure, but this is followed by a loss of mental and physical power, an irresistible desire to sleep, and dependency.

The homeopathic preparation is made by dissolving opium in alcohol and succussing.

GENERAL SYMPTOMS

Eyes glassy. **Face** dark red or blue. **Faintness**: after excitement; after fright. **Pains** absent. **Pupils** contracted. **Shock** from injury. **Sweat**: profuse; hot; on single part of the body; from fright.
Worse for alcohol; during sleep; on getting up; for warmth of bed.

Opium is characterised by an abnormal lack of pain, as if the senses have been blunted. After a shock, people needing *Opium* appear glassy eyed and stupefied, and suffer from great inertia. They feel faint, numb and/or trembly. Their faces go red and become drawn, sunken and old looking, possibly with a bluish tinge. Children who have just experienced a fright or shock will be unable to urinate.

Generally, there is profuse sweating with scanty urination and in a fever *Opium* types will become heated in bed and feel worse for the heat and the sweating and will kick off the covers.

The shock that follows alcohol poisoning with these symptoms may well call for *Opium* – this is only useful in an unusual, mistaken accident and not for habitual drinkers.

EMOTIONAL/MENTAL SYMPTOMS

Apathetic during fever. **Complaints from:** anger; reprimands; shock. **Confused. Dreamy. Drowsy. Exhilarated. Expression** sleepy. **Indifferent** during a fever. **Lively. Senses:** dull; acute. **Sensitive** to noise. **Stupor.**

In an acute illness like a fever, *Opium* patients are dull and apathetic, duller than any other remedy – to the point of stupor. They don't complain or even ask for anything and may be overwhelmingly sleepy. Before reaching this state of stupor, however, they may become exhilarated and delirious and imagine they see things, especially on closing their eyes.

People who have become stuck into a state of fear after a bad fright or shock may benefit from *Opium*. They look similar to *Aconite* (that is, enormously shocked) but they are also in a dream-like state that they cannot snap out of. This is common after an operation and *Opium* will help people after a general anaesthetic where they feel 'spaced out' and drowsy to get back to their normal states. The *Opium* person will recreate the image or situation that caused the shock, but during waking hours; he will not have bad dreams. *Arnica* types, on the other hand, will be fine during the day but will have bad dreams relating to the fright.

Children who have been severely told off sometimes develop an *Opium* 'acute'.

PHYSICAL COMPLAINTS

Constipation

Symptoms DESIRE TO PASS STOOL absent. STOOLS: black; hard; small balls; like sheep's dung/droppings; 'shy' (recede). With UNFINISHED FEELING.
The stool will lie in the bowel and the person has no desire to pass it. Nor is there any pain that would normally be associated with such constipation. The constipation may be acute after an operation. It may alternate with diarrhoea, which may come on after sudden joy or after fright.

Cough

Symptoms BREATHING difficult; slow; snoring.
Worse during sleep; on falling asleep; on waking.
The breathing slows down during sleep and when the fever is strong; it becomes irregular and laboured, like a waking snoring. This aspect is very marked in this remedy picture and needs to be present for it to work successfully.

Fever

Symptoms HEAT: burning; intense. With DEEP SLEEP; SWEATING (see General Symptoms).
Better for uncovering.
Worse during sleep; for sweating.
A person with this fever will experience overpowering sleepiness and yawning, will fall asleep and then breathe slowly and loudly as if snoring. Heat comes on during sleep, and sweating which does not relieve the symptoms. If woken, the person will be dazed and confused, will want to uncover, and is either delirious and excitable or stupefied and semi-conscious during the fever.

Insomnia

Symptoms With SLEEPINESS.
Sleeps lightly and restlessly and hears every sound. Is sleepy but cannot fall asleep, and the bed may feel hot.

Retention of urine

Causes shock.
After a shock or fright the person is unable to pass urine.

PETROLEUM (Petr.)

Other names: petra-rock; oleum oil; coal oil; rock oil

The word 'petroleum' originates from the Latin for 'rock' (*Petra*) and 'oil' (*Oleum*). The term commonly refers to the liquid crude oil which comes from beneath the earth's surface, although petroleum also occurs in the earth in gaseous or solid forms, and a few petroleum lakes or tar pits are known throughout the world. It is formed over millions of years from the remains of marine plant and animal life deposited under the sea, where they decompose without oxygen; heat, pressure and time convert this into petroleum.

Petroleum was known to many ancient peoples, who referred to it as 'burning water' and used it in the form of bitumen to caulk ships and build roads as well as to give light. More recently, it has provided us with heating and a fuel for this century's machinery. It is refined and processed into numerous products, such as solvents, paints, asphalt, plastics, cleansing agents, waxes and jellies, medicines, explosives and fertilisers. The crude oil has been used for the treatment of wounds.

The homeopathic preparation is made from purified oil or from crude oil from which a tincture is prepared and then diluted and succussed in the normal way.

GENERAL SYMPTOMS

Dislikes: meat; fatty, rich food. **Sweat:** one-sided; smelly.
Worse for fresh air; during the morning; travelling (boat, car, train, bus, etc.)

This is a small remedy that I have included because of its uses in travel sickness and nausea during pregnancy. There is a general dislike of fresh air which also aggravates the nausea.

EMOTIONAL/MENTAL SYMPTOMS

Confused in fresh air. **Forgetful. Irritable. Quarrelsome.**

People needing *Petroleum* will be generally worse for and also mentally confused out in the fresh air. They may not recognise well-known streets and may make mistakes in finding their way.

PHYSICAL COMPLAINTS
Chilblains

Symptoms CHILBLAINS: on feet, hands, toes; inflamed.

Feet become cold and 'fall asleep' easily, and the hands become cold and chapped. The chilblains are painful and itching, and occur in the winter during cold weather.

Diarrhoea

Symptoms DIARRHOEA during the day only. PAINS pressing. With ravenous APPETITE.
This is a very specific diarrhoea that occurs only during the day and is not accompanied by a loss of appetite.

Headache

Symptoms PAINS: in back of head; pressing. With HEAVINESS; NAUSEA (see below).
The headache usually comes on when travelling and accompanies the nausea.

Nausea

Symptoms With DIZZINESS.
Worse for fresh air.
This nausea is usually accompanied by dizziness and/or headache.

Travel sickness

Symptoms With HEADACHE (see above); NAUSEA (see above); VOMITING.
Worse for fresh air.
Causes travelling.
Petroleum is one of the main travel sickness remedies and is indicated where fresh air actually aggravates. (It is the opposite of *Tabacum*, which has nausea but is better for fresh air.) This symptom should help to differentiate between the various travel sickness remedies.

PHOSPHORIC ACID (Pho-ac.)

Other name: glacial phosphoric acid

Phosphoric acid occurs either as a clear, colourless, sparkling liquid or as a transparent crystalline solid – depending on its temperature. It is used in the manufacture of fertilisers, soft drinks (giving them a fruity, acidic flavour), pharmaceuticals, gelatin, animal feeds, waxes, polishes, dental cements and detergents. It is also used in the processes of sugar refining and rustproofing metals, and in other industrial uses.
  Medicinally it is occasionally taken as a tonic to stimulate the secretion of gastric juices, in combination with quinine and strychnine (that is, with our friends *Nux vomica* and *China*!).

The homeopathic remedy is made from pulverised phosphate rock which is dissolved in sulphuric acid and then diluted by succussion.

GENERAL SYMPTOMS

Complaints from: loss of body fluids. **Eyes** glassy. **Face** pale. **Likes:** fruit; refreshing things. **Pains** in bones. **Sweat:** clammy; profuse. **Symptoms** one-sided. **Thirstless.**
Better after sleep.
Worse for cold; for sweating; during the evening; during the morning; on one side of body.

Phosphoric acid benefits those who have become weak and tired from studying too much or from losing a lot of body fluids, for example after diarrhoea, a heavy period, bleeding or vomiting. This picture occurs in young people with bone pains who have grown too fast, in people who are acutely depressed or those who are convalescing from an illness where they have lost a lot of their own fluids. They may look pale and sickly with dark rings around their eyes and they sweat a lot. They want refreshing food to eat, such as fruit and vegetables (in order to replace the liquids), but may not be especially thirsty and will often feel tired after eating. They are generally worse for cold and better for a sleep, even a short nap.

EMOTIONAL/MENTAL SYMPTOMS

Apathetic. Complaints from: disappointed love; excitement; fright; grief; humiliation; shock. **Depressed. Forgetful. Homesick. Indifferent** during a fever. **Irritable. Uncommunicative.**

These are people in whom the acute emotional trauma has an obvious cause such as disappointment in love, shock and homesickness, and this causes mental apathy; they do not want to talk, to think or to answer because they cannot concentrate, and they may even forget words while they are speaking. They appear to be quite indifferent to everything, especially during a fever. They do not weep; there is a tranquillity about them, a very still depressiveness.

PHYSICAL COMPLAINTS
Cough

Symptoms COUGH: dry; tickling; violent.

Diarrhoea

Symptoms BELLY/STOMACH: rumbling. STOOLS: profuse; thin; watery; white. Without WEAKNESS.
Worse after eating solid/dry food.
Causes summer; hot weather.

NB   SEE ALSO PAGES 203–26 FOR GENERAL ADVICE, DOS AND DON'TS.

This is a profuse summer diarrhoea. It is not as exhausting as you might expect (an unusual and therefore helpful symptom), although exhaustion may set in after the diarrhoea has stopped. The person may pass an involuntary stool at the same time as passing flatulence. There may be gurgling and cramping, gripping pains and a bloated, full feeling in the belly, although it is usually painless.

Exhaustion

Symptoms EXHAUSTION: nervous; paralytic.
Worse after eating; in the morning on getting up; for slightest exertion; for walking
Causes breastfeeding; loss of body fluids; flu.

Hair loss

Symptoms HAIR falls out.
Causes grief.

Headache

Symptoms IN SCHOOLCHILDREN. EYES smarting. HEAD feels heavy. PAINS: in top of head; in back of head; at nape of neck; one-sided; pressing.
Better for excitement.
Worse for getting up from lying down.
Causes eye strain; grief; mental strain, especially in schoolchildren.
These headaches occur in schoolchildren who have worked too hard and who are suffering from mental strain as a result. The head feels heavy.

Insomnia

Symptoms SLEEP unrefreshing. WAKING: frequent; after midnight.

Shock

Causes emotional trauma.
The *Phosphoric acid* shock is one that has been caused by an emotional trauma and is accompanied by the typical emotional symptoms.

PHOSPHORUS (Phos.)

Other name: white phosphorus

This element has a number of forms. The most common, the yellow solid called white phosphorus, is a non-metallic, poisonous element widely found in nature. It is highly flammable and glows in the dark. It bursts into a brilliant white flame on contact with air and is kept under water or in alcohol. It is unique among the non-radioactive substances in that in the process of oxidation it spontaneously gives off light without heat. When heated, white phosphorus turns into a powder called red phosphorus, which is less poisonous and is used to make matches. Industrial poisoning in the manufacture of matches led to a complaint known as 'phossy jaw' where the bone of the jaw died off.

Phosphorus is an element essential to life – both vegetable and animal – and much of the food we eat contains phosphate. Large amounts of it are mined and used as fertilisers.

Medicinally, phosphorus was used until the nineteenth century, when it fell out of use because of its highly poisonous nature, the symptoms of which are violent burning pains in the chest and stomach, vomiting and diarrhoea, prostration, haemorrhaging and death – either within a few days or a few months. It has been used as a rat poison and an insecticide.

The homeopathic remedy is prepared from the element itself by trituration.

GENERAL SYMPTOMS

Anaemia. Bleeding: occurs easily; bright red; profuse. **Complaints from:** any change of weather; getting chilled. **Discharges** blood-streaked. **Dislikes** hot food. **Face** red in spots. **Hair loss. Haemorrhages. Heavy feeling. Hot flushes. Likes:** cold drinks; cold food; spicy food; ice-cream; milk; chocolate; salt. **Pains:** in glands; burning. **Sweat:** on single parts of the body; from slightest physical exertion; clammy. **Taste:** mouth tastes sour. **Thirsty:** unquenchable for ice-cold drinks; for water. **Tongue** red-coated. **Better** after sleep; for cold drinks; for massage. **Worse** for cold; before eating; for change of weather; during the evening; during the morning; for wind.

Phosphorus types are usually tall and slim with long dark eyelashes, or red-haired with freckles. Despite being thin they are always hungry and burn up their food quickly; they therefore need to eat often. They are also very thirsty and want cold or iced drinks (especially cold milk). They may be warm blooded but more often they are chilly individuals who feel worse for changes in the weather and for getting cold, and who hate the wind.

They bleed easily and copiously, producing a lot of bright red blood which is slow to coagulate. Small cuts or tooth extractions will bleed a lot, and they suffer heavy periods and nosebleeds. They are therefore prone to anaemia; if they are anaemic, their hair may fall out, probably in handfuls.

Phosphorus patients are weak, delicate and chesty. Their weakness is often due to nervous exhaustion, and they are then prone to feeling heavy and cold; feet and hands become icy cold, especially in bed and from mental strain. Legs fall asleep easily. Sleep, however brief, and massage make them feel better. They prefer sleeping on the right side.

Phosphorus pains are usually burning pains, wherever they are. Mornings and evenings, between dusk and midnight, are their worst times of day.

EMOTIONAL/MENTAL SYMPTOMS

Affectionate. Anxious. Apathetic. Desires company. **Excitable. Fearful:** generally; of being alone; of the dark; of death; during a storm. **Jumpy. Irritable. Sensitive:** generally; to pain; to light. **Slowness. Sympathetic. Uncommunicative.**

In health these individuals are lively, affectionate and excitable – although they may also have the classic *Phosphorus* fears. They hate to be alone, especially in the dark at night when their vivid imaginations conjure up all sorts of ghosts and monsters creeping out of the shadows. They are also scared of thunderstorms, and jump with each thunderclap, but as they grow older they may find the lightning exciting. These are people who want company, who feel things strongly and are very sensitive, but, being highly strung, they are very easily startled.

When sick, all this changes. They become irritable and sluggish mentally (like *Phosphoric acid*) and apathetic and they don't want to think, talk or work. Illness debilitates these types; though their energy may flare up in excited bursts, this will be followed by a return to their exhausted states. They need sympathy when ill, and, despite being fearful and prone to becoming irritable if tired or upset, they are easily comforted and reassured. They love massage, touch and affection.

PHYSICAL COMPLAINTS

Backache

Symptoms PAINS: between shoulder blades; in lower back; as if broken; burning.
Better for rubbing/massage.
Worse on getting up from sitting.

Bleeding gums

Causes tooth extraction.

Common cold

Symptoms NASAL CATARRH: blood-streaked; profuse; one-sided; dry. SENSE OF TASTE/SMELL lost. With HOARSENESS; SORE THROAT (see below).
The nose may run profusely or be blocked (when it will

feel very dry and there will be no discharge). The catarrh is usually blood-streaked.

Cough

Symptoms BREATHING: difficult; fast. COUGH: dry at night; during fever; hacking; irritating; racking; tickling; tight; violent; from tickling in larynx; wakens person at night; person must sit up. LARYNX raw. MUCUS: tastes sweet; salty; transparent; white; yellow; green; copious; bloody. PAIN IN CHEST: burning. With SWEATING.
Better for heat.
Worse for change of temperature from warm to cold or cold to warm; for cold air; for fresh air; during fever; for lying on left side; during the morning after getting up; during the evening until midnight; reading aloud.
There is a feeling of a weight on, and burning pains in, the chest, which are both worse for coughing. The airways feel irritated and the tickling in the chest is worse for cold air. The person will wake from sleep with the cough and will then have to sit up to cough. He will cough up copious quantities of sputum, especially in the morning, which is usually blood-streaked and ranges in colour from clear to white to yellow or green.

Croup

Symptoms of COUGH (see above).

Diarrhoea

Symptoms STOOLS: blood-streaked; frequent; painless; profuse; watery. With ICY-COLD HANDS AND FEET.
Better after eating cold food.
Worse during the morning; getting chilled.
The abdomen may be bloated and gurgling, and the stools blood-streaked. The person may feel better for cold drinks.

Exhaustion

Symptoms EXHAUSTION: nervous; paralytic. With FEVER (see below).
Worse for slightest exertion; for walking.
Causes diarrhoea; fever; sweating.
The patient is so tired during an acute illness that he cannot even stay sitting upright in bed but continually slides down.

Fever

Symptoms Increased APPETITE. HEAT: dry; burning at night; one-sided; worse on the right side.
Worse in the afternoon/evening/night.
The person with this fever will have an unquenchable thirst for cold drinks and a bigger appetite than

normal. Children with a high fever may play normally and appear quite well in themselves (with rosy cheeks) and even eat well.

Hair loss

Symptoms HAIR falls out in handfuls.
Causes acute illness.

Headache

Symptoms HUNGER before/during headache. PAINS: in forehead; in sides of head; burning; bursting; pressing; throbbing.
Better after sleep; for cold; for cold compresses; for fresh air; on getting up; for massage; for walking.
Worse for getting cold; for coughing; for daylight; for hot drinks; in a stuffy room; for wrapping up head.
Causes before a thunderstorm.
During this nervous headache, the head feels heavy and is worse for being wrapped up warmly. The eyes water in the cold air. The person usually feels very hungry before and during the headache, and the sense of smell is often very acute.

Hoarseness

Symptoms PAINFUL.
Causes over-using voice.

Indigestion

Symptoms PAINS: in the stomach; burning; sore; bruised.
Worse after eating.

Injuries

Symptoms CUTS/WOUNDS: bleed freely; bright red; slow to clot.

Insomnia

Symptoms Anxious DREAMS. With SLEEPINESS.
The person will sleep on her right side – she cannot fall asleep when lying on her left side, especially if she has a chest infection or a cough. Has anxious, vivid dreams.

Nausea

Symptoms BELLY/STOMACH feels empty. BELCHES sour.
Worse for putting hands in warm water; for hot drinks; for drinking water.
The empty feeling in the stomach is not relieved by eating.

Nosebleeds

Symptoms BLOOD: bright red; persistent. With SWEATING.
Worse for blowing nose.

Sore throat

Symptoms PAINS: raw; sore. TONSILS swollen. VOICE hoarse.
Worse for breathing in; for coughing; during the morning/evening; for pressure; for talking.
These sore throats in a *Phosphorus* type often accompany a cold. The patient can't talk as the throat is so painfully hoarse, and the larynx is sensitive to touch and feels irritated and tickly.

Voice lost

Symptoms IN SINGERS; PAINLESS.

Vomiting

Symptoms Burning PAINS IN STOMACH. VOMIT: bile; mucus; bitter; yellow. VOMITING violent.
Worse after drinking/eating.
The patient vomits food and drink – even the smallest quantity – as soon as it becomes warm in the stomach. There may be burning pains in the stomach or a bruised soreness. This often accompanies a stomach bug, or occurs when the stomach is especially sensitive for some reason, often emotional.

PHYTOLACCA DECANDRA (Phyt.)

Family name: Phytolaccaceae
Other names: Virginian poke; poke-root; target weed; pigeon berry; American nightshade

This perennial plant grows in moist ground along hedges and road-sides in the United States, North Africa and China, and it is also common in Mediterranean countries. It is a striking bush with fine, dark reddish-purple stems; numerous small whitish flowers appear from July to September which give way to long clusters of dark purple berries similar to blackberries. The stems when young and green can be cooked and eaten rather like asparagus, and the berries are loved by birds.
Phytolacca has an unusually high potassium content and the ashes, which contain over 45 per cent caustic potash, have been used by country folk as a salve for ulcers and cancerous growths. It was well known to the Indian tribes as a useful medicinal plant for its purgative qualities and for the treatment of rheumatism.

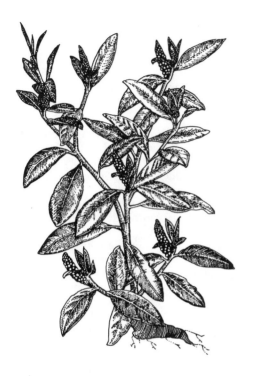

A decoction of the roots has been used for dosing cattle suffering from mastitis.

For the homeopathic preparation the fresh root is chopped and pounded to a pulp, added to alcohol and left to stand before being strained and succussed.

GENERAL SYMPTOMS

Breath smells. **Pains** shoot upwards. **Tongue** red-tipped.

The main action of *Phytolacca* is on the throat and the breast, on the muscular tissues and on the joints. It is a wonderful remedy for breast abscesses and cracked nipples in breastfeeding mothers.

Phytolacca types will usually feel exhausted, stiff and worn out, and unable to think. Smelly breath accompanies many of the complaints. *Phytolacca* pains characteristically appear and disappear suddenly and shoot up the body.

EMOTIONAL/MENTAL SYMPTOMS

The emotional/mental symptoms of this remedy are not strongly marked but there may be some depression with tearfulness and/or irritability accompanied by not wanting to think or work.

PHYSICAL COMPLAINTS
Breastfeeding problems

Symptoms BREASTS: inflamed; lumpy. ABSCESSES. NIPPLES: cracked; raw, sore. PAIN while nursing.
Many homeopaths regard this remedy as a specific for sore, cracked nipples where there is pain from the nipple radiating all over the body. It is also useful for infections and for abscesses where the breast is hard, nodular and lumpy; or if a lump in the breast becomes painful and an abscess is therefore threatening. This remedy can take twelve to twenty-four hours to act (unlike the quick action of *Aconite* or *Belladonna*).

Mumps

Symptoms GLANDS: hard; painful; swollen. PAINS spread to breasts, ovaries, testicles. With COPIOUS SALIVA/SWEATING; SORE THROAT (see below).

Sore throat

Symptoms THROAT dark red. TONSILS swollen.
Better for cold drinks.
Worse for hot drinks.
The throat is dry and dark red. Swallowing is difficult and causes the pains to shoot through both ears (in *Belladonna* sore throats the pains only shoot up to the right ear on swallowing). The throat may also hurt on sticking out the tongue; this is an unusual symptom, and therefore useful to look out for when prescribing.

Teething

Symptoms PAINFUL IN CHILDREN.
Better for biting gums together hard.
Teething babies have an irresistible urge to bite their teeth (or gums) together – on anything and everything!

PODOPHYLLUM (Podo.)

Family name: Berberidaceae
Common names: May apple; mandrake; duck's-foot; ground lemon

The American mandrake is a small herb that grows in wet meadows and in damp, open woods in the north and east of the USA and in Canada. It grows up to two feet high and produces a dropping foul-smelling white flower in May, which is followed by a rosehip-type fruit measuring 1 to 2 inches. Its name is derived from the Latin *podos* ('foot'), and *phyllon* ('leaf'), as its leaves resemble the webbed feet of a duck; hence also its nickname duck's-foot.

NB   SEE ALSO PAGES 203–26 FOR GENERAL ADVICE, DOS AND DON'TS.

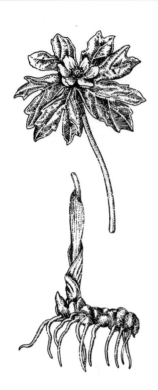

It was well known to the North American Indians as a remedy to kill parasites or intestinal worms, as an emetic (to induce vomiting) and as a purgative (a drastic laxative). This use spread to early American immigrants who used it as a chief component in 'cathartic' pills for cleansing the gut.

Podophyllum has been used by herbalists as a stimulant for the liver and bowels where there is congestion (though great care is taken not to use large doses which can poison the system and cause severe inflammation of the stomach and intestines). It was used for colic, usually in combination with other herbs such as colocynthis, and was found to stimulate the glandular system when given in small doses.

For the homeopathic preparation the fresh root is gathered before the fruit is ripe and chopped and pounded to a pulp, then left to stand in alcohol before being strained and succussed.

GENERAL SYMPTOMS

Discharges watery.
Worse after midnight; mid-morning.

Podophyllum is used mainly for treating diarrhoea where the patient feels weak and faint after the stool (see below). Generally speaking, these people often feel at their worst and/or the diarrhoea is at its worst in the early hours of the morning or mid-morning.

EMOTIONAL/MENTAL SYMPTOMS

This remedy does not have strong emotional symptoms, though patients may be talkative, excitable and restless, especially at night; and may moan during their sleep.

PHYSICAL COMPLAINTS
Diarrhoea

Symptoms IN CHILDREN. BELLY/STOMACH: gurgling; rumbling. ALTERNATING WITH constipation/headache. STOOLS: frequent; gushing; involuntary; painless; profuse; smelly; sudden. With EXHAUSTION after passing stool.
Worse after drinking water; immediately after drinking; after eating; for hot weather; mid-morning; around 4 a.m.; at night.

This diarrhoea may alternate with other symptoms such as a headache or even constipation. There is much rumbling and gurgling in the abdomen before a stool, and there may be dull aches or cramping pains accompanying the gurgling. The stools are usually painless, and are profuse and watery and literally shoot out. They may be frothy and of a changeable colour and consistency, that is, white, yellow or green. They are usually accompanied by loud wind. These 'evacuations' leave a person feeling completely drained, faint and weak. The guts soon fill up again and another stool must be passed, so that people suffering from this type of diarrhoea will need to visit the toilet frequently. They may think that they are going to pass wind (whilst sitting on the toilet) but diarrhoea shoots out involuntarily. It often comes on immediately after drinking water.

Teething children sometimes produce this type of diarrhoea.

Flatulence

Symptoms BELLY/STOMACH gurgling before a stool. WIND loud during stool.

PULSATILLA NIGRICANS (Puls.)

Family name: Ranunculaceae
Other names: meadow anemone; pasque flower; wind flower; anemone pratensis

Pulsatilla nigricans grows in open fields in central and northern Europe. It is a perennial plant which flowers in May and again in August or September, and reaches a height of six to eight inches. The flower petals are a blackish-purple colour, and they and the smooth

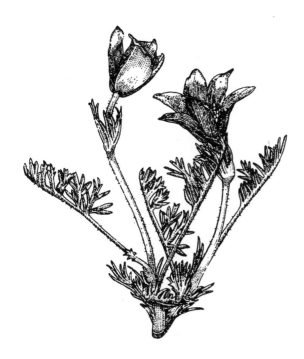

stems are covered with soft, downy hairs. It resembles the *Anemone pulsatilla*, but the *nigricans* has a smaller flower and deeper purple petals.

The plant has an extremely acrid taste when chewed, and will burn the tongue and throat as well as cause blisters on the skin. In ancient times so many marvellous cures were attributed to it that it eventually fell into disrepute. Its main uses, however, were as an external remedy for ulcers and for inflammations of the eyes.

For the homeopathic remedy, the whole fresh plant is gathered when in flower, then chopped and pounded to a pulp, mixed with alcohol and left to stand for a time before being strained and succussed.

GENERAL SYMPTOMS

Anaemia. Breath smells. **Complaints from/after** measles; getting wet; getting feet wet. **Discharges:** thick; yellow; bland. **Dislikes:** bread; hot food/drinks; fatty, rich food; meat. **Faintness** in a warm room. **Glands** swollen. **Lips** dry. **Mouth** dry. **Sweat:** smelly; single parts of the body; one-sided; worse at night. **Thirstless. Tongue** coated white/yellow. **Pains** on parts lain on; wandering. **Symptoms:** right-sided; changeable. **Taste:** mouth tastes bad in the morning. *Better* for bathing; for fresh air; for movement; for pressure; for walking in fresh air; for crying. *Worse* for getting cold; for exposure to sun; for fatty food; for getting feet wet; for heat; in stuffy rooms; at twilight; for wet weather; for wind.

Pulsatilla has such a wide range of action in all age groups that it has been called the Queen of Homeopathic Remedies (*Sulphur* being the King).

Pulsatilla types have dry mouths and lips and an absence of thirst. They may be chilly, with cold hands and feet, but they actually dislike the heat, becoming quickly flushed, and they hate stuffy rooms. They will always feel better out in the fresh air, where their moods lift and their symptoms (especially the coughs) disappear, returning only when in a warm, stuffy room again. However, they *are* sensitive to getting wet or to being exposed to wet, windy weather, and they may well start a cough or cold after becoming cold and wet. They and their moods are changeable.

Pulsatillas hate rich, fatty food, which gives them indigestion and nausea. They may, however, have such a strong craving for butter that *Pulsatilla* children will often scoop it straight from the bowl.

Their chests and joints are worse for rest and better for moving about, especially in the fresh air; twilight is a time of general aggravation.

Pulsatilla is especially useful for babies and children whose pictures fit both the physical and the general and emotional symptoms. It is a wonderful remedy for teething children who are weepy and whiny and better for fresh air. Since a large percentage of babies start out the *Pulsatilla* way – wanting to be carried, and weeping if they don't get what they want – it is a must for every new mother's homeopathic first-aid kit!

It is also useful in pregnancy where the anaemia in a *Pulsatilla* type may actually result from an excess of ordinary iron pills, so stopping the iron is essential (see *Ferrum metallicum*).

EMOTIONAL/MENTAL SYMPTOMS

Affectionate. Anxious: at night; indoors. **Changeable. Clingy. Complaints from:** fright; grief; shock. **Depressed:** worse before menstrual period; in a stuffy room; in the evening; from suppressed grief; better for fresh air. **Excitable. Fearful:** at twilight; during the evening. **Desires** to be carried (infants). **Introspective. Irritable. Jealous. Lonely. Gentle. Moody. Sensitive. Shy. Tearful:** during a fever; better for fresh air. **Whiny.**

Pulsatilla types have a gentle, yielding, mild disposition and are easily moved to laughter or tears; they are highly emotional and can cry at every little thing. They are clingy and dependent, particularly so when sick, when they also become irritable and whiny. Children will want to be carried and will cling to their mothers' skirts. They often say 'It's not fair!' in a whiny way. These types usually elicit sympathy and compassion from those around them, because they are responsive to affection, and are so needy and clingy. *Most* parents will feel sorry for them and protective towards them. However, if the parent is, for example, an *Arsenicum* – someone who cannot stand being clung to – then he or she will feel intensely irritated by the child's behaviour, which will make their symptoms worse.

Pulsatillas are affectionate creatures who love animals and who cannot bear to see films where animals are hurt. They too are easily hurt but may suppress it and become introspective, moody and even irritable.

Their depression will be better for fresh air, and worse during the evening and in warm, stuffy rooms. A breastfeeding mother will weep while nursing. Generally, these types moan and weep during a fever, and cry when talking about their illnesses.

PHYSICAL COMPLAINTS

Backache

Symptoms PAINS: in lower back; in small of back; aching; pressing.
Better for gentle exercise; for walking slowly.
Worse on beginning to move; before/during a menstrual period; on getting up from sitting.
The back feels weak and tired. Getting up after a long period of sitting or bending down (for example after gardening) is almost impossible. The back may actually feel sprained.

Bedwetting
These are children who wet the bed when sick who were formerly dry at night.

Breastfeeding problems

Symptoms MILK SUPPLY over-abundant.
If the general and emotional/mental symptoms fit, this is a useful remedy for post-natal depression, especially in women suffering from post-natal 'weeps'.

Chicken pox

Symptoms With COUGH (see above).
There is normally a low fever and typical *Pulsatilla* symptoms, i.e., weeping, clinging and lack of thirst. The itching is worse for heat.

Chilblains

Symptoms CHILBLAINS: on feet, hands, toes; inflamed; itching.

Common cold

Symptoms NASAL CATARRH: dirty yellow; green; yellow-green; bland (non-irritating); smelly; thick; dry alternating with profuse; watery in the fresh air. SENSE OF SMELL/TASTE lost. With SNEEZING in a stuffy room.
Better for fresh air.
Worse in a stuffy room.
The nose is watery in the fresh air, and is better (that is, blocked up) in the evenings, and in a warm room, though there will be much sneezing then too. The patient's sense of taste is lost altogether or there is a bitter taste before and after eating.

Cough

Symptoms COUGH: constant during the evening; dry at night; loose during the morning; exhausting; irritating; racking; in fits; violent; disturbs sleep. MUCUS: yellow; green; yellow-green; copious; sticky; difficult to cough up (must sit up). With NAUSEA (see below); RETCHING.
Better for fresh air; for sitting up.
Worse for getting hot; for exertion; for heat; for lying down; during the morning; at night/evening; in a stuffy room; in bed (once warm).
Causes after measles.
The *Pulsatilla* cough disturbs sleep – the patient will be woken by the cough and will need to sit up in bed to cough; it may then prevent the person getting back to sleep. There will be loud rattling/breathing in sleep. The cough is nearly always dry at night and loose in the mornings. The sputum is characteristically thick and yellow-greenish, and difficult to cough up; it may taste unpleasant and be worse in the morning on getting up.

Cystitis

Symptoms DESIRE TO URINATE: frequent; ineffectual; urgent. Spasmodic PAINS. Frequent URINATION. URINE copious.
Worse after urination.
Causes getting cold and wet.
The person has frequent urges to urinate and has to hurry to the lavatory to prevent urine escaping; but once on the lavatory the urine dribbles slowly. Kidneys may feel sore and bruised.

Diarrhoea

Symptoms IN CHILDREN. STOOLS: changeable; greenish-yellow; slimy; watery.
Better for fresh air.
Worse after eating; after eating starchy or rich food; at night; for getting overheated; in a stuffy room.
Causes rich food; fruit.

Earache

Symptoms DISCHARGE: smelly; thick; yellow; yellow-green. EAR (external) red; EAR (internal) feels blocked.

PAINS: aching; pressing; pressing outwards; stitching; tearing; throbbing. With DEAFNESS; ITCHING; NOISES IN THE EAR.
Worse at night.
Causes after common cold; after measles.

Exhaustion

Symptoms EXHAUSTION nervous.
Worse for heat of sun; in a stuffy room; mental exertion; morning in bed.
Pulsatilla types wilt in the heat and can't think!

Eye inflammation

Symptoms IN BABIES. DISCHARGE: purulent; smelly; thick; yellow. EYES: aching; burning; itching; watering. EYELIDS itching in the evening. With symptoms of COMMON COLD (see above).
Better for cold bathing; for fresh air; for cold.
Worse during the evening; in a warm room.
In the mornings the eyes are sticky and the inner corners discharge. They ache and burn, especially in a warm room, and they water in cold air or wind and/or with a cough.
   Sticky eyes in newborn babies commonly need *Pulsatilla*.

Fever

Symptoms HEAT: burning; dry during the evening; one-sided. With CHILLINESS.
Better for uncovering.
Worse for heat; for washing; in the afternoon; in the evening; at night; in the morning in bed; for warm covers; in a stuffy room; for being uncovered.
The patient wants to be covered for some of the time but at other times dislikes it. The heat may be on one side of the body only and is often worse (hotter) in the early afternoon; this is followed by a chill around 4 p.m. Sweating may also be one-sided (usually the left) or it may be localised to a part. The person will sweat while asleep and wake up chilled, and will then find it difficult to get back to sleep. *Pulsatilla* types generally moan and whine during a fever.

Flatulence

Symptoms   BELLY/STOMACH: rumbling/gurgling. WIND: smelly; obstructed (difficult to expel).
Better for passing wind.

Food poisoning

Causes rotten meat; rotten fish.

Hayfever

Symptoms of COMMON COLD (see above).

Headache

Symptoms HEADACHE nervous. PAINS: in forehead; one-sided; pressing; sore, bruised; throbbing.
Better for firm pressure; for fresh air; for lying with head high; for walking in fresh air.
Worse after eating; for bending down; for blowing nose; for hot drinks; for running; for standing; in a stuffy room; in heat.
Causes excitement; ice-cream; running.
Pulsatilla types are prone to nervous headaches over the eyes, usually on one side, and these are worse for movement and better for fresh air. They are caused by a variety of factors, from too much sun (remember that *Pulsatillas* wilt in the sun) to eating too much rich food.

Indigestion

Symptoms BELCHES: bitter; empty; tasting of food just eaten. BELLY/STOMACH feels empty. PAINS: in stomach; pressing. With HEARTBURN.
Worse at night; for rich, fatty foods.
Causes rich, fatty food (ice-cream, fats, pork, etc.).
The belly/stomach gurgles and rumbles during the evening.

Insomnia

Symptoms Anxious DREAMING. SLEEP restless. With SLEEPINESS. WAKING: from cold; frequently.
Worse before midnight.
Causes over-active mind; repeating thoughts.
Pulsatilla insomniacs like to sleep on their backs, with their arms above their heads, and they poke their feet out of bed because they become hot. They sleep restlessly, with twitchy arms and legs, and have anxious dreams and nightmares. They wake frequently and can't get back to sleep because of over-active minds and 'stuck record' thoughts. Children kick the covers off because they are too hot and then they cool down and wake because they have become cold.

Joint pain

Symptoms PAINS: in bones; in joints; pulling; sore, bruised; wandering.
Better for cold compresses; for fresh air; for gentle movement; for walking.
Worse after common cold; on beginning to move; for heat; for warmth of bed; for wet weather.

Labour pains

Symptoms PAINS: irregular; weak; in the back; stop altogether; ineffectual.
With characteristic general and emotional/mental symptoms.

NB   SEE ALSO PAGES 203–26 FOR GENERAL ADVICE, DOS AND DON'TS.

Measles

Symptoms With cough (see above); common cold (see above); eye inflammation (see above).
With characteristic weepiness and lack of thirst.

Mumps

Symptoms Glands: swollen/painful. Pains: spread to breasts, ovaries or testicles. With fever (see above).
The characteristic *Pulsatilla* general and emotional/mental symptoms will be present.

Nausea

Worse after drinking/eating; during cough; during the morning; for hot drinks.
Causes rich food; ice-cream.

Period problems

Symptoms Period: late; painful. Bleeding during the day only. Pains: aching; dull; wandering.
Better for doubling up.
Worse before/during the period.
The pains cause the person to cry out and bend double. The period may flow only during the day, and be consistently late.

Sciatica

Better for fresh air.
Worse in a warm room.

Sore throat

Symptoms Throat dry. Larynx: irritated; tickling. Pains: raw; scraping; stitching.
Worse for heat.
The larynx feels as though there is dust in it; it feels rough, and raw from coughing. The patient chokes when swallowing solid food.

Styes

Symptoms Styes.
Worse on upper eyelids.

Teething

Symptoms Painful in children.
Better for cold water; a walk in fresh air.
Worse for heat of bed, warm food/drinks.

Toothache

Symptoms Pains: gnawing; pulling; stitching.
Better for cold water; for fresh air.
Worse in a stuffy room; for heat; for warmth of bed.
Causes teething.
Holding cold water in the mouth greatly relieves the pains. The nerves feel stretched.

Varicose veins

Symptoms Varicose veins painful.
Worse during pregnancy.
Limbs lain on become numb and cold; this is an indication of poor circulation.

PYROGEN (Pyr.)

Other names: pyrexin; sepsin; pyrogenium

The homeopathic remedy *Pyrogen* is a product of decomposed beef. It is defined as 'a chemical non-living substance formed by living bacteria, but also by living pus-corpuscles, or the living blood- or tissue-protoplasms from which these corpuscles spring.'

Though used initially for treating typhoid fever and diphtheria, it became an indispensable treatment for blood poisoning, especially poisoning from bacterial products. It was later found to be effective in various different conditions such as ulcers and flus.

The remedy is prepared by mixing chopped lean beef with water and leaving it in the sun to decompose for two weeks. It is then potentised by succussion.

GENERAL SYMPTOMS

Discharges (breath, pus, sweat) smelly. **Pains:** in parts lain on; sore, bruised. **Pulse:** rapid. **Thirsty.**
Better for movement.
Worse for cold; for cold, wet weather.

Pyrogen is mainly for chronic complaints or for very severe acute complaints such as blood poisoning, both of which need the care of a professional homeopath. It is, however, useful for a particular type of flu and I have therefore included it here. I have also given the indications for blood poisoning in the (I hope unlikely) event that you need this emergency treatment. If indicated it will work quickly and make the need of antibiotic treatment unnecessary.

EMOTIONAL/MENTAL SYMPTOMS

This is a small remedy with few strong emotional/mental symptoms, although in the acute fever you may see anxiety and an unusual degree of talkativeness.

PHYSICAL COMPLAINTS
Blood poisoning

Symptoms With fever (see below); extreme chilliness.
Worse for cold.

Causes after childbirth; after surgery; from infected wounds.

Give *Pyrogen* every five minutes and seek emergency help. A keynote for the use of *Pyrogen* is the rotten-smelling discharges of the body (*Pyrogen* itself is of course a product of rotten meat). The urine may be clear.

Fever

Symptoms HEAT. With CHILLINESS: internal; extreme; SWEATING; SHAKING.
Worse for being uncovered.
During a fever parts lain on feel sore and bruised (like *Arnica*) and the bed may therefore feel hard. A low fever is usually accompanied by a fast pulse and is not a cause for immediate concern. If however the fever is high and the pulse slow this may indicate acute blood poisoning. If *Pyrogen* is called for the pulse is fast out of all proportion to the fever, or the reverse – unusually slow. The patient will be extremely chilly, and will be unable to get warm.

Flu

Symptoms PAINS: aching; in bones of legs. With FEVER (see above); extreme THIRST; CHILLS in back/SHIVERING.
Better for movement; for walking; for warmth of bed.
Worse during chilly stage; for sitting.

RHEUM (Rhe.)

Family name: Polygonaceae
Other names: rhubarbarum; China rhubarb; East India rhubarb; Turkey rhubarb; palmated rhubarb; rheum palmatum

This is a perennial herbaceous plant that flowers from June to July and is indigenous to north-west China and north-east Tibet. It has been cultivated in European gardens as an ornamental plant since the mid-eighteenth century, and is distinguishable from our familiar garden rhubarb by its much larger size, its height of up to 11 feet, and its distinctively shaped leaves. Its different names reflect its origins and the routes it has taken to reach the European market.

It was used medicinally by the Arabian physicians for dropsy, obstructions of the spleen, and for jaundice. It has always been recognised for its purgative qualities; in humans small doses act as an astringent tonic to the digestive organs and larger doses act as a mild laxative. The name is said to have come from the

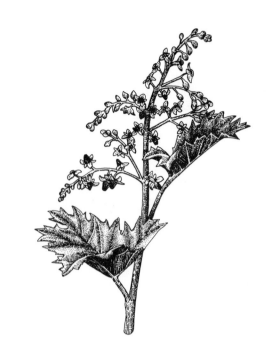

Greek *rheo* meaning 'to flow', alluding, apparently, to the purgative properties of the root!

The homeopathic tincture is prepared from the dried root.

GENERAL SYMPTOMS

Discharges (stools, sweat, etc.) sour.

These are pale children who have a hard time assimilating their food when they are producing (or trying to produce) teeth. Sourness is the keynote of this remedy. The whole child may smell sour, despite frequent washing. Even the scalp smells of sour sweat.

EMOTIONAL/MENTAL SYMPTOMS

Capricious. Indifferent in children to playing. **Irritable.**

Rheum is for teething children who are colicky. They will be irritable, difficult children who are peevish and restless and who don't want to play.

PHYSICAL COMPLAINTS
Diarrhoea

Symptoms IN TEETHING CHILDREN. STOOLS: sour; pasty.
Causes teething.

The child may eat a lot, without appearing to enjoy it. Food is not assimilated well and the colicky pains cause the child to cry and toss about at night.

Teething

Symptoms PAINFUL IN CHILDREN. With DIARRHOEA (see above).
The general and emotional/mental symptoms should also be present.

RHODODENDRON (Rhod.)

Family name: Ericaceae
Other names: yellow snow rose; rosebay; rosage alpenrose; rhododendron chrysanthum; Siberian rhododendron

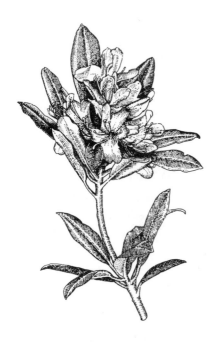

This species of rhododendron is indigenous to the mountains of Siberia, and is now cultivated worldwide. It is a small bush that grows to a height of 1–1½ feet, and has golden flowers.
  Though not widely known in general medicine, it was much used in its native Siberia as a remedy for rheumatism, gout and syphilis. The growing conditions of the plant – it survives the storms, winds and rain of the Siberian mountains – indicate its keynote as a homeopathic remedy; that is, a sensitivity to stormy and changeable weather.
  For the homeopathic preparation, the leaves are gathered when the seed capsules have ripened, and a tincture is made from them.

GENERAL SYMPTOMS

Complaints from change of weather to stormy.
Better for movement.
Worse for cold; for cold, wet weather; for stormy weather; before thunderstorms; for wind.

Rhododendron types are extremely sensitive to the change in pressure that precedes a storm; their symptoms come on then or are generally worse. They are also sensitive to changes in the weather, particularly to cold, wet and windy weather, and are worse during the seasons of change – spring and autumn. Their symptoms may abate either during or after the storm has broken.

EMOTIONAL/MENTAL SYMPTOMS

Fearful of thunderstorm.

This is a small remedy with very few strong emotional symptoms but the aggravation that occurs before a thunderstorm is emotional as well as physical. These people may feel apprehensive, fearful or just 'unwell' before and, to a certain extent, during a storm. They may also be particularly afraid of thunder.

PHYSICAL COMPLAINTS
Backache

Symptoms PAINS: in lower back; in neck; rheumatic; sore, bruised.
Better for movement.
Worse for wet weather.

Headache

Symptoms PAINS tearing.
Better for getting up; for walking; for walking in fresh air; for wrapping up the head.
Worse before/during a storm; for damp weather.
The pains are in the face and eyes and are always worse before and during a storm.

Joint pain

Symptoms PAINS: in arms/legs/shoulders; drawing; tearing.
Better for movement; for stretching limb.
Worse for change of weather; for sitting down; for stormy weather; for wet weather.

Toothache

Symptoms PAINS: spreading to the ear; grumbling.
Better after eating; for heat; warm compresses.
Worse before a storm.

RHUS TOXICODENDRON (Rhus-t.)

Family name: Anacardiaceae
Common names: poison ivy; mercury vine; poison
ash; poison vine; pubescent poison oak; trailing
sumach

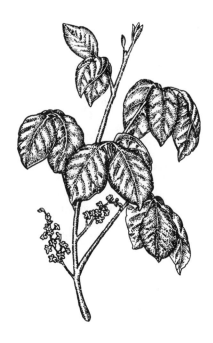

This deciduous shrub grows in fields, woods and
along fences all over North America. The root sends
up many stems which divide into woody branches and
trail along the ground until they meet with support –
for example a wall, or a tree – which they will climb.
The plant produces a milky juice which turns black on
exposure to the air and is highly poisonous.

Poison ivy's medicinal properties were first noted in
1798 by a French doctor who observed that after an
accidental poisoning by the plant a patient of his was
cured of a long-standing herpetic eruption (rash) on
his wrist. He went on to use the ivy to cure similar skin
diseases as well as to treat paralysis and rheumatism
with some degree of success.

In places where the plant grows freely, accidental
poisonings are common; symptoms begin with an
extremely nasty rash, often with a violent fever, loss of
appetite, nausea, headache and delirium followed by
swollen glands and ulcers of the mouth and tongue.
The rash is hot, itches violently and blisters painfully.

For the homeopathic preparation the fresh leaves
are collected when the poison is most active: before it
flowers, during the night (it is thought to be almost
innocuous when exposed to sunlight) and in damp
weather (see General Symptoms). The leaves are
chopped and pounded to a pulp, then left to stand in
alcohol before being strained and succussed.

GENERAL SYMPTOMS

Complaints from: getting wet; change of weather
to cold/to damp; getting chilled. **Face** red. **Glands**
swollen. **Likes** milk. **Lips** dry. **Pains:** burning;
pressing; shooting; sore, bruised. **Sweat:** worse for
lying down and uncovering; worse for slightest
physical exertion. **Taste:** mouth tastes metallic.
Tongue red-tipped.
Better for changing position; for fresh air; for movement; for sweating; for warmth of bed; for hot drinks.
Worse in the autumn; for change of weather; for
cloudy weather; for cold; for cold/wet weather;
for foggy weather; for cold drinks/food; for damp; for
draughts; on beginning to move; for lying down;
for being uncovered; swimming in cold water.

Rhus tox is one of the main mumps remedies, indicated
by the hard, swollen glands that often feature in *Rhus
tox* acute illnesses. The tongue is coated white or
yellowy white and has a triangular red tip to it that
may be sore.

These people feel better generally for sweating,
especially during a fever, but getting chilled whilst
sweating will aggravate their conditions and produce
a cough or cold. They are extremely chilly – they hate
the cold in any form: cold food or drink, swimming or
washing in cold water, and cold and wet weather in
any form (cloudy, foggy or damp). They are so sensitive to cold that touching cold things can aggravate,
and putting a hand out of bed into the cold air can
make them feel worse. Even eating ice-cream on a hot
day when a person is overheated can bring on an
aggravation of symptoms. They feel as if the coldness
is running through their blood vessels, although this
may alternate with a feeling of heat in the vessels if
there is an accompanying fever. Not surprisingly, they
feel better for the heat, for warm, dry compresses (heat
packs) and for hot baths.

They are also very sensitive to the damp, so that
when autumn comes, bringing a damp atmosphere,
those with *Rhus tox* rheumatism will start to moan
and complain. This is one of the most important
homeopathic rheumatic/arthritic remedies, so long as
the general symptoms agree.

NB   SEE ALSO PAGES 203–26 FOR GENERAL ADVICE, DOS AND DON'TS.

Rhus tox pains are typically aching, sore and bruised with tearing or stitching pains that are worse on first moving after a rest. These ease off after the joint has been gently exercised by, for example, gentle walking. But after a while the person will feel tired, the pains may start up again and they will need to rest once more, only to feel that they need to move after a short period of sitting. And so the cycle continues. The patients suffer a terrible torture of not being comfortable in any position; they are restless, and need to be constantly on the move. Their pains cause them to get up at night, preventing sleep. Lying on a hard floor may help.

Like *Arnica*, it is also a remedy for the sort of physical strain that can come on after a period of 'overdoing it', (for example, gardening or spring cleaning). However, with *Rhus tox* the stiffness, aches and pains actually improve after a bit of gentle exercise whereas *Arnica* types stay sore and bruised in spite of any moving about (though of course with *Rhus tox* there is the characteristic aggravation on beginning to move, which then wears off).

They have a fear of flying, mainly because of having to keep still for so long without fresh air.

EMOTIONAL/MENTAL SYMPTOMS

Anxious: indoors; in bed. **Confused. Depressed. Irritable. Restless** in bed. **Tearful.**

This is one of the most restless remedies; these people cannot get comfortable in any position and are therefore constantly on the move. The restlessness is caused by physical pain, but it is also a nervous restlessness, which will drive a person out of bed at night. It can be seen during an acute illness with a fever where a person just cannot keep still but tosses and turns and has to get up. The anxiety is worse in bed at night because of having to be still then, especially after midnight when the mind will dwell on unpleasant past events.

They feel worse in other ways at night, being irritable and fearful then, and they may actually feel a bit better for a walk in the fresh air.

The patients may suffer from depression, which, though not very deep, may be constant, and they may suddenly and involuntarily burst into tears without knowing why, and they will usually say so.

PHYSICAL COMPLAINTS

Backache

Symptoms PAINS: in lower back; in small of back; in neck; aching; sore, bruised; rheumatic. With STIFFNESS.

Better for lying on a hard surface; for movement; for walking; for heat.
Worse on beginning to move; on getting up from sitting; for reaching up; for wet weather.
Causes damp weather; draughts; injury; lifting; sprains.

The back feels weak, lame and tired, and the pains compel a constant moving about in bed. Getting up after sitting down for a long time is extremely difficult. The pain may result from sitting in a draught or from lifting, or from a sprain, or it may be rheumaticky pain in damp, wet weather, but there is always improvement from warmth, and an aggravation on first movement.

Chicken pox

Symptoms SKIN RASH itches severely.

There will be great restlessness with the itching, and also the characteristic *Rhus tox* red-tipped tongue.

Cold sores

Symptoms SORES on lips.

Cough

Symptoms COUGH: irritating; short; tickling.
Better for hot drinks.
Worse for getting cold; for being uncovered; on single parts of the body; for uncovering hands.
Causes swimming in cold water.

This cough is aggravated if any single part of the body is uncovered and consequently becomes cold.

Diarrhoea

Symptoms STOOLS: mushy; watery.
Causes getting wet; getting feet wet.

Exhaustion

Symptoms EXHAUSTION nervous. With HEAVINESS; RESTLESSNESS.
Better for walking in the fresh air.
Worse for slightest exertion; for sitting down.

The exhaustion is so strong that the slightest exertion, including getting up and walking about, is an effort. However, a gentle walk out in the fresh air will actually help. It will be accompanied by the characteristic *Rhus tox* restlessness.

Eye inflammation

Symptoms EYES: sensitive to light; sore; watering. EYELIDS: glued together; itching; swollen.
Worse for moving eyes.
Causes cold, wet weather.

The eyelids are stuck together in the mornings.

Fever

Symptoms HEAT: alternating with chills; dry; burning.
Better for hot drinks.
Worse at night/evening/mid morning; for movement; cold drinks; for being uncovered.
The patient sweats from the slightest exertion, as well as when lying in bed and when asleep, and will sweat over the whole body except for the head. Will also urinate frequently while sweating. He may get chilled after being hot and sweaty; any movement also brings on chilliness as does uncovering when in bed. Warmth will help the chilliness. The fever may be one-sided (that is, one side may be hot while the other side is cold). It may feel as though there is hot water running through the blood vessels.

Flu

Symptoms PAINS; in bones; in joints; in legs; aching; shooting; sore, bruised. With EXHAUSTION (see above); FEVER (see above); SNEEZING.

Headache

Symptoms PAINS: in back of head; rheumatic; violent.
Better for gentle walking; for wrapping up head; for movement.
Causes change of weather; cold air/wind; damp weather; getting wet; lifting.

Hives

Symptoms RASH: burning; itching; stinging. With JOINT PAIN (see below).
Worse for cold; after scratching.
Causes getting wet/chilled; cold air; during a fever.

Hoarseness

Causes over-using voice.

Insomnia

Symptoms SLEEP: restless; sleepless after midnight.
The person has vivid, work-related dreams, caused by strain from working too hard.

Joint pain

Symptoms PAINS: aching, sore, bruised; shooting; tearing. With HEAVINESS; LAMENESS. STIFFNESS.
Better for continued movement; for external heat; for walking; for warm compresses; for warmth of bed.
Worse for damp weather; during a fever; on beginning to move; at night; for sitting; when chilled.
The pains are worse for rest and on beginning to move; they improve temporarily but the patient soon gets tired again (see General Symptoms). The pains can also be brought about by over-exertion, for example spring cleaning or gardening.

Mumps

Symptoms GLANDS swollen/painful. With FEVER (see above).
Better for heat.
Worse for cold; on left side of body.
This is one of the most important mumps remedies, *providing the characteristic general symptoms agree*. The typical glands are affected and it is often the left side that becomes swollen first.

Sciatica

Better for movement; for walking; for heat.
Worse for cold; for cold compresses; on beginning to move; for lying on painful part; for washing in cold water; for wet weather.

Sore throat

Symptoms THROAT dry. Tickling in LARYNX. VOICE hoarse.
Worse for cold drinks; for swallowing; for uncovering throat.
Causes straining voice.
The voice is hoarse, or strained, from too much talking or singing but it improves after continued use (as do *Rhus tox* joints!).

Sprains

Symptoms PAIN. With STIFFNESS; TREMBLING.
Causes falling; lifting; twisting.
It is important to use *Arnica* first after an injury or a sprain in order to deal with any bruising and possible swelling. Then give *Rhus tox* if the sprain is accompanied by the typical general symptoms. A sprained wrist will be accompanied by an inability to grip anything properly and strongly.

Stiff neck

Causes draughts; getting chilled; lifting.

Strains

Symptoms With STIFFNESS; TREMBLING.
Better for continued movement.
Worse for beginning to move.
Gardening or spring cleaning can cause this stiffness in the joints. It is worse when getting up after a rest, and better for gentle exercise (whereas *Arnica* stiffness and soreness *stays* in spite of gentle exercise).

Toothache

Better for heat; for warm compresses.
Worse for cold drinks; in winter.
Causes cold, damp weather.

This toothache is one that always comes on after getting cold and chilled; it is sensitive to cold and better for heat, for example lying on a hot water bottle or drinking warm drinks.

RUMEX CRISPUS (Rumex)

Family name: Polygonaceae
Other names: Narrow-leafed/sour/curled/yellow dock; garden patience

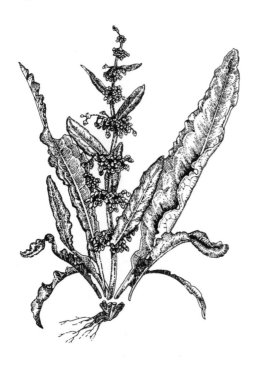

The yellow dock is a common weed that grows in arable farmland, on roadsides, in ditches and on waste ground throughout the world. Its leaves are narrow and curled at the edges, and the root is deep yellow, odourless and bitter tasting.

The root is the useful part of the plant: it has been used since ancient times as a mild tonic and laxative (its laxative action is very similar to that of rhubarb but it is less powerful); it has also been used to treat many diseases including diphtheria, cancer, rheumatism, piles, jaundice and obstinate skin diseases, especially ulcers, and it is widely regarded as a blood cleanser.

For the homeopathic preparation the fresh root is gathered at the end of the autumn before the frost has touched the plant. The tincture is made by chopping and pounding the root to a pulp and then mixing it with alcohol, before straining and succussing.

GENERAL SYMPTOMS

This remedy is only useful in acute prescribing for a particular type of cough, but it is very effective so I have included it here. The general symptoms are the same as the specific symptoms for the cough itself.

There are no notable emotional/mental symptoms.

PHYSICAL COMPLAINTS

Cough

Symptoms COUGH: in fits; constant; dry; irritating; tickling. PAINS IN CHEST: burning; sore, bruised; stitching. LARYNX raw.
Worse for lying down; for breathing in cold air; for fresh air; for change of temperature from warm to cold; for becoming cold; for cold air; on left side of body; in morning on waking; for talking; for being uncovered; for walking in the cold air.
The cough causes pains in the chest, usually on the left side or in the left lung, or under the sternum. These pains are worse on breathing in cold air, and patients will usually cover their heads/mouths with scarves so that only warm air is breathed. There is a feeling of rawness and tickling in the larynx and this makes the cough worse. Patients hawk up mucus from the back of the throat, where it gets stuck.

Sore throat

Symptoms THROAT: raw; sore; irritated. AIR PASSAGES irritated. VOICE lost.
Worse for breathing in cold air.

RUTA GRAVEOLENS (Ruta.)

Family name: Rutaceae
Common names: common rue; bitter herb; countryman's treacle

Rue is an evergreen, shrubby plant that thrives in poor soil in full sun. Indigenous to southern Europe, it was first cultivated in this country in the gardens of monks and is now found in herb gardens throughout the world.

The name *Ruta* is derived from the Greek *reuo* ('to set free'), because this herb was useful in so many diseases. Country people treated many complaints with it – coughs, croup, colic, and headaches, to name but a few. At one time it was used as a powerful defence against witches, and the Greeks used it for the indigestion they suffered when eating with strangers which they attributed to witchcraft. It was also highly thought of as a remedy that protected against

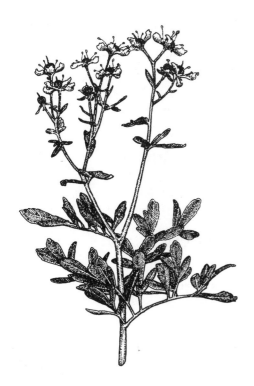

infections and poisoning. In ancient times rue seed drunk in wine was used to antidote the poison from mushrooms, toadstools, snakebites and the stings of scorpions, bees, hornets and wasps. Houses were sprinkled with water infused with rue in order to rid them of fleas. Engravers and painters ate rue to relieve their eyes when they were weak from overwork.

The homeopathic remedy is prepared from the fresh herb which is gathered in June, shortly before blooming, then chopped and pounded to a pulp. The expressed juice is left to stand in alcohol and succussed.

GENERAL SYMPTOMS

Pains: in bones; in parts lain on; sore, bruised.
Better for movement.
Worse for lying on painful part.

Like *Rhus toxicodendron*, *Ruta* is a remedy for sprains; the difference is that *Rhus tox* is indicated for damaged ligaments and *Ruta* is for injuries to the tendons and the periosteum (the covering of the bones). It can be very hard to differentiate between *Rhus tox* and *Ruta* in a sprain, and usually it will be *Rhus tox*'s clear general symptoms that guide you. *Ruta* is indicated where there are sore, bruised joint pains which feel worse when lying on the affected part of the body. There may be restlessness but not nearly so marked as in *Rhus tox*.

EMOTIONAL/MENTAL SYMPTOMS

Fearful of dying. **Weary**.

The emotional symptoms are not strongly marked, but during a fever the patient will feel scared, and may also be irritable and a little depressed.

PHYSICAL COMPLAINTS
Backache

Symptoms PAINS sore, bruised. With LAMENESS.
Better for lying on back.

Eye strain

Symptoms EYESIGHT: dim; weak. PAINS: aching; burning; strained.
Worse during the evening; at night; for poor light; for using eyes; for close work.
Causes too much close work; overstraining eyes.
Ruta will stimulate and strengthen the eye muscles and restore the sight where eyesight has become weak and dim after straining the eyes with fine work or too much reading (when the letters on the page seem to run together). This particular weakness of the eye occurs in people who do a great deal of close work for prolonged periods of time. It is not a remedy for inflammations of the eye.

Headache

Symptoms PAINS: in sides of head; sore, bruised. With EYE STRAIN (see above).
Causes eye strain
The head feels as if it has been beaten or crushed.

Injuries

Symptoms BRUISES on shins. PAINS bruised, sore.
Ruta is indicated for bruises to the covering of the bone (the periosteum), in particular bruises on the shins. These can be very painful injuries.

Joint pain

Symptoms PAINS: in hands; in feet; in lower back; in parts lain on; in bones; sore, bruised. With LAMENESS.
Worse for walking.

Sprains

Symptoms PAINS: bruised; constant; in ankle; in wrist. With EXHAUSTION; LAMENESS.
Worse for exercise; for pressure; for standing; for walking.
Used after *Arnica* has dealt with the swelling and bruising of sprains and strains, *Ruta* will finish off the

NB   SEE ALSO PAGES 203–26 FOR GENERAL ADVICE, DOS AND DON'TS.

healing. Hands and feet feel cold. The injured part feels lame and as if bruised and the pains are constant – there is no relief of pain from continued movement. Pressure is also painful. The person feels weak and weary.

Tennis elbow

Symptoms PAINS bruised, sore. With LAMENESS.
Worse for exercise.

These are potentially difficult injuries to deal with and should always be given a lot of time to heal in case the tendon itself is partially detached. *Ruta* will help to heal a damaged tendon, provided the joint is bandaged tightly and completely rested.

SARSAPARILLA (Sars.)

Family name: Liliaceae
Other names: wild liquorice; shot bush; small spikeard; rabbit root

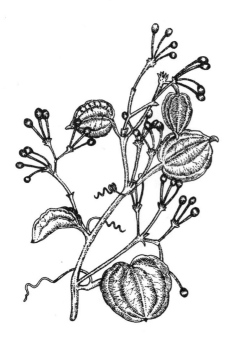

Sarsaparilla is a perennial climber found in certain parts of north and south America. It has long, slender, bitter-tasting rootlets which are poisonous if taken in large quantity, producing nausea, vomiting and a temporary loss of appetite.

The plant was brought to Europe in the mid-sixteenth century by explorers of the 'New World' and afterwards soon became a popular remedy to treat chronic rheumatism and obstinate skin diseases. The Moroccans used it in the treatment of leprosy. It was also regarded as a tonic and a blood purifier. It is one of the major flavouring ingredients of root beer.

The homeopathic preparation is made from the dried and powdered root, which is added to alcohol and succussed in the usual way.

GENERAL AND EMOTIONAL/ MENTAL SYMPTOMS

Sarsaparilla is a small remedy that has no marked general or emotional symptoms, but it is often needed for cystitis and I have therefore included it here.

PHYSICAL COMPLAINTS
Breastfeeding problems

Symptoms NIPPLES inverted.
This makes it very difficult to establish breastfeeding.

Cystitis

Symptoms DESIRE TO URINATE: ineffectual. PAINS cutting. URINATION: slow; dribbling; can only pass urine while standing. URINE: green; pale; with mucus; with sediment.
Worse at end of urination; during a menstrual period.
Causes getting chilled; cold, wet weather.
The person may pass urine without feeling it, but will experience unbearable pain at the end of urinating, and will yell with the pain. Urinating is difficult while sitting down, and the person may only be able to urinate freely while standing up. Even then she may only manage a feeble stream. Children with cystitis cry out before peeing because of the anticipated pain. The kidneys may also be painful (the right more so than the left) and inflamed (with cutting pains) – it is advisable to seek professional help before this point, but *Sarsaparilla* will help to relieve the pain in the meantime.

SEPIA (Sep.)

Family name: Dibranchiata
Other names: squid, cuttlefish

Cuttlefish are molluscs related to the octopus and squid, and are found most commonly in the Mediterranean and other European seas. Unlike most molluscs, which have shells outside their bodies, cuttlefish have soft, gelatinous bodies with tiny shells *inside*. They grow to one to two feet long, and swim

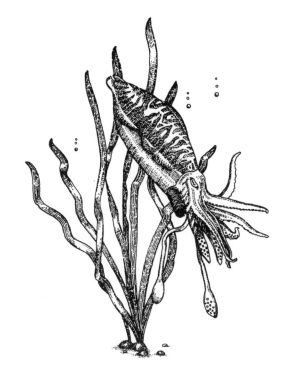

about rapidly by squirting jets of water from their bodies. They can change colour and squirt jets of ink as a protective, camouflaging device.

Sepia is the name given to the dried brownish-black ink, which is used as an artists' pigment; the raw ink is not fit for medicinal use and indeed was unknown to medicine until Hahnemann observed that a sickly artist friend of his licked his paintbrush frequently as he worked. He made a potency of the 'sepia' ink and cured the artist of his complaints.

For the homeopathic preparation the pure pigment is triturated.

GENERAL SYMPTOMS

Catches colds easily. Complaints from getting wet. **Craves** vinegar. **Discharges** yellow. **Dislikes** meat. **Face** pasty. **Pains** pressing. **Sweat:** cold; hot; profuse; smelly; sour; from slightest physical exertion; from mental exertion; from pain; on single parts of the body. **Symptoms** left-sided.
Better after eating; for vigorous exercise; for running; for fast walking.
Worse before/during/after menstrual period; at night; for cold; for fasting; for getting wet; for rest; for frosty air; for sweating; for touch; for walking in the wind; for mental/physical exertion; for writing.

Sepia is a remedy that has a profound effect on the female hormones and is therefore often needed during and after pregnancy, around the time of the menopause, and for problems with periods or problems that are exacerbated around the time of the menstrual period.

The typical *Sepia* face is yellow, earthy and pale, with a marked yellowness running across the saddle of the nose and dark rings under the eyes.

These are chilly types, with cold hands and feet, who are extremely sensitive to the cold in almost any shape or form. They sweat easily and profusely, when experiencing strong emotions or with any exertion of either the body or the mind. Coughing can also make them sweat. The sweat will smell sour and will make them feel worse and aggravate their symptoms.

They feel exhausted and run down. They have no muscle tone and they feel and look saggy; they feel as though there is something heavy inside that is dragging them down. This is a marvellous remedy for prolapse of the uterus, whatever the cause (though this is usually too many children too close together), and means that the trauma of an operation can be avoided. However, this condition does always require careful prescribing by a professional homeopath. Despite *Sepia* types' weakness, they are generally worse for rest, and exercising vigorously will energise their sluggish state. Eating will help temporarily (they are much worse for missing meals). They do not want to be touched or massaged.

EMOTIONAL/MENTAL SYMPTOMS

Angry from contradiction. **Anxious:** during a fever; during the evening. **Confused. Depressed. Desires** to be alone. **Dislikes** company; consolation; contradiction. **Forgetful. Indifferent:** to own children; to family; to loved ones; to work. **Irritable. Sensitive:** to music; to noise; to pain. **Sluggish. Tearful. Weepy.**

Sepia types are prone to dreadful emotional states, where they become sluggish, indifferent, irritable, weepy and depressed. *Sepia* has been found to be more useful for women than for men and is especially needed for the typical worn-out-mother-without-any-support syndrome, for women who are worn down by the cares of life and too many children with not enough time between them for their bodies to recover. This is the classical *Sepia* picture, though women may also be simply worn out from having too much to do and not enough personal resources to see them through it.

When in this depressed state, *Sepias* sag, mentally and physically. They sit silently, feeling empty and enjoying nothing in their lives, and feeling indifferent to all those things that formerly gave them enjoyment – such as their children and family, and their work.

They do not want any help and will respond badly to sympathy, preferring to be alone to avoid any further stress. Because thinking is so difficult and their brains seem to have ground to a halt the only thing they want to do is to be quiet and alone.

They will feel very much better if they drag themselves out of their torpor to do something strenuous, such as exercise, aerobics, dancing or spring cleaning. It is as if the circulation has slowed right down and the exercise gets it moving again. This is the only remedy that has this symptom to this degree. Children who need *Sepia* may be negative and sulky and indifferent to *their* work, that is, to playing! They may be afraid of being alone, of the dark (because of ghosts) but they will not want to be handled either. They become lazy and do not want to do anything, but once they have actually got going, or have, for example, arrived at the party, they are quite happy and have a good time.

PHYSICAL COMPLAINTS

Backache

Symptoms PAINS: in lower back; aching; dragging down.
Better for pressure.
Worse during the afternoon; at night; before/during menstrual period; for bending down; for sitting.
The lower back feels weak and tired and as if it has been hit with a hammer.

Cold sores

Symptoms SORES on lips.

Common cold

Symptoms NASAL CATARRH: green; dirty yellow; yellow-green; drips down back of throat. SENSE OF SMELL lost.

Constipation

Symptoms BELLY/STOMACH feels full. STOOLS: hard; large. STRAINING ineffectual.
Worse during a menstrual period.
Causes pregnancy.
This is for the type of acute constipation that can accompany pregnancy or a woman's periods. The person will strain to pass a large, hard stool but will be unable to.

Cough

Symptoms BREATHING fast. COUGH: constant at night; dry; exhausting; hacking; irritating; loose; must sit up to cough; rattling; short; disturbs sleep; tickling; violent; wakes from the cough at night. MUCUS: copious; yellow; white; tastes salty.

Better for sitting up.
Worse at night; during the evening in bed; for lying down.
The patient coughs up lots of salty white or yellow mucus. Chest feels constricted (tight) or oppressed and the ribs may hurt from coughing. The air passages feel irritated and the cough seems to come from the stomach and is very violent, especially after lying down at night. Patient sweats after coughing and feels worse for it.

Cystitis

Symptoms DESIRE TO URINATE: constant dragging down in pelvis; urgent. PAINS pressing. URINATION frequent; slow (has to wait a long time for it to start). URINE: cloudy; dark brown; red; scanty; smelly; with sediment.
This cystitis is common after childbirth. The patient will have a constant dragging-down sensation in the pelvis, and she will have to rush to pass urine or it will escape involuntarily, because of saggy muscles in the pelvic area. She may then have to wait for it to start once sitting on the toilet.

Exhaustion

Symptoms EXHAUSTION: nervous; sudden.
Worse on getting up in the morning; during a menstrual period; for sweating; for walking.
Causes sweating.
The legs feel stiff and weak. This often accompanies the *Sepia* hot flushes, or pregnancy.

Eye inflammation

Symptoms EYES: burning. EYELIDS: glued together; swollen.
Worse after a walk; during the evening; for reading.
The eyes feel sore, as if there were sand in them.

Faintness

Symptoms HEAT with faintness. COLDNESS after faint.
Worse for exercise; during a fever; during menstrual period; in a stuffy room.
Sepia types can easily feel faint and are always generally worse for standing for any length of time.

Fever

Symptoms With SWEATING (see General Symptoms).
Worse in the autumn; for sweating; for being covered.
Causes anger.
Sepia may be needed in a flu or any other infection where the characteristic general and emotional symptoms are also present. The accompanying fever is often severe with external heat and internal chilliness.

The feeling of heat is followed by chills with shaking and no thirst. Being covered up warmly makes patients feel uneasy (which is an unusual and helpful symptom); they do not want to be covered even when chilled.

Hair loss

Symptoms HAIR falls out.
Causes menopause.

Headache

Symptoms EXTREMITIES icy cold. PAINS: in bones; bursting; pressing; shooting; tearing; throbbing; in waves.
Better after eating; for fresh air.
Worse for bending down; during menstrual period; for getting head cold; for travelling.
Causes artificial light.
Pains can be almost anywhere in the head, although the left side will often be more affected than the right.

Hot flushes

Symptoms FLUSH moves up the body.
Worse during the afternoon/evening; after sweating.
The hot flush feels as if warm water were being poured over the body, and/or the flush starts in the body and moves upwards.

Insomnia

Symptoms WAKING after 3 a.m. With SLEEPINESS.
The person wakes in the night and can't get back to sleep, and may lie awake thinking dismal thoughts. In the morning he or she feels exhausted.

Labour pains

Symptoms PAINS: distressing; severe.
The pains drag down and are much better for vigorous exercise. *Sepia* characteristic emotional symptoms will be present.

Nausea

Symptoms BELLY/STOMACH feel empty. PAINS gnawing.
Worse after eating; before breakfast; during the morning; for milk; for pork.
Causes pregnancy.
There is an empty, sinking feeling in the stomach that is only temporarily relieved while eating, is often accompanied by a headache and is worse when thinking about food or eating.

Period problems

Symptoms PERIODS painful. PAINS: aching; dragging down; dull; pressing; sore, bruised.
Better for crossing the legs.
Worse between 9 a.m. and 6 p.m.; during the afternoon/morning; during the period; for standing; for walking.
The insides of the pelvis feel as if they will fall out. This feeling is often worse when urinating. The periods may be very short.

Thrush (genital)

Symptoms DISCHARGE: burning; copious; like cottage cheese; like egg white; smelly; yellow. With DRYNESS; ITCHING.
Worse before/between menstrual periods; during pregnancy.
The simple thrush that occurs during pregnancy, where the woman feels exhausted and worn down, will respond well to *Sepia*.

Toothache

Symptoms PAINS: radiate to the ears; pulling; stitching; tearing; throbbing.
Worse for biting teeth together; for cold drinks/food; during menstrual period; during pregnancy; for touch; for hot drinks.

Travel sickness

Symptoms With BILIOUSNESS; HEADACHE (see above); NAUSEA (see above).
Worse after eating; during the morning.
Causes pregnancy.

Vomiting

Symptoms VOMIT: bile; smelly.
Worse after eating.
Causes pregnancy.
The person may feel better for eating, but the improvement will be temporary.

SILICA (Sil.)

Other names: rock crystal; pure flint; silex

Silica is the most common mineral in the Earth's crust. It is the main constituent of most rocks, and comes in many forms, for example sand, quartz, agate and opal. *Silica* sand is used industrially to make portland cement, concrete, mortar and sandstone. It is also used in grinding and polishing glass and stone; in

NB   SEE ALSO PAGES 203–26 FOR GENERAL ADVICE, DOS AND DON'TS.

foundry moulds; in the manufacture of glass, ceramics, enamelware and paper. *Silica* is an essential element of the supporting structures of many plants such as the stalks of grain or grass. Normal body tissues contain only traces of the element, but it is a component of teeth, nails, hair and connective tissues.

It is almost unknown as a medicine outside homeopathy, as it was thought to be inert. The homeopathic preparation is made in a number of ways: Hahnemann, who first proved it, obtained it from mountain crystal; and a British method dilutes *silica* powder with sodium carbonate by trituration.

GENERAL SYMPTOMS

Catch colds easily. Complaints from: getting feet wet; change of weather to cold. **Dislikes** meat. **Glands** swollen. **Pains** stinging. **Sweat:** at night, during sleep; profuse; smelly; sour. **Thirsty. Ankles** weak.
Better for heat; for wrapping up head.
Worse for change of weather; for cold; for damp; for draughts; for fresh air; for getting feet wet; for touch; for being uncovered; for wet weather.

Silica types feel the cold intensely and have icy-cold hands and feet. They are easily tired and chilled; if they go out into the cold after a swim, or if they get wet and chilled in the rain they become sick, with a cold or cough. They are also sensitive to draughts and changes of weather, and are always better for warmth and being wrapped up well, especially the head.

Silica individuals sweat at night, particularly on the back of the head and neck (like *Calcarea carbonica*, though not so profuse). The sweat smells sour and their feet are characteristically sweaty and smelly, to the point of eating holes in their socks. The feet may smell even without sweating.

They have trouble assimilating their food and therefore their bones do not form as well as in other children. They have weak ankles and are slow in learning to walk and slow to teethe. Their fontanelles close slowly. There are white spots on the nails, and the nails themselves do not grow strong and healthily but split easily. The skin is often dry and the mouth may crack at the corners.

EMOTIONAL/MENTAL SYMPTOMS

Anxious. Complaints from: mental strain; shock. Poor **concentration. Confused. Conscientious. Dislikes** consolation. **Irritable. Jumpy. Mild. Sensitive** to noise; to pain. **Restless.** Lack of **self-confidence. Shy. Sluggish.**
Worse for being consoled.

These are people who typically lack stamina both mentally and physically – who lack 'grit' (flintiness). They become worn out easily from too much work (usually mental) because they do not have the stamina to keep going under stress.

Alternatively they can be very 'gritty' – able to work all hours under pressure, extremely conscientious and able to sustain superhuman feats of endurance. They collapse only when the job in hand has been completed.

They are very shy and exceedingly anxious about appearing in public because they fear they will fail or do badly. They are unassertive, lacking in confidence and will give way rather than take a position and fight for it, although conversely they can be stubborn and wilful and develop fixed ideas.

They become irritable if they are consoled when feeling low. They feel restless and nervous inside and become over-sensitive to noise, especially small noises, and will startle easily from unexpected noises. **NB.** A '*Silica* type' may well need *Pulsatilla* if he or she develops an acute illness, and conversely *Silica* is often needed after *Pulsatilla* has worked well but some symptoms remain, for example the cough (see below).

PHYSICAL COMPLAINTS

Abscesses

Symptoms ABSCESSES of glands; of roots of teeth.
Silica will bring to a head abscesses that are in the process of forming.

Athlete's foot

Symptoms CRACKS between toes. With SWEAT: on feet; profuse; smelly.

Backache

Symptoms PAINS: sore, bruised; stitching. With LAMENESS; STIFFNESS; WEAKNESS.
Worse on getting up from sitting; at night; for pressure; for sitting.
Causes a fall onto the back; injury to coccyx; manual labour.

Bedwetting

Causes injury to back; worms.
For children who wet the bed after a fall or after an attack of worms.

Breastfeeding problems

Symptoms BREASTS: inflamed; painful; lumpy. NIPPLES: cracked, inverted. PAINS: in breast; cutting; stitching. BREAST ABSCESSES.

Worse while nursing; in left breast.
The mother experiences sudden sharp pains while the child is nursing. The back may ache while nursing.

Broken bones

Symptoms BONES slow to mend.

Common cold

Symptoms NASAL CATARRH: dry; hard crusts; smelly; thick. SINUSES painful. SENSE OF SMELL/TASTE lost. SNEEZING difficult.
Sinuses become blocked up; the nose is dry and blocked and the nostrils become sore and ulcerated.

Constipation

Symptoms Ineffectual STRAINING. PAIN burning after stool. STOOL: hard; knotty; large; 'shy'.
Worse before/during menstrual period.
The muscles in the bowels are weak, making it difficult to pass stools; the stools are partially expelled and then slip back.

Corns

Symptoms CORNS inflamed; soft. PAINS: sore; tearing.

Cough

Symptoms COUGH irritating. MUCUS: lumpy; thick; yellow.
Better for hot drinks.
Worse in morning on waking; for getting cold; for uncovering feet or head.
Silica is especially useful for lingering winter coughs that start after getting chilled, or wet and chilled, and that do not clear up easily with the indicated or constitutional remedy.

Diarrhoea

Symptoms IN TEETHING CHILDREN. FLATULENCE: wind smelly.
Better for heat; for wrapping up warmly; for warmth of bed.
Causes teething.

Earache

Symptoms EAR: feels blocked; itching in the ears. PAINS: behind the ear; tearing.
The Eustachian tube is itchy and full of mucus. If there is a discharge it will be bloody, smelly and thick.

Exhaustion

Symptoms EXHAUSTION nervous.
Causes diarrhoea.

Eye inflammation

Symptoms DISCHARGE yellow. EYE sore.
Worse for cold air.
Causes a foreign body in the eye.
This soreness and inflammation is caused by a foreign body in the eye. If the foreign body is still lodged in the eye, *Silica* taken internally will help to expel it.

Fever

Worse for movement; for being uncovered; in the evening; at night.
The patient feels icy cold and shivery all day, and this may be one-sided. The sweat is profuse and sour smelling, and if it is suppressed in any way this will exacerbate the general (and specific) condition.

Fingernails

Symptoms NAILS: split easily; weak. With WHITE SPOTS.

Flatulence

Symptoms WIND: smelly; obstructed (difficult to expel).

Gum boils

Simple gum boils with no other symptoms respond very well to a short course of *Silica*.

Headache

Symptoms PAINS: in back of head; in forehead; spreading to top of head/to eyes/to right eye; in sinuses; burning; hammering; pressing; sore, bruised; throbbing; violent.
Better for closing eyes; for lying in a quiet, dark room; for heat; for wrapping up head.
Worse for getting chilled; for getting feet/head cold; for daylight; for getting up from lying down; for jarring; for walking up stairs/heavily.
Causes cold air; damp weather; draughts; eye strain; overwork; working in artificial light; travelling (car, coach, train, etc.).
This headache is often a result of sinus catarrh; it settles over the eyes and the forehead feels heavy. The head and feet will feel cold.

Injuries

Symptoms CUTS/WOUNDS: slow to heal; inflamed; painful; with pus; with foreign body; suppurate. SCARS: become lumpy; break open; painful.
Causes splinter.
Silica cuts and wounds become infected easily and heal slowly; the skin looks unhealthy.

Insomnia

Symptoms Vivid NIGHTMARES. SLEEP restless.
Worse after midnight; after waking.

Mumps

Symptoms GLANDS: painful; swollen.
Better for heat.
Worse for cold.

Sore throat

Symptoms THROAT dry. GLANDS swollen. PAINS stitching. TONSILS: swollen/inflamed. With HAIR SENSATION at back of tongue.
Worse for getting cold; for swallowing; for uncovering throat.

Splinters

Symptoms WOUND inflamed.
Silica taken internally will help to push out foreign bodies from the skin, especially if the wound has become inflamed. It heals wounds once the pus has started discharging.

Teething

Symptoms PAINFUL IN CHILDREN. DIFFICULT. SLOW. With DIARRHOEA (see above); TOOTHACHE (see below). *Silica* children can take years to produce teeth and will get coughs, colds and diarrhoea during this time. *Silica* will help with the infections and with the teeth.

Toothache

Symptoms SWELLING: of face; of glands.
Better for wrapping up head.
Worse in winter.
Causes teething; abscess; winter.

Vomiting

Symptoms IN BREASTFED BABIES.
Worse for milk.
This vomiting occurs in babies who refuse their mothers' milk and/or vomit it up. Reconstituted milk may be no better.

SPONGIA TOSTA (Spo.)

Family name: Ceratospongiae
Other name: sea sponge

Sponges are one of the most primitive forms of life known to man and are found in seas worldwide. They

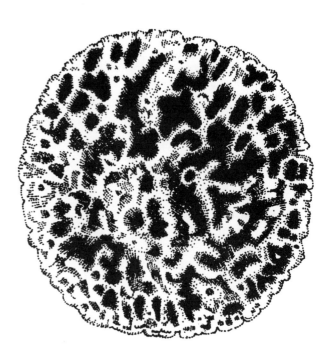

attach themselves to rocks and were regarded by early naturalists as plants because of their branching form and lack of movement, but they actually contain both DNA and RNA as well as many other substances common to all animal life. Sponges have remarkable powers of regeneration: any piece cut or broken from an adult sponge will attach to a suitable surface and re-form into a new plant.

A commercial sponge is simply the 'skeleton' that surrounds the numerous cells of the animal. The sponge was a familiar household item in ancient Greece and Rome, where they were used as mops and to apply paint, amongst other things. During the Middle Ages powdered burnt sponge was used medicinally for many complaints.

To prepare the homeopathic preparation, the sponge is roasted brown, covered with alcohol and left to stand, and then strained and succussed.

GENERAL SYMPTOMS

Worse after sleep; for cold wind; for movement; for wearing tight clothing; for tobacco.

Spongia is a specific for certain types of cough, croup and sore throat. Patients feel worse when they become excited or exert themselves. They wake from sleep with a sense of suffocation and much anxiety, finding difficulty in catching their breath. They are intolerant of tight clothing because of their difficulty in breathing. *Spongia* is often indicated in cases where *Aconite* has been given but failed to help.

EMOTIONAL/MENTAL SYMPTOMS

Anxious on waking. **Tearful** during a fever.

This is a smallish remedy with few strong emotional symptoms. The patients feel worse on waking, and will wake up with a start and be anxious and fearful, and sometimes depressed. May wake in the night with the same symptoms.

PHYSICAL COMPLAINTS

Cough

Symptoms Cough: barking; constant; dry; hollow; in fits; irritating; tickling. Breathing: difficult; rough. Pains in Chest: burning; sore, bruised. Voice hoarse.
Better for eating and drinking.
Worse during the day; for excitement.
The cough is worse for excitement and may even have been caused by too much excitement. Eating sweets may aggravate the cough but it is generally better for eating and drinking, especially warm things. The chest is sore and bruised from coughing. Breathing is difficult and may sound loud between bouts of coughing. This difficulty is worse after a sleep and for exercise, and sometimes talking can aggravate also. The voice is hoarse, crowing and hollow. The bronchial tubes are inflamed (bronchitis).

Croup

Symptoms With cough (see above).
This is one of the main croup remedies. It is usually accompanied by *Spongia* general symptoms, though it may be difficult to differentiate between an *Aconite* croup and a *Spongia* croup as they both have the acute anxiety, and *Spongia* croup is worse at night, around midnight, as is *Aconite* croup. If *Aconite* is indicated and fails to help then *Spongia* will do the trick.

Exhaustion

Worse for slightest exertion; for movement.

Sore throat

Symptoms Throat dry. Pains: burning; sore. Voice hoarse.
Worse for coughing; for singing; for swallowing; for sweet food/drinks; for talking; for touch.
The larynx is sore and sensitive to touch and the voice is hoarse and hollow sounding. Throat feels raw, rough and sore, especially when coughing; it is swollen and feels as if there is a plug in it.

STAPHYSAGRIA (Stap.)

Family name: Ranunculaceae
Other names: stavesacre; palmated larkspur; Delphinium Staphysagria

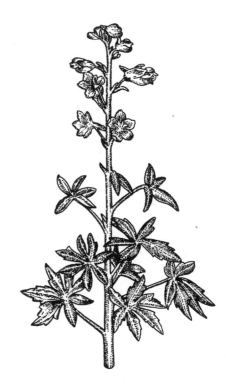

This is a biennial plant that flourishes in poor soils in southern Europe. It grows to a height of one to two feet, has large leaves resembling a grape vine and produces blue-purple flowers from April to August.

Staphysagria is an ancient remedy employed in medicine as early as the time of Hippocrates. It was used to cause vomiting and purging, even though it was known that its internal use was dangerous. Externally, it was used for warts, lice and for itches. It was also used for toothaches and other painful conditions of the throat and gums, as the seeds produced a strong salivation on being chewed. The herbalist Gerard says, 'The seed . . . chewed in the mouth draweth forth much moisture from the head, and cleanseth the braine.'

The poisonings produce symptoms of excitement followed by depression and extreme sensitivity of all the nerves, which give way to paralysis, a slowing down of the pulse and finally death caused by asphyxia.

The homeopathic remedy is made from the seeds by trituration.

NB SEE ALSO PAGES 203–26 FOR GENERAL ADVICE, DOS AND DON'TS.

GENERAL SYMPTOMS

Anaemia. Sweat from mental exertion.
Worse for exertion; for fasting; for tobacco; for touch.

These individuals are extremely sensitive, both physically and emotionally, and they suffer pain more acutely than others. Wounds and cuts are unusually painful and sensitive to touch, especially if there is a feeling of having been assaulted, with resultant indignation.

They feel generally worse for exercise, smoky rooms and missing meals, and are especially irritable after an afternoon nap.

EMOTIONAL/MENTAL SYMPTOMS

Violently **angry. Apathetic. Capricious. Complaints from:** disappointed love; grief; humiliation; indignation; mental strain; reprimands; suppressed anger/emotions. **Forgetful. Irritable. Sensitive:** to pain; to rudeness.

This is a remedy for sensitive, touchy people – adults and children – who are very easily offended. They cannot tolerate rudeness in others although they may well be rude themselves. They suppress their feelings, brooding and letting little out. In particular, anger will be suppressed; they will fume inside and may even appear sweet and compliant on the surface. Afterwards, they quickly become exhausted and will say that they feel shaky and cannot sleep, work or speak; and they may well get a headache.

This suppression of angry feelings can turn into an active and acid resentment. Any complaint that has been caused by or accompanied by a sense of violation with ensuing indignation and resentment will call for *Staphysagria*. Children may become ill after they have been told off or you may notice them ailing after having been bullied or humiliated, even though they appear to have taken it well. *Staphysagria* will be indicated for adults who have suffered at the hands of an angry boss or spouse, or are in any situation where they feel violated while seething inside. They do not want to be touched when they are feeling low or upset.

These people cannot say no. They are accommodating and they allow the pressure to build up inside; this ends in a violent outburst of rage or getting sick or both. When in this state they will often throw things (as do *Chamomillas*).

PHYSICAL COMPLAINTS

Bites/stings

The bites are very painful and sensitive to touch.

Colic

Symptoms PAINS cramping.
Worse after drinking.
Causes indigestion; vexation.
Children (or adults!) who are told off and do not stand up for themselves sometimes produce stomach-aches as a result. They may not admit to the 'event' that sparked off the pains unless questioned closely.

Cough

Symptoms COUGH tickling.
Causes suppressed anger.
The larynx and air passages feel irritated with this cough.

Cystitis

Symptoms DESIRE TO URINATE frequent. URINATION: frequent; involuntary. URINE scanty.
This cystitis often follows a sense of being assaulted either physically or emotionally, where the person's own feelings and/or needs were not expressed.

Exhaustion

Symptoms EXHAUSTION nervous. TREMBLING.
This is for people who become worn out, anaemic, trembly and exhausted from suppressing their feelings.

Eye injuries

Symptoms WOUND punctured; very sensitive to touch.

Headache

Symptoms PAINS: in back of head; in forehead; pulling; pressing; sore, bruised.
Worse for touch.
Causes emotions; excitement; grief; vexation.
These are headaches of people who cannot cope with stressful emotions. They usually suppress their anger, and become resentful.

Injuries

Symptoms CUTS/WOUNDS: painful; to nerve-rich parts. PAINS tearing.
Worse for touch.
Causes accident; childbirth; episiotomy; surgery.
Staphysagria is for wounds or injuries where there are feelings of humiliation, indignation and anger. This might be caused by an operation to a sphincter (anus, urethra, stomach, etc.), after any operation, especially if more was done than expected, after a mechanical childbirth with pain afterwards and possibly stitches,

or it may simply be pain following an unpleasant examination.

Staphysagria wounds are typically caused by sharp, cutting instruments such as glass; the pains (and those following surgery) are stinging, smarting. Injuries to the eyes or eyelids where there is inflammation can call for *Staphysagria* as long as the accompanying emotional symptoms are present.

Styes

These are sensitive to touch and are often accompanied by *Staphysagria* emotional symptoms.

Toothache

Symptoms PAINS: spread to the ears; gnawing; tearing; in decayed teeth. IN CHILDREN.
Worse after eating; for cold drinks; during menstrual period.
This is for people whose teeth decayed and turned black early, and who have toothache in the decayed teeth, especially with drinking cold drinks.

Travel sickness

Staphysagria is the remedy to prescribe for travel sickness where the individual is extremely difficult, stroppy and indignant that this should be 'happening to him or her'.

SULPHUR (Sul.)

Other names: brimstone; flowers of sulphur

Sulphur occurs naturally and is an essential chemical constituent of all living tissue. It is one of the substances thrown out by a volcanic eruption; the sulphur dries round the edge of the volcano, and this is similar to a 'sulphur eruption' where the pus is aggravated by heat, oozes out and then forms crusts on the skin.

Its wide commercial application includes its use in the manufacture of gunpowder, dyes, fungicides and insecticides, to harden rubber and to make sulphuric acid.

It has a long history in medicine. It was considered a preventive for epidemic illnesses, and 'Flowers of sulphur' were burned to fumigate rooms occupied by people suffering from infectious diseases (the burning sulphur produces sulphur dioxide, a powerful disinfectant). It was taken regularly, along with molasses, to 'cleanse' the gut, and has been used for more than 2000 years to treat skin diseases, including acne and scabies; other uses in orthodox medicine include its use as a laxative, for chronic bronchial catarrh and for rheumatism.

The homeopathic preparation is made from pure sulphur (a fine yellow-greenish, gritty powder) either by trituration or as a tincture in strong alcohol.

GENERAL SYMPTOMS

Anaemia. Breath smells. **Complaints from** change of weather from cold to warm. **Discharges** smelly; sour; watery. **Dislikes** meat. **Face:** red; sallow; red in spots. **Glands** swollen. **Likes:** spicy food; sweets. **Lips:** cracked; dry; red. **Pains** burning. **Sweat:** profuse; smelly; sour; from slightest physical exertion. **Symptoms** left-sided. **Taste:** mouth tastes bitter; bad. **Thirsty:** extreme; for large quantities; for water. **Tongue:** white-coated; red edges and tip.
Better for fresh air.
Worse for bathing; for change of weather to warm; for draughts; for exertion; for fasting; for heat; for milk; around 10–11 a.m.; for standing; in stuffy rooms; for warmth of bed.

Sulphur types come in all shapes and sizes, but they seem always to look untidy and/or unwashed, especially the children, no matter how often they wash or change clothes. In fact, their manner of dress will usually give them away – there is always something missing such as an odd sock, or a hem coming down, or a collar escaped from inside a jumper (things no self-respecting *Arsenicum* would put up with!). They are either completely indifferent to how they look or do not notice if they are dirty. They have hot feet, and so can easily wear sandals the whole year round. They are lazy and they hate to wash; they often feel worse for it and do not in fact look much cleaner for it. They slump when sitting and stoop when walking and are always worse for having to stand up for long – they make straight for a bar stool in a pub!

They have markedly red faces and red lips which can become dry and cracked when they fall ill. The tongue is often white coated with red edges and tip. They are extremely thirsty types who will consume large quantities of tap water whether sick or well.

These people are sensitive to heat and are always worse for being in a stuffy room and getting overheated; they are better for fresh air. Their discharges are usually hot, smelly and burning. They sweat profusely and feel worse while sweating. Hot flushes during the menopause will respond well to *Sulphur*, providing the general and emotional/mental symptoms fit.
NB. This remedy is hailed for its effect on eczema and skin rashes, but I strongly advise you not to prescribe for these complaints without consulting a professional homeopath, as the aggravations can be severe and need to be monitored carefully.

EMOTIONAL/MENTAL SYMPTOMS

Angry. Anxious in the evening. **Confused. Critical. Depressed. Discontented. Impatient. Indifferent** to personal appearance. **Irritable. Lazy. Quarrelsome. Restless. Sluggish** in children.

Sulphur children are curious and bright and drive their parents mad asking endless questions, mostly preceded with 'Why. . . ?' As they grow older they develop into people with many ideas who find it difficult to bring these ideas from the land of dreams into the land of reality. At one extreme they are successful academics and at the other they are unrealistic dreamers, or the so-called 'ragged philosophers'. The nearest to this in modern terms are the hippies with their endless ideals and theories, bare feet and unkempt appearances. They may start many things and never finish anything, and the further away they are from realising their ideas, the sicker they become.

These individuals are sloppy, lazy and disorganised; they feel constantly rushed and hurried and would really rather not work at all if they can avoid it. Mess doesn't bother them, although they may get periodical cravings for a sort of limited external order. They are hoarders and cannot throw anything away. However, despite their untidiness and sloppiness, they may have a strong feeling of self-disgust for their own bodily functions. Other remedies have this symptom but it is curious in such a slob!

Sulphur types are basically self centred, impatient, irritable and critical of others and how they run their lives; they have lots of ideas and theories of how they themselves could do it better. They suffer from all sorts of worries which plague them in the evening and stop them sleeping at night.

PHYSICAL COMPLAINTS

Backache

Symptoms BACK: feels weak/tired. PAINS: in lower spine; aching; sore, bruised. With STIFFNESS; WEAKNESS.
Worse after period of long sitting; for bending down; during a menstrual period; on getting up from sitting; at night; for standing; for walking.

Bedwetting

These are children who are generally dry at night but start bedwetting when they fall ill.

Boils

Symptoms BOILS itching.

Breastfeeding problems

Symptoms BREAST ABSCESS: inflamed. BREASTS red. The breasts may be itchy.

Chicken pox *see* Measles

Common cold

Symptoms NASAL CATARRH: smelly; dirty yellow. NOSE: dry; itching. With frequent SNEEZING; EYE INFLAMMATION (see below).
The nose is dry and itchy and the tip is red. It may bleed when blown. The person may smell unpleasant smells.

Cough

Symptoms BREATHING fast. COUGH: disturbs sleep; dry during the evening/at night, loose during the day/morning; painful; irritating; racking; suffocative. CHEST congested. LARYNX raw. MUCUS green.
Worse for coughing; during evening in bed; during the morning; at night; for lying down.
The person will wake from the cough and his or her sides will hurt from coughing. The larynx feels irritated and raw, as if there were dust in it. The patient may have difficulty breathing in a warm room and be better for fresh air; usually wants the windows to be open.

Cramp

Symptoms CRAMP: in the thighs; in legs; in calves; in soles of feet.
Worse at night; in bed; while walking.
These cramps should be accompanied by the *Sulphur* general and emotional symptoms.

Cystitis

Symptoms DESIRE TO URINATE: frequent; urgent. PAINS burning. URINE: burning; brown (like beer); copious; scanty; smelly.
Worse on getting up in the morning; at night; during urination.
The patient has to hurry to pass water to prevent it escaping, but will then pass only a few drops and dribbles each time.

Diarrhoea

Symptoms IN CHILDREN. DIARRHOEA: during the morning only; drives person out of bed; painless. FLATULENCE: smelly. PAINS: burning; cramping. STOOLS: slimy; smelly; sour; watery.
Better for passing wind.
Worse around 5 a.m.; in the morning; at night; for standing.
Causes beer.

The person wakes up early with a sudden urge to pass a stool, or has the urge just after getting up. There is rumbling before, and pains are felt in the belly before, during and even after passing a stool. The anus becomes sore and red after passing a stool, especially in children.

Earache

Symptoms PAINS: aching; lacerating; stitching; tearing. With painful NOISES IN EAR.
Worse in left ear; for noises.
There are roaring and ringing noises in the ear, which are more noticeable when the person is in bed. The external parts of the ear itch.

Exhaustion

Worse during the afternoon; for the heat of the sun; for talking.
Causes hunger; talking; walking.

Eye inflammation

Symptoms EYES: burning; gritty; sensitive to light; itching; watering. EYELIDS: itching in daytime only; burning; red.
Worse for washing eyes.
The eyes are glued together in the mornings. They may be dry, as if there were sand in them. They water easily in the fresh air and are sensitive to bright sunlight.

Fever

Symptoms HEAT alternating with chills. With SWEATING (see General Symptoms); SHIVERING.
Worse at night; for thinking.
The person feels alternately chilled and hot. Fever with sweating comes on after waking or it may be bad in the night if the person is unable to sleep. He or she feels worse whilst sweating, and hot, especially on the soles of the feet, which are poked out of the bed.

Flatulence

Symptoms BELLY/STOMACH: bloated; gurgling; rumbling. WIND: smelly; of rotten eggs.
Better for passing wind.

Hair loss

Symptoms HAIR falls out.
Causes childbirth.

Hayfever

Symptoms With COMMON COLD (see above); EYE INFLAMMATION (see above).

Headache

Symptoms HEAD: feels constricted; feels full/hot. PAINS: in forehead; burning; bursting; hammering; pressing; in top of head; throbbing. With NAUSEA.
Better for cold.
Worse after eating; for bending down; for blowing nose; for coughing; on getting up; during the morning; for sneezing.
Causes damp weather; excited conversation; winter.
There is a feeling of constriction or tightness, as if a band or hoop or string were tied around the head. The head feels full and hot, especially in bed or in a stuffy room. The headache may recur weekly, especially on a Sunday when the person tries to relax!

Indigestion

Symptoms BELLY/STOMACH bloated; feels empty around 11 a.m. BELCHING: empty; sour. FLATULENCE: wind smells of rotten eggs. PAINS burning.
Worse after eating; after drinking milk.
The person may suddenly feel very hungry mid morning, after not wanting to eat breakfast, and will need to eat to avoid feeling faint, weak and headachey. The appetite may, however, vanish at the sight of food. The stomach feels full and heavy after eating, and rumbles and gurgles.

Insomnia

Symptoms Unpleasant DREAMS. SLEEP: disturbed; unrefreshing; restless. WAKING: frequent; late.
Better for short naps.
Worse after 3, 4 or 5 a.m.
The *Sulphur* insomniac always wakes tired, however much she sleeps. She feels sleepy in the daytime and will be refreshed then by a short catnap. At night her feet get hot and burn in bed; she has to poke them out of bed to cool them down so she can sleep. Wakes in the early hours of the morning, often from cold, and may be unable to get back to sleep. She is very restless, and has nightmares when lying on her back. She may have to get out of bed around 5 a.m. to pass a stool.

Joint pain

Symptoms PAINS: burning; tearing.
Worse for walking; for warmth of bed.
There is a feeling of heat in the joints, and a general restlessness.

Measles

Symptoms SKIN RASH: red; burning; itching maddeningly. With COUGH (see above); FEVER (see above).
Worse for heat.
Sulphur is often needed where recovery is slow from a

NB   SEE ALSO PAGES 203–26 FOR GENERAL ADVICE, DOS AND DON'TS.

childhood illness. It can help to relieve the itching of measles, German measles or chicken pox if it is severe, very red, and much worse for heat (of bed or a hot bath). The children will be restless, feverish and sweaty, and should fit the general picture. They will be thirsty and hungry but will eat very little. Chicken pox rash becomes crusty, smelly and weeps after scratching.

Nosebleeds

Worse for blowing the nose.

Prickly heat

Symptoms With *Sulphur* general and emotional/mental symptoms.

Sore throat

Symptoms THROAT dry; raw. CHOKING sensation. PAINS: burning; raw; sore; stitching. TONSILS swollen. VOICE hoarse.
Worse for coughing; for swallowing.
The larynx is dry, as if there were dust in it. The pain and rawness in the throat are worse for coughing, and the voice is most hoarse in the mornings.

Toothache

Symptoms PAINS: spreading to the ears; throbbing.
Worse for cold air; for washing with cold water; for fresh air; at night in bed.
Causes draughts.

SULPHURIC ACID (Sul-ac.)

Common name: oil of vitriol

Sulphuric acid is a dense, oily liquid, colourless or brown, made by combining sulphur water and oxygen; it exists in its natural free state only in the Rio Vinagre in South America. It is strongly corrosive, able to dissolve most metals, and it is also highly reactive.

Sulphuric acid is considered to be one of the most important industrial chemicals, as it is employed in the manufacture of practically all industrial products.

Medicinally this powerful acid was used in the Middle Ages for treating ulcers in the mouth and the throat, but its terrible burning side effects led to it being abandoned as a medicine soon afterwards. It has been used as an astringent for diarrhoea and was occasionally prescribed to stimulate the appetite. 'Sulphuric acid lemonade' has been used by lead workers as a preventive of plumbism (lead poisoning).

The homeopathic preparation is made from sulphuric acid diluted with water and then succussed.

GENERAL SYMPTOMS

Anaemia.
Worse for alcohol; for heat; during the evening; mid morning.

Sulphuric acid people are anaemic, chilly types who feel hurried and trembly inside. They usually feel worse after drinking anything alcoholic, and their worst times are mornings and evenings.

EMOTIONAL/MENTAL SYMPTOMS

Irritable. Feeling of being **hurried**: while eating; at work; while writing; while walking. **Moody.**

In spite of feeling absolutely exhausted, *Sulphuric acid* types feel rushed and hurried inside and do everything 'at a pace'. They bolt their food, walk quickly, and work in a frantic way, including writing quickly. They feel driven inside and cannot do things fast enough. Their moods may be changeable, swinging from being reasonable and agreeable to being irritable.

PHYSICAL COMPLAINTS

Bruises

Symptoms BRUISES: bluish-black; slow to heal.
Sulphuric acid will finish the healing of bruises that turn bluish-black and do not clear up in spite of having been given *Arnica* and/or *Ledum*.

Diarrhoea

Symptoms BELCHING sour. STOOLS: soft; stringy; yellow. VOMIT sour.
Stools are bright yellowy-orange, like saffron, and there will be a feeling of emptiness and weakness after passing a stool. If the stomach is upset, there will be sour burps and vomiting.

Exhaustion

Symptoms With TREMBLING.
Worse after passing a stool.
People needing *Sulphuric acid* suffer from extreme lassitude and, although this may not be visible on the surface, they feel trembly inside.

Hot flushes

Causes Menopause.
These hot flushes are accompanied by the typical *Sulphuric acid* emotional and general symptoms.

Thrush (oral)

Symptoms In children. Of tongue/gums.

SYMPHYTUM (Symph.)

Family name: Boraginaceae
Common names: comfrey; knitbone; boneset; bruise-wort; blackwort; gum plant; healing plant

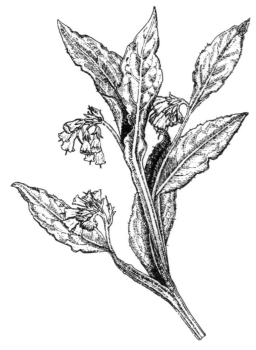

Comfrey is a handsome plant found in damp, wet places throughout Europe, Western Asia and the USA. Its tall flowering stem sprouts in June and July from low, large hairy leaves; the plant can grow to a height of four feet.

Comfrey has long been grown in the gardens of country folk for its well-known healing powers. The name 'comfrey' comes from the Latin *con firma*, 'to form' or 'to unite', and *Symphytum* is from the Greek *Sympho*, also 'to unite'. The plant in fact contains a substance called allantoin which stimulates cells to heal faster. Culpeper quotes it as being so 'powerful to consolidate and knit together, that if they [the leaves] be boiled with dissevered pieces of flesh in a pot, it will join them together again.' It has been used externally to heal broken bones, wounds, burns, piles, scalds, ulcers, sprains and gouty joints. The young leaves can be eaten rather like spinach, and nowadays the dried roots are ground, along with chicory and dandelion to make a caffeine-free 'coffee'.

For the homeopathic preparation the fresh root is gathered before the plant blooms. It is chopped and pounded to a pulp then left to stand in alcohol before being strained and succussed.

GENERAL AND EMOTIONAL/MENTAL SYMPTOMS

This is a very small remedy that has not been well proved but is of such enormous value as a first-aid treatment for injuries to the eye and for broken bones that I have included it here.

PHYSICAL COMPLAINTS

Broken bones

Symptoms Bones painful; sticking.
Symphytum eases the pain and speeds up the healing of broken and fractured bones.

Eye injuries

Symptoms Pains: in eyeball; sore, bruised.
Causes a direct blow to eyeball.
Symphytum is a specific for injury to the eyeball itself or to the bones surrounding the eye (resulting from, for example, a stray fist or tennis ball) where pain persists after *Arnica* has been given and has dealt with the swelling.

TABACUM (Tab.)

Family name: Solanaceae
Common names: Nicotiana Tabacum; tobacco; tabacca

Tobacco is an annual plant with large, hairy, bitter-tasting leaves. It was first known to and smoked by the Indians of South America and the Mississippi Valley. In 1559 the Spaniards brought it to Europe, and the plant was introduced into England by Sir Walter Raleigh in 1586, when it met with violent opposition. Kings prohibited it, Popes pronounced against it in Bulls, and in the East Sultans condemned tobacco smokers to cruel deaths. Three hundred years later, in 1885, the leaves were official in the British Pharmacopoeia.

Tobacco contains a volatile oil called nicotine, which is a virulent poison, producing nausea, vomiting, sweating, palpitations and weakness.

Medicinally it has been used as a powder in the form of snuff to cause sneezing and therefore increase the 'healthy' secretion of mucus. When chewed, it increases the flow of saliva, also considered beneficial at one time, and Culpeper cites some of the uses of

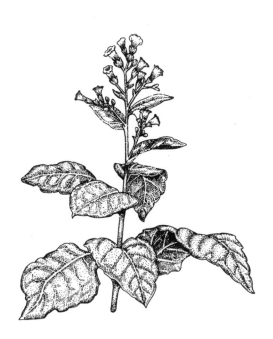

tobacco as a herbal remedy, for piles, to kill lice and worms, as a laxative and 'for the recovery of persons apparently drowned'.

The homeopathic preparation is made from the dried leaves which are cut up and left to stand in alcohol before being strained and succussed.

GENERAL SYMPTOMS

Face pale.
Worse before breakfast; for fasting.

EMOTIONAL/MENTAL SYMPTOMS

This is a small remedy with no strong emotional symptoms, although these people may be sluggish and confused and have difficulty in concentrating. They may be anxious and restless, and may start on falling asleep or during their sleep.

PHYSICAL COMPLAINTS

Nausea

Symptoms NAUSEA: deathly; intermittent; violent.
Better for fresh air.
Worse in a stuffy room.
Causes pregnancy; travelling.
The nausea is better in the fresh air, although the feeling of dizziness is worse for it. There is an empty, sinking feeling in the stomach.

Travel sickness

Symptoms With NAUSEA (see above); VOMITING (see below).
Better for fresh air.
Worse for a stuffy room; for movement; for tobacco.
The nausea is more acute when travelling by boat and the vomiting when travelling by car or train (although vomiting on a boat is also quite possible!).

Vomiting

Symptoms VOMITING: exhausting; sour; violent.
Worse before breakfast; for movement.
Causes travelling; pregnancy.
The face is pale and drawn.

THUJA OCCIDENTALIS (Thu.)

Other names: Arbor vitae; tree of life; white cedar; false white cedar

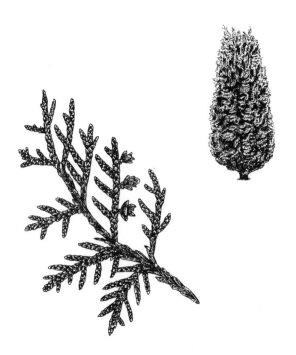

The white cedar is a graceful, thickly branched tree which grows in swamps and wetlands of North America and Canada. It grows very slowly, taking over 150 years to reach a height of fifty feet.

The name 'Thuja' derives from the Greek *thero* which means 'fumigate' or 'sacrifice', for in ancient times this fragrant wood was burnt at sacrifices. It was used by the Egyptians in embalming and employed medicinally by the American Indians for a variety of diseases including malaria, coughs, gout and rheumatism. The leaves and twigs, boiled with lard, were made into a salve for muscular aches and pains.

The homeopathic remedy is prepared from the leaves and twigs, which are gathered when the tree is flowering, chopped and pounded to a pulp and left to stand in alcohol before being strained and succussed.

GENERAL SYMPTOMS

I have included *Thuja* in this Materia Medica as it is available in most chemists and whole food shops that stock homeopathic medicines, but it is a deep-acting remedy that ideally needs to be prescribed by a competent homeopath.

PHYSICAL SYMPTOMS
Warts

Symptoms WARTS: bleeding; large; stinging.
Thuja is indicated for a certain type of wart that grows in a 'cauliflower' shape. These warts can appear anywhere on the body (hands, feet, face, etc.). Use the remedy cautiously and do not take it for longer than up to a week at a time; one week on and then one week resting would be ideal for a couple of months. If there is no reaction – no alleviation of the symptoms – you should seek professional help.

URTICA URENS (Urt-u.)

Family name: Urticaceae
Other names: common nettle; dwarf stinging nettle

The common nettle is a familiar annual plant found in gardens and fields throughout the world. It grows to a height of one foot and it flowers from June to September. The whole plant is covered with fine, hollow hairs that act rather like insects' stings: the hairs' sharp points pierce the skin on pressure and poisonous fluid is injected, causing inflammation and irritation.

The nettle plant's uses are manifold. In Ancient Egypt oil expressed from the seeds was burned in lamps, and the Russians extract a beautiful green dye from the leaves and a bright yellow one from the roots. At one time nettle leaves were given as a food supplement to pigs and poultry, and the juice was used as a tonic for hair loss and to whiten the hands. In certain parts of Europe young nettle shoots are regarded as a fine tonic and are eaten as a vegetable or a soup to cleanse the blood (cooking renders the poison inert). Nettle fibres (from the stems) have been used by

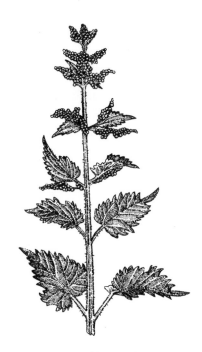

fishermen around the world to make ropes and nets, and during the First World War they were used to make a rough cloth and various types of paper.

Medicinally, the plant was used in ancient times to flay paralysed limbs and so bring muscles back to life. This treatment also eased the pains in rheumatic joints. It has been used internally as a herbal remedy to treat piles, gastric disorders, diabetes and nosebleeds.

The homeopathic preparation is made from the fresh plant which is gathered when in flower; it is chopped and pounded to a pulp, left to steep in alcohol and then strained and succussed.

GENERAL AND EMOTIONAL/ MENTAL SYMPTOMS

This is a very small remedy that has no strong general or emotional/mental symptoms; its use is limited to a few physical complaints but as it has such an important place in the first-aid box it is included here.

PHYSICAL COMPLAINTS
Bites/stings

Symptoms BITES/STINGS: biting; burning; itching; stinging.

Breastfeeding problems

Symptoms MILK: supply low; supply over-abundant.
Urtica is useful as a remedy to help establish a good

NB   SEE ALSO PAGES 203–26 FOR GENERAL ADVICE, DOS AND DON'TS.

supply of milk in the early days of feeding where this seems slow, and there is no obvious cause. Give where there are no obvious general or emotional/mental symptoms that would guide you to another remedy. It can also help where there is an over-abundance of milk and the mother does not want to express and store but wishes her supply to be geared more to the demand.

Burns

Symptoms BURNS minor. PAINS: burning; stinging.
Useful in everyday minor scalds and burns, especially where there are burning, stinging pains afterwards.

Food poisoning

Causes rotten shellfish.

Hives

Symptoms RASH: biting; burning; itching; stinging.
With JOINT PAIN.
Better for rubbing.
Worse at night; for heat; for exercise.
Causes stinging nettles; insects.
This rash will appear as red, raised blotches. It may accompany a rheumatic flare-up, or it may be a reaction to eating shellfish. There is a constant desire to rub the skin.

Prickly heat

Symptoms With symptoms of HIVES (see above).
Feels as though stung by stinging nettles.

VERATRUM ALBUM (Ver-a.)

Family name: Liliaceae
Common names: white-flowered Veratrum; white hellebore; European hellebore

Veratrum album is a hardy perennial plant found in moist, grassy spots in mountainous parts of Europe, though not in the British Isles. It grows up to five feet high, has hairy branches and produces large greenish-white flower heads from June to August.

It is one of the oldest known poisons, apparently used by the Gauls and others on arrows and daggers in their fight against the Romans. The poisonings cause terrible suffering to all animals: the whole gastric tract becomes irritated, causing violent vomiting, painful (often bloody) diarrhoea, abdominal, griping pains, burning sensations in the mouth, throat, stomach and bowels, small pulse, faintness, cold sweats, trembling, dizziness, dilated pupils, and finally loss of

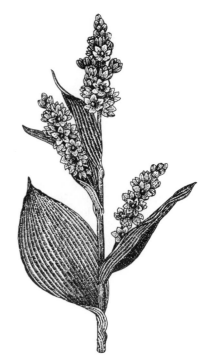

voice, loss of sight, convulsions, unconsciousness and death.

It has occasionally been administered externally for stubborn cases of scabies or lice but this practice is fraught with danger and rarely used. It has been used traditionally from Hippocrates' time as a cure for cholera; more recently homeopaths have prescribed it successfully for certain types of cholera, especially the third stage where there is terrible, continual vomiting, an unquenchable thirst and collapse.

The homeopathic preparation is made from the root which is collected in June, powdered coarsely and left to stand in alcohol before being strained and succussed.

GENERAL SYMPTOMS

Breath cold. **Collapse** after diarrhoea. **Expression:** anxious. **Face** blue; pale. **Likes:** cold drinks; fruit; ice-cream; refreshing things; sour foods. **Saliva** increased. **Sweat:** cold; clammy; profuse; sour. **Thirsty** for large quantities. **Tongue** cold.
Worse after eating fruit.

Veratrum album is indicated for the type of exhaustion with faintness that may accompany an acute illness, usually a 'tummy bug', for example gastro-enteritis, dysentery, food poisoning. Acute illnesses that can be helped by *Veratrum album* will be accompanied by a general coldness – of the breath, the tongue and the skin (which is cold to touch.) Icy-cold sweat is another general symptom, and these types feel worse while sweating. There will also be an increase of saliva in the mouth and a ferocious thirst for large quantities of cold or icy-cold drinks. These may be vomited immediately in gastric troubles. Eating fruit causes a general worsening.

EMOTIONAL/MENTAL SYMPTOMS

Broody. Forgetful. Tearful. Uncommunicative.

Veratrum album types may appear very distressed, and restless (they *have* to be up and doing something), and may be prone to weeping and wailing and incessant talking. Alternatively, they may be totally withdrawn, silent and inactive.

PHYSICAL COMPLAINTS

Cough

Symptoms COUGH: deep; hollow.
Breathing is difficult and may be louder than usual. There is a feeling of tightness in the chest, and the cough is accompanied by the characteristic *Veratrum* cold sweat.

Diarrhoea

Symptoms DIARRHOEA: exhausting; involuntary; violent. PAINS: burning; cutting; dull/aching.
STOOLS: copious; frequent; green; watery. With ICY-COLD HANDS AND FEET; SWEATING (see General Symptoms) during and after passing a stool; VOMITING (see below).
Worse after drinking; during a menstrual period; for movement.
Causes fruit; getting chilled.
This diarrhoea may be accompanied by a ravenous appetite, with a feeling of emptiness which is not relieved by eating. The person has trouble passing wind, and when is able to do so may pass an involuntary stool. Stools shoot out, and the person has to pass them frequently. Hands and feet are icy cold.

Exhaustion

Symptoms EXHAUSTION: paralytic; sudden. With COLD EXTREMITIES.
Worse after passing a stool.
Causes diarrhoea.

Fever

Symptoms With SWEATING (see General Symptoms).
Worse for sweating.
The skin is pale and icy cold to touch, either over the whole body or in spots or patches. If there is diarrhoea

the sweating will be worse (during and after passing stools), and the patient will feel generally worse while sweating.

Vomiting

Symptoms BELLY/STOMACH feels cold. PAINS: cramping/griping. VOMIT: of bile; of mucus; sour, watery; yellow. VOMITING violent. With DIARRHOEA (see above); DIZZINESS; HICCUPING after vomiting.
Worse after eating; after drinking.
This often accompanies *Veratrum album* diarrhoea and is one of the most severe forms of diarrhoea and vomiting. The person may vomit and pass diarrhoea simultaneously.

ZINCUM METALLICUM (Zinc.)

Other name: zinc

Zinc is a soft, blue-white metal of moderate hardness. It doesn't rust and is therefore used to 'galvanise' metals or protect them from corrosion, as well as to make alloys such as brass (zinc plus copper). It has many uses, for example in dry batteries, radios, zips, car parts, electrical fuses, roofing and guttering, cable wrappings and organ pipes.

Zinc as a trace element is essential for both plants and animals and is found in most foods. Zinc deficiency in humans causes loss of appetite and sense of taste, and slow healing. Zinc ointments to promote healing have long been known in medicine. It is mildly astringent and protective to the skin and is used in dusting powders and lotions such as calamine, where it is combined with iron.

The homeopathic preparation is made by heating pure zinc and then grinding it to a fine powder. It is then triturated and diluted by succussion.

GENERAL SYMPTOMS

Face pale. White spots on **fingernails. Twitchy. Trembling.**
Worse after eating; during the evening; at night; for wine.

Zinc acts well in people of any age who are weary and run down from stress and overwork. They may tremble, twitch and jerk. Their symptoms tend to be worse at night, from drinking wine and after eating, although they may feel better while actually eating. Like *Sulphur* types they have an empty feeling in the stomach around 11 a.m.

Though there is a general twitchiness with these

types, a keynote symptom is restless, twitchy legs; *Zincum* types will feel exhausted but fidgety, and they will feel that they must keep their legs constantly on the move. This is worse in the evenings in bed, and the legs will carry on twitching in the sleep.

In a childhood illness like measles where the rash does not appear properly the child may be left feeling weak and low *and* twitchy, and possibly chesty. *Zincum* will be of help, if this is the case.

EMOTIONAL/MENTAL SYMPTOMS

Depressed. Irritable. Moody. Sensitive to noise. **Sluggish. Uncommunicative.**

People needing *Zinc* have difficulty thinking because of nervous exhaustion. Their thoughts wander and they may be slow to answer, perhaps repeating your question before answering, or forgetting what they are saying halfway through their conversation with you. They are depressed, irritable and generally worn out.

PHYSICAL COMPLAINTS

Backache

Symptoms PAINS in coccyx; in neck; in spine; aching; sore, bruised. With WEAKNESS.

Worse for sitting, for writing.
The whole back feels sore and weak from too much stress.

Exhaustion

Symptoms LEGS: restless; weak.
The legs feel weak and twitchy, especially in bed at night.

Eye inflammation

Symptoms EYES: sore; gritty; burning.
Worse during the evening; at night; after drinking wine.
The eyes feel sore and gritty, particularly the inner corners, as if there were sand in them. There is a general aggravation during the evening and at night, when the eyes may water.

Headache

Symptoms HEADACHE nervous. PAINS: in forehead; in sides of head; in temples; bursting; tearing.
Better for fresh air.
Worse after drinking wine.
Causes overwork.
The headache may be on both sides or on one side only of the head.

INTERNAL REPERTORY

Abscesses   *Calc-c., Hep-s., Merc-s., Sil.*
   Discharging pus: *Calc-s.*
   Pains see **Pains**
   Of glands: *Calc-s., Hep-s., Merc-s., Sil.*
   Of roots of teeth: *Hep-s., Merc-s., Sil.*
Absent-minded   (see also **Confused**; **Forgetful**)
   Caust., Nat-m.
Affectionate   *Phos., Puls.*
Afraid   see **Fearful**
Anaemia   *Calc-c., Calc-p., Chin., Ferr-m., Kali-c.,*
   Kali-p., Merc-s., Nat-m., Nit-ac., Phos., Puls.,
   Stap., Sul., Sul-ac.
   After acute illness: *Calc-p.*
   Lips pale: *Ferr-m.*
   With exhaustion: *Calc-p., Ferr-m.*
   Causes:
      loss of blood (haemorrhage, heavy periods,
         etc.): *Chin., Ferr-m.*
      pregnancy: *Ferr-m.*
Angry   (see also **Complaints from** anger; **Irritable**)
   Ars., Bell., Bry., Cham., Hep-s., Ign., Kali-c.,
   Kali-s., Lyc., Nat-m., Nit-ac., Nux-v., Sep.,
   Stap., Sul.
   From contradiction: *Ign., Lyc., Sep.*
   Raging: *Bell., Cham.*
   Violently: *Cham., Hep-s., Nit-ac., Nux-v., Stap.*
   When has to answer: *Nux-v.*
Ankles   weak *Carb-a., Nat-c., Sil.*
   Children learning to walk: *Carb-an.*
Antisocial   see **Dislikes** company
Anxious   *Aco., Arg-n., Ars., Bell., Bry., Calc-c.,*
   Calc-p., Calc-s., Carb-v., Caust., Chin., Cocc.,
   Con., Kali-c., Kali-p., Kali-s., Lyc., Mag-m.,
   Nat-c., Nit-ac., Phos., Puls., Rhus-t., Sep.,
   Spo., Sul.
   Anticipatory (see **Exam nerves**, **Fearful** public
      speaking): *Arg-n., Gels., Lyc.*
   During a fever: *Aco., Ars., Bar-c., Ip., Sep.*
   On waking: *Lach., Spo.*

   When chilled: *Aco.*
   When indoors: *Kali-s.*
   When overheated: *Kali-s.*
   Better:
      fresh air: *Kali-s., Puls.*
   Worse:
      after midnight: *Ars.*
      around 3 a.m.: *Ars.*
      evening: *Calc-c., Calc-s., Carb-v., Sep., Sul.*
      in bed: *Ars., Carb-v., Mag-c., Rhus-t.*
      when alone: *Ars., Phos.*
      from downward motion: *Bor.*
      heat: *Kali-s.*
      indoors: *Lyc., Puls., Rhus-t.*
      night: *Ars., Puls.*
      on waking: *Ars., Lach., Spo.*
Apathetic   (see also **Sluggish**) *Ap., Carb-v., Chin.,*
   Nat-c., Nat-m., Nat-p., Op., Pho-ac., Phos.,
   Puls., Stap., Sep.
   During fever: *Op.*
Appetite
   Alternating with hunger: *Ferr-m.*
   Lost: *Chin., Ferr-m.*
Apprehensive   see **Anxious** anticipatory
Argumentative   see **Quarrelsome**
Arthritis   see **Joint pain**
Athlete's foot   *Sil.*
   Cracks between toes: *Sil.*
   With profuse/smelly sweat: *Sil.*
Awkward   see **Clumsy**
Backache   *Bry., Calc-c., Calc-f., Dulc., Ferr-m., Hyp.,*
   Kali-c., Kali-p., Lyc., Merc-s., Nat-m., Nat-s.,
   Nux-v., Phos., Puls., Rhod., Rhus-t., Ruta.,
   Sep., Sil., Sul., Zinc.
   Between shoulder blades: *Phos.*
   Coccyx: *Hyp., Zinc.*
   Lower back: *Bry., Calc-c., Calc-f., Dulc., Ferr-m.,*
      Hyp., Kali-c., Lyc., Merc-s., Nat-m., Nux-v.,
      Phos., Puls., Rhod., Rhus-t., Sep., Sul.

Neck: *Rhod., Rhus-t., Zinc.*
Small of back: *Puls., Rhus-t.*
Spine: *Kali-p., Zinc.*
Pains:
 aching: *Calc-c., Dulc., Nat-m., Nux-v., Puls.,*
  Rhus-t., Sep., Sul., Zinc.
 back feels broken: *Nat-m., Phos.*
 burning: *Merc-s., Phos.*
 dragging down: *Sep.*
 pressing: *Nux-v., Puls.*
 rheumatic: *Rhod., Rhus-t.*
 shooting: *Hyp., Merc-s.*
 sore, bruised: *Dulc., Hyp., Kali-c., Kali-p.,*
  Nat-m., Nat-s., Nux-v., Rhod., Rhus-t.,
  Ruta., Sil., Sul., Zinc.
 feels sprained: *Calc-c.*
 stitching: *Bry., Kali-c., Sil.*
 tearing: *Hyp.*
With:
 lameness: *Dulc., Ruta., Sil.*
 stiffness: *Lyc., Rhus-t., Sil., Sul.*
 weakness: *Sil., Sul., Zinc.*
Better for:
 continued movement: *Calc-f.*
 gentle exercise: *Puls.*
 heat: *Rhus-t.*
 lying on back: *Ruta.*
 lying on a hard surface: *Kali-c., Nat-m.,*
  Rhus-t.
 massage: *Phos.*
 movement: *Dulc., Kali-p., Lyc., Rhod.,*
  Rhus-t.
 passing wind: *Lyc.*
 pressure: *Kali-c., Sep.*
 rubbing: *Phos.*
 urinating: *Lyc.*
 walking: *Dulc., Rhus-t.*
 walking slowly: *Ferr-m., Puls.*
Worse:
 afternoon: *Sep.*
 around 3 a.m.: *Kali-c.*
 in bed: *Nux-v.*
 bending down: *Sep., Sul.*
 beginning to move: *Calc-f., Ferr-m., Lyc.,*
  Puls., Rhus-t.
 breathing: *Merc-s.*
 coughing: *Bry., Merc-s.*
 damp: *Calc-c.*
 before a menstrual period: *Kali-c., Puls., Sep.*
 during a menstrual period: *Bry., Puls., Sep.,*
  Sul.
 morning: *Nux-v.*
 movement: *Nux-v.*
 slightest movement: *Bry.*
 night: *Sep., Sil., Sul.*
 passing a stool: *Lyc.*

 pressure: *Sil.*
 reaching up: *Rhus-t.*
 sitting: *Sep., Sil., Zinc.*
 after long sitting: *Kali-c., Sul.*
 getting up from sitting: *Calc-c., Lyc., Merc-s.,*
  Phos., Puls., Rhus-t., Sil., Sul.
 standing: *Sul.*
 sweating: *Merc-s.*
 walking: *Kali-c., Sul.*
 wet weather: *Dulc., Rhod., Rhus-t.*
 writing: *Zinc.*
Causes:
 change of weather: *Dulc.*
 childbirth: *Hyp.*
 damp weather: *Dulc., Rhus-t.*
 draughts: *Rhus-t.*
 epidural: *Hyp.*
 forceps delivery (childbirth): *Hyp.*
 falling on the back: *Sil.*
 getting cold: *Dulc., Nux-v.*
 getting wet: *Dulc.*
 injury: *Rhus-t.*
 injury to coccyx: *Hyp., Sil.*
 injury to spine: *Hyp., Nat-s.*
 lifting: *Calc-c., Lyc., Rhus-t.*
 manual labour: *Nat-m., Sil.*
 sprain: *Rhus-t.*

Back injuries see **Backache**
Bad tempered see **Angry**; **Irritable**
Bedwetting *Bell., Caust., Puls., Sil., Sul.*
 Child sleeps too deeply to wake: *Bell.*
 During first sleep: *Caust.*
 Causes:
  injury to back: *Sil.*
  worms: *Sil.*

Better (generally)
 Bathing: *Puls.*
 Changing position: *Rhus-t.*
 Cold applications: *Glon.*
 Cold bathing: *Led.*
 Cold drinks: *Caust., Cupr., Phos.*
 Company: *Arg-n.*
 Constipation: *Calc-c.*
 Crying: *Puls.*
 Damp: *Caust.*
 After eating: *Ign., Nat-c., Phos., Sep.*
 While eating: *Lach.*
 Fanning: *Carb-v.*
 Firm pressure: *Bry., Chin., Mag-p.*
 Fresh air: *Aco., Arg-n., Carb-v., Kali-s., Lach., Lyc.,*
  Mag-c., Mag-m., Nat-s., Puls., Rhus-t., Sul.
 Heat: *Ars., Calc-c., Caust., Hep-s., Ign., Kali-p.,*
  Mag-p., Nux-v., Sil.
 Hot drinks: *Ars., Nux-v., Rhus-t.*
 Lying down: *Ars., Bell., Calc-c., Cocc., Nat-m.,*
  Nit-ac., Nux-v.

Lying still: *Bry.*
Massage: *Nat-c.*, *Phos.*
Movement: *Dulc.*, *Phos.*, *Puls.*, *Pyr.*, *Rhod.*,
    Rhus-t., *Ruta.*
Pressure: *Mag-m.*, *Puls.*
Rest: *Kali-p.*
After a rest: *Nat-m.*
After a good sleep: *Pho-ac.*, *Phos.*
Running: *Sep.*
Sitting down: *Colch.*, *Con.*, *Nux-v.*
Sweating: *Gels.*, *Nat-m.*, *Rhus-t.*
Urinating: *Gels.*
Vigorous exercise: *Sep.*
Walking: *Dulc.*
Walking fast: *Sep.*
Walking in fresh air: *Puls.*
Walking slowly: *Ferr-m.*
Warmth of bed: *Ars.*, *Caust.*, *Hep-s.*, *Kali-c.*, *Lyc.*,
    Rhus-t.
Wrapping up: *Hep-s.*
Wrapping up the head: *Sil.*

Bites/stings   *Ap.*, *Hyp.*, *Lach.*, *Led.*, *Stap.*, *Urt-u.*
Blue: *Lach.*
Inflamed: *Hyp.*
Itching: *Ap.*, *Urt-u.*
Pains:
    biting: *Urt-u.*
    burning: *Ap.*, *Urt-u.*
    shooting: *Hyp.*
    stinging: *Ap.*, *Urt-u.*
    tearing: *Hyp.*
Red: *Ap.*
Swollen: *Ap.*
Better for:
    cold: *Ap.*, *Led.*, *Lach.*
Worse for:
    heat: *Ap.*, *Led.*, *Lach.*
Causes:
    animal/insect bites: *Hyp.*, *Lach.*, *Led.*

Bleeding
Bright red: *Phos.*
Occurs easily: *Phos.*
Profuse: *Phos.*

Bleeding gums   see **Gums**, bleeding
Black eye   *Led.*
Blisters   *Caust.*, *Lyc.*, *Nat-m.*
Burning: *Lyc.*
Painful: *Caust.*
Tip of tongue: *Caust.*, *Lyc.*, *Nat-m.*

Bloated   see **Indigestion**
Blood blisters   *Arn.*
Caused by a blow or injury: *Arn.*
Blood poisoning   *Pyr.*
Extreme chilliness with fever: *Pyr.*
Worse:
    for cold: *Pyr.*

Causes:
    childbirth/surgery/infected wound: *Pyr.*
Boils   *Arn.*, *Ars.*, *Hep-s.*, *Sul.*
Inflamed: *Hep-s.*
Itching: *Sul.*
Pains:
    burning: *Ars.*
Small/sore: *Arn.*
Breastfeeding problems
Breast abscess (Mastitis): *Hep-s.*, *Merc-s.*, *Phyt.*,
    Sil., *Sul.*
Breasts:
    engorged: *Bell.*, *Bry.*
    hard: *Bell.*, *Bry.*
    hot: *Bell.*, *Bry.*
    inflamed: *Bell.*, *Bry.*, *Hep-s.*, *Phyt.*, *Sil.*, *Sul.*
    lumpy: *Con.*, *Phyt.*, *Sil.*
        worse in right breast: *Con.*
    painful: *Bell.*, *Bry.*, *Merc-s.*, *Sil.*
    pains:
        aching after nursing: *Bor.*
        while nursing: *Phyt.*
        cutting: *Sil.*
        stitching: *Sil.*
        in opposite breast whilst nursing: *Bor.*
        slightest movement: *Bry.*
        throbbing: *Bell.*
    pale: *Bry.*
    red: *Sul.*
    red-streaked: *Bell.*
Milk supply:
    low: *Dulc.*, *Urt-u.*
        in chilly women: *Dulc.*
    over-abundant: *Bell.*, *Bry.*, *Calc-c.*, *Puls.*,
        Urt-u.
Nipples:
    cracked: *Phyt.*, *Sil.*
    inverted (retracted): *Sars.*, *Sil.*
    raw, sore: *Phyt.*
Worse:
    left breast: *Sil.*
    while nursing: *Sil.*
Breath
Cold: *Ver-a.*
Smelly: *Arn.*, *Carb-v.*, *Lach.*, *Merc-c.*, *Merc-s.*,
    Nit-ac., *Phyt.*, *Puls.*, *Sul.*
Broken bones   *Arn.*, *Bry.*, *Calc-c.*, *Calc-p.*, *Sil.*,
    Symph.
Pains:
    sticking: *Symph.*
    stitching: *Bry.*
Slow to mend: *Calc-c.*, *Calc-p.*, *Sil.*
With swelling/bruising: *Arn.*
Worse:
    slightest movement: *Bry.*
Broody   (see also **Introspective**; **Moody**) *Ign.*, *Ver-a.*

Bruises   (see also **Injuries**) *Arn., Bell-p., Led., Sul-ac.*
   Bluish-black: *Sul-ac.*
   Pains:
      sore, bruised: *Arn., Bell-p.*
   Slow to heal: *Sul-ac.*
   With:
      bumps, lumps remaining: *Bell-p.*
      discolouration: *Led.*
      swelling (no discolouration): *Arn.*
   Causes:
      childbirth: *Arn., Bell-p.*
      injury: *Arn., Bell-p., Led.*
      over-exertion: *Bell-p.*
      surgery: *Arn., Bell-p.*
Burns   *Ars., Canth., Caust., Kali-b., Urt-u.*
   Deep: *Kali-b.*
   Minor: *Urt-u.*
   Pains:
      burning: *Ars., Canth., Caust., Urt-u.*
      stinging: *Urt-u.*
   Second degree: *Canth.*
   Slow to heal: *Kali-b.*
   Third degree: *Caust.*
   With blisters: *Ars., Canth., Caust.*
   Better for:
      cold compresses: *Canth.*
      heat: *Ars.*
Capricious   *Bry., Cham., Cina, Ip., Rhe., Stap.*
Carried   see **Desires** to be
Catches colds easily   *Ars., Bar-c., Calc-c., Calc-p.,*
      Dulc., Hep-s., Kali-c., Nat-m., Nux-v., Sep., Sil.
Changeable   see **Moody**
Cheerful   *Coff., Lach., Nat-c.*
Chicken pox   *Aco., Ant-c., Ant-t., Bell., Merc-s.,*
      Puls., Rhus-t., Sul.
   First Stage: *Aco.*
   Skin rash:
      itches maddeningly: *Rhus-t., Sul.*
      slow in coming out: *Ant-t.*
      suppurates: *Merc-s.*
   With:
      cough: *Ant-c., Ant-t., Puls.*
      fever: *Aco., Bell.*
      headache: *Bell.*
Chilblains   *Agar., Petr., Puls.*
   Feet, hands, toes: *Petr., Puls.*
   Burning: *Agar.*
   Inflamed: *Petr., Puls.*
   Itching: *Agar., Puls.*
   Red: *Agar.*
   Worse:
      for cold: *Agar.*
Childish   *Bar-c.*
Clingy   *Puls.*
Clumsy   *Agar., Apis., Calc-c., Caust.*
   Drops things: *Ap.*

Trips easily while walking: *Agar., Caust.*
Cold sores   *Nat-m., Rhus-t., Sep.*
   Sores:
      on lips: *Nat-m., Rhus-t., Sep.*
      around mouth: *Nat-m.*
   Causes:
      exposure to sun: *Nat-m.*
      grief: *Nat-m.*
Colic   (see also **Indigestion, Heartburn**) *Coloc.,*
      Cupr., Dios., Ip., Mag-m., Mag-p., Nat-p.,
      Nat-s., Nux-v., Stap.
   In babies: *Coloc., Dios.*
   Belly:
      bloated: *Coloc., Nat-p.*
      rumbling: *Dios.*
      windy: *Dios.*
   Pains:
      aching: *Ip.*
      around the navel: *Dios.*
      cramping: *Cupr., Dios., Ip., Mag-m., Mag-p.,*
         Nux-v., Stap.
      cutting: *Coloc., Dios.*
      drawing: *Mag-p.*
      griping: *Coloc., Dios., Ip., Nux-v.*
      pressing: *Nux-v.*
      sore, bruised: *Mag-m., Nux-v.*
      tearing: *Coloc.*
      twisting: *Dios.*
      violent: *Coloc., Cupr.*
      in waves: *Coloc.*
   With:
      constipation: *Mag-m.*
      diarrhoea: *Coloc., Mag-m.*
      indigestion: *Mag-m., Nat-s.*
      nausea: *Coloc., Cupr.*
      vomiting: *Coloc., Cupr.*
      sour vomit: *Nat-p.*
   Better:
      bending back: *Dios.*
      bending double: *Coloc., Mag-p.*
      hot drinks: *Nux-v.*
      passing a stool: *Coloc., Nux-v.*
      passing wind: *Nux-v.*
      pressure: *Coloc.*
      stretching out: *Dios.*
      warmth: *Mag-p.*
      warmth of bed: *Nux-v.*
   Worse:
      after drinking: *Coloc., Stap.*
      bending forward: *Dios.*
      cold drinks when overheated: *Coloc.*
      coughing: *Nux-v.*
      after eating: *Nux-v.*
      during a fever: *Nux-v.*
      before a stool: *Coloc.*
      fruit: *Coloc.*

after drinking milk: *Mag-m.*
in the morning: *Dios., Nux-v.*
for movement: *Ip.*
tight clothing: *Nux-v.*
Causes:
anger: *Coloc.*
excitement: *Coloc.*
fruit: *Coloc.*
drinking milk: *Mag-m.*
indignation: *Stap.*
teething: *Mag-m.*
vexation: *Coloc., Stap.*

Collapse
After diarrhoea: *Ver-a.*

Common cold   *All-c., Ars., Bar-c., Bell, Bry., Calc-c.,*
Calc-f., Calc-s., Carb-v., Euphr., Hep-s.,
Kali-b., Kali-m., Kali-s., Lyc., Mag-m., Merc-s.,
Nat-c., Nat-m., Nit-ac., Nux-v., Pho-ac., Puls.,
Sep., Sil., Sul.

Eyes:
dry: *Ars.*
burning: *Ars.*
streaming: *Euphr.*
Discharge from eyes:
burning: *Euphr.*
watery: *Nat-m., Nux-v.*
Eyelids:
red: *Ars.*
puffy: *Ars.*
Glands:
swollen: *Bar-c.*
Nasal catarrh:
bland (not irritating): *Euphr., Puls.*
blood-streaked: *Calc-s., Phos.*
bloody: *Merc-s., Nit-ac.*
burning: *All-c., Ars., Merc-s., Nit-ac., Nux-v.*
crusty: *Kali-b.*
drips down back of throat: *Hep-s., Kali-b.,*
Nat-c., Nat-m., Sep.
dry (stuffed up/congested without
discharge): *Calc-c., Calc-f., Kali-b., Phos., Sil.*
dry at night, profuse during the day: *Nux-v.*
dry alternating with profuse: *Puls.*
like egg white: *Nat-m.*
green: *Kali-b., Merc-s., Puls., Sep.*
hard crusts: *Kali-b., Sil.*
one-sided: *All-c., Phos.*
profuse: *All-c., Ars., Kali-s., Nat-m., Phos.*
smelly: *Calc-c., Calc-s., Hep-s., Kali-b.,*
Merc-s., Nat-c., Puls., Sil., Sul.
sticky/stringy: *Kali-b.*
thick: *Calc-s., Kali-b., Kali-s., Nat-c., Puls.,*
Sil.
thin: *Nit-ac.*
watery: *All-c., Ars., Eupr., Merc-s., Nit-ac.,*
Nux-v.

watery, alternating with blocked up nose:
Nat-m.
watery in the fresh air: *Nit-ac., Puls.*
white: *Kali-m., Nat-m.*
yellow: *Calc-c., Calc-s., Hep-s., Kali-b., Kali-s.,*
Lyc., Merc-s.
dirty yellow: *Nit-ac., Puls., Sep., Sul.*
yellow-green: *Kali-b., Merc-s., Puls., Sep.*
Nose:
blocked: *Calc-c., Carb-v., Lyc., Nat-c.*
dry: *Bar-c., Lyc., Sul.*
itching: *Sul.*
runs during day, blocked at night: *num-v.*
Sinuses:
blocked/painful: *Kali-b., Lyc., Merc-s., Sil.*
Sneezing: *All-c., Ars., Bry., Carb-v., Eup-p.,*
Hep-s., Merc-s., Nux-v., Puls., Sul.
better for sneezing: *Calc-f.*
frequent sneezing: *Ars., Carb-v., Merc-s.,*
Nux-v., Sul.
difficult sneezing: *Calc-f., Carb-v., Sil.*
in a stuffy room: *Puls.*
slightest uncovering: *Hep-s.*
With:
cough: *Euphr.*
dry throat: *Kali-b.*
eye inflammation: *Euphr., Sul.*
headache: *Aco., All-c., Bell., Bry., Lyc.,*
Merc-s., Nux-v.
fever: *Bell., Merc-s.*
hoarseness: *Calc-c., Carb-v., Merc-s., Phos.*
itching throat: *Carb-v.*
painless hoarseness: *Calc-c.*
loss of smell: *Bell., Calc-c., Calc-s., Merc-s.,*
Nat-m., Phos., Puls., Sep., Sil.
loss of taste: *Bell., Nat-m., Phos., Puls., Sil.*
sneezing: *All-c.*
sore throat: *All-c., Merc-s., Nux-v., Phos.*
Better:
fresh air: *All-c., Kali-s., Nux-v., Puls.*
Worse:
cold and heat: *Merc-s.*
after eating: *Nux-v.*
fresh air: *Nit-ac.*
after getting up: *Nux-v.*
morning: *Calc-c., Nux-v.*
evening: *Ars.*
night: *Merc-s., Nit-ac.*
on the right: *Ars., Lyc.*
for drinking milk: *Calc-s.*
stuffy room: *All-c., Kali-s., Puls.*
uncovering: *Hep-s.*
Causes:
getting chilled: *Aco., Bell.*
getting chilled when overheated: *Ars.*
cold wind: *All-c.*

cold, dry wind: *Aco.*
draughts: *Nux-v.*
getting head wet: *Bell.*
getting wet feet: *All-c.*
swimming in the sea: *Mag-m.*

Complaints from/after (see also **Worse**)
Accident/injury: *Arn., Bell-p., Con., Hyp., Nat-s.*
Anger: *Cham., Cocc., Colch., Coloc., Ign., Ip., Nux-v., Op.*
   suppressed anger: *Stap.*
   anger with anxiety: *Ars., Ign., Nux-v.*
Bad news: *Gels.*
Getting chilled: *Aco., Bry., Merc-s., Nux-v., Phos., Rhus-t.*
   when overheated: *Bell-p.*
Change of weather: *Bry., Caust., Dulc., Kali-s., Phos., Rhod., Rhus-t., Sil., Sul.*
   any change: *Phos.*
   from cold to warm: *Bry., Kali-s., Sul.*
   to cold: *Rhus-t., Sil.*
   to damp: *Dulc., Rhus-t.*
   to dry (especially dry cold): *Caust.*
   to stormy: *Rhod.*
Coffee: *Cham.*
Cold wind: *Aco., Bell., Hep-s., Nux-v., Spo.*
Disappointed love: *Ign., Nat-m., Pho-ac., Stap.*
Excitement: *Coff., Gels., Pho-ac., Puls., Stap.*
Fear: *Aco.*
Fright: *Ign., Pho-ac., Puls.*
Grief: *Caust., Cocc., Ign., Lach., Nat-m., Pho-ac., Puls., Stap.*
Humiliation (wounded pride): *Coloc., Ign., Lyc., Nat-m., Pho-ac., Stap.*
Indignation: *Colch., Coloc., Stap.*
Injuries to nerves/coccyx: *Hyp.*
Joy: *Coff.*
Loss of body fluids: *Calc-p., Carb-v., Chin., Pho-ac.*
Measles: *Carb-v., Puls.*
Mental strain: *Arg-n., Kali-p., Lach., Lyc., Nat-c., Sil., Stap.*
Over-eating: *Ant-c.*
Overwork: *Kali-p.*
Reprimands: *Ign., Op., Stap.*
Shock: *Aco., Arn., Ign., Op., Pho-ac., Puls., Sil.*
Sprains: *Calc-c.*
Sunstroke: *Glon., Nat-c.*
Suppression of emotions: *Ign., Nat-m., Stap.*
Surgery: *Arn., Bell-p., Hyp., Stap.*
Teething: *Cham.*
Vexation: *Ip.*
Getting wet: *Calc-c., Caust., Puls., Rhus-t., Sep.*
Getting feet wet: *Puls., Sil.*
Getting head wet: *Bell.*

Concentration
Poor: *Bar-c., Caust., Lyc., Nux-v., Sil.*

Confidence see **Self-confidence, Lack of**
Confused (see also **Absent-minded; Forgetful**)
Arg-n., Bell., Calc-c., Carb-v., Cocc., Glon., Lach., Merc-s., Nat-c., Nat-m., Op., Petr., Rhus-t., Sep., Sil., Sul.
In the fresh air: *Petr.*
Conjunctivitis see **Eye inflammation**
Conscientious *Ign., Sil.*
Constipation *Calc-c., Caust., Hep-s., Lyc., Mag-m., Nat-m., Nux-v., Op., Sep., Sil.*
Alternates with diarrhoea: *Nux-v.*
Belly/stomach feels full: *Sep.*
Desire to pass stool:
   absent: *Op.*
   constant: *Nux-v.*
   ineffectual: *Caust., Lyc., Mag-m., Nat-m., Nux-v., Sep., Sil.*
Pains:
   burning after stool: *Sil.*
   stitching: *Caust.*
Stools:
   black balls: *Op.*
   crumbling: *Mag-m., Nat-m.*
   hard: *Lyc., Mag-m., Nux-v., Op., Sep., Sil.*
   hard at first: *Calc-c.*
   knotty: *Lyc., Mag-m., Sil.*
   large: *Calc-c., Mag-m., Nux-v., Sep., Sil.*
   pale: *Calc-c.*
   passed with difficulty: *Mag-m.*
   rabbits'/sheep's droppings: *Mag-m., Nat-m., Op.*
   'shy' (they recede): *Op., Sil.*
   small balls: *Mag-m., Nat-m., Op.*
   soft: *Hep-s.*
   sour smelling: *Calc-c.*
With:
   ineffectual straining: *Mag-m., Nat-m., Sep., Sil.*
   unfinished feeling: *Nat-m., Nux-v., Op.*
Better:
   being constipated: *Calc-c.*
   passing a stool when standing: *Caust.*
Worse:
   before a menstrual period: *Sil.*
   during a menstrual period: *Nat-m., Sep., Sil.*
Causes:
   alcohol: *Nux-v.*
   drinking milk: *Mag-m.*
   over-eating: *Nux-v.*
   pregnancy: *Nux-v., Sep.*
   sedentary habits: *Nux-v.*
Convulsions *Bell., Cina, Cupr.*
With:
   blue lips: *Cupr.*
   coldness of hands and feet: *Cupr.*

Causes:
    worms: *Cina*
    teething children: *Bell., Cina, Cupr.*
    vexation: *Cupr.*

Corns   *Ant-c., Lyc., Sil.*
On soles of feet: *Ant-c.*
Under nails: *Ant-c.*
Horny: *Ant-c.*
Inflamed: *Ant-c., Lyc., Sil.*
Soft: *Sil.*
Pains:
    pressing: *Ant-c., Lyc.*
    sore: *Lyc., Sil.*
    tearing: *Lyc., Sil.*

Cough   *Aco., All-c., Ant-t., Arn., Ars., Bar-c., Bell., Bry., Calc-c., Calc-p., Calc-s., Carb-v., Caust., Cham., Cina, Cocc-c., Con., Cupr., Dros., Dulc., Euphr., Ferr-m., Hep-s., Ign., Ip., Kali-b., Kali-c., Kali-m., Kali-s., Lach., Lyc., Merc-s., Nat-m., Nat-s., Nux-v., Op., Pho-ac., Phos., Puls., Rhus-t., Rumex., Sep., Sil., Spo., Stap., Sul., Ver-a.*
In elderly people: *Bar-c.*
Breathing:
    asthmatic: *Ant-t.*
    abdominal/difficult: *Ant-t.*
    difficult: *Ant-t., Ars., Cupr., Dros., Ip., Lyc., Nux-v., Op., Phos., Spo.*
    fast: *Aco., Ant-t., Ars., Bell., Bry., Carb-v., Cupr., Dros., Ip., Lyc., Phos., Sep., Sul.*
    rattling: *Ant-t., Dulc.*
    rough: *Spo.*
    slow: *Bell., Op.*
    snoring: *Op.*
    wheezing: *Ars., Carb-v., Ip., Kali-c.*
Cough:
    barking: *Aco., Bell., Dros., Hep-s., Kali-m., Spo.*
    choking: *Cocc-c., Ip.*
      as soon as falls into a deep sleep: *Lach.*
    constant: *Caust., Lyc., Rumex., Spo.*
      when lying down at night: *Sep.*
      in the evening: *Puls.*
    croupy see **Croup**
    deep: *Dros., Ver-a.*
    disturbs sleep: *Bry., Lyc., Puls., Sep., Sul.*
    distressing: *Caust., Nux-v.*
    dry: *Aco., Ars., Bell., Bry., Calc-c., Calc-s., Con., Dros., Hep-s., Ign., Ip., Kali-c., Lach., Lyc., Nat-m., Nux-v., Pho-ac., Phos., Rumex., Sep., Spo., Sul.*
    dry in the evening, loose in the morning: *Calc-c., Hep-s., Sul.*
    dry at night: *Ars., Calc-c., Cham., Dros., Hep-s., Phos., Puls., Sul.*
      loose by day: *Sul.*

loose in the morning: *Puls.*
dry during fever: *Aco., Phos., Puls.*
exhausting: *Ars., Bell., Caust., Sep.*
    night: *Puls.*
hacking: *All-c., Ars., Dros., Lach., Nat-m., Phos., Sep.*
    evening in bed after lying down: *Ign., Sep.*
    worse cold air: *All-c.*
    worse after dinner: *Hep-s.*
    from tickling in the larynx: *All-c., Ars., Dros., Lach., Nat-m., Phos.*
hard: *Bell., Kali-c., Kali-m.*
hollow: *Bell., Caust., Spo., Ver-a.*
in fits: *Bell., Bry., Carb-v., Cina, Cocc., Cocc-c., Ferr-m., Ip., Puls., Rumex., Spo.*
in long fits at irregular intervals: *Cupr.*
irritating: *Aco., All-c., Bell., Bry., Cham., Cocc-c., Con., Dros., Hep-s., Ign., Ip., Kali-c., Lach., Lyc., Nat-m., Nux-v., Pho-ac., Phos., Puls., Rhus-t., Rumex., Sep., Sil., Spo., Stap., Sul.*
loud: *Ant-t.*
loose: *Ars., Kali-c., Sep.*
painful: *All-c., Bry., Lyc., Sul.*
racking: *Bell., Bry., Carb-v., Caust., Cocc-c., Ign., Kali-c., Merc-s., Nux-v., Phos., Puls., Sul.*
rattling: *Ant-t., Caust., Dulc., Ip., Kali-s., Sep.*
short: *Aco., Ign., Kali-m., Rhus-t., Sep.*
suffocative: *Carb-v., Cina, Cupr., Dros., Hep-s., Lach., Nux-v., Sul.*
tickling see irritating
tight: *Phos.*
tormenting: *Ars., Bell., Caust., Dros., Ip.*
uninterrupted: *Cupr.*
violent: *Bell., Carb-v., Caust., Cocc-c., Con., Cupr., Hep-s., Ign., Kali-c., Lach., Pho-ac., Phos., Puls., Sep.*
violent fits: *Dros., Nux-v.*
voice hoarse: *Aco., All-c., Bell., Carb-v., Caust., Dros., Hep-s., Kali-b.*
vomiting with or after cough: *Ant-t., Bry., Dros., Hep-s., Ip., Kali-c.*
wakens from the cough at night: *Caust., Kali-c., Phos., Sep., Sul.*
whooping: *Ant-t., Arn., Carb-v., Cocc-c., Cupr., Dros., Ip., Kali-s.*
Chest congested: *Sul.*
Daytime only: *Euphr., Nat-s.*
Expectoration see Mucus
Larynx:
    raw: *Nux-v., Phos., Rumex., Sul.*
    tickling: *All-c., Ars., Cocc-c., Dros., Nat-m., Phos.*
Mucus:
    bloody: *Ip., Phos.*

copious: *Ars., Calc-c., Calc-s., Cocc-c., Euphr.,*
   Hep-s., Lyc., Phos., Puls., Sep.
     after each coughing fit: *Cocc-c.*
     in elderly people: *Bar-c.*
difficult to cough up: *Caust., Con., Ip.,*
   Kali-b., Kali-s., Puls.
     has to swallow what comes up: *Caust.,*
       Con., Kali-s.
egg white: *Nat-m.*
frothy: *Ars.*
green: *Carb-v., Lyc., Merc-s., Nat-s., Phos.,*
   Puls., Sul.
lumpy: *Calc-s., Sil.*
smelly: *Calc-c.*
sticky: *Cocc-c., Hep-s., Kali-b., Puls.*
ropy/stringy: *Kali-b.*
tastes:
     bitter: *Cham., Puls.*
     sour: *Calc-c., Nux-v.*
     sweet: *Calc-c., Phos.*
     salty: *Ars., Lyc., Phos., Puls., Sep.*
thick: *Hep-s., Kali-b., Sil.*
tough: *Calc-c., Hep-s., Kali-b.*
transparent: *Nat-m., Phos.*
white: *Lyc., Nat-m., Phos., Sep.*
yellow: *Calc-c., Calc-p., Calc-s., Hep-s., Lyc.,*
   Phos., Puls., Sep., Sil.
yellow-green: *Puls.*
Pain in chest: *Arn., Bell., Bry., Caust., Dros., Ign.,*
   Kali-b., Kali-c., Phos., Spo.
burning: *Phos., Rumex., Spo.*
cutting: *Kali-c.*
must hold chest to cough: *Arn., Bry., Dros.*
racking: *Ign.*
raw: *Caust.*
sharp: *Bell.*
short: *Ign.*
sore, bruised: *Arn., Kali-b., Rumex., Spo.*
stitching: *Bry., Ign., Kali-c., Rumex.*
Pain in stomach: *Bry.*
With:
bloodshot eyes: *Arn.*
blue face: *Dros., Ip.*
dry throat: *Cocc-c.*
lump sensation in the throat: *Lach.*
nausea: *Ip., Kali-c., Puls.*
nosebleeds: *Arn., Dros., Ip.*
retching: *Carb-v., Cina, Dros., Hep-s., Ip.,*
   Puls.
sleepiness: *Ant-t.*
splitting headache: *Bry.*
sweating: *Ars., Hep-s., Phos.*
vomiting: *Ant-t., Bry., Dros., Hep-s., Ip.,*
   Kali-c.
     when hawking up mucus: *Nux-v.*
vomiting of mucus: *Dros.*

voice hoarse: *Aco., Bell., Caust., Dros.,*
   Hep-s., Kali-b., Spo.
Better:
drinking/eating: *Spo.*
fresh air: *Bry., Cocc-c., Puls.*
heat: *Phos.*
hot drinks: *Ars., Lyc., Nux-v., Rhus-t., Sil.*
lying down: *Euphr.*
lying on painful side: *Bry.*
pressure: *Dros.*
for sips of cold water: *Caust., Cupr.*
sitting up: *Puls., Sep.*
     must sit up: *Ars., Con., Phos., Puls., Sep.*
     must sit up as soon as cough starts, to
       cough up mucus and then can rest:
       Con.
walking slowly: *Ferr-m.*
Worse:
around 11.30 p.m.: *Cocc-c.*
around 3 a.m.: *Kali-c.*
getting warm in bed: *Caust., Puls.*
bending head forward: *Caust.*
breathing in cold air: *Caust., Rumex.*
change of temperature: *Phos.*
   from warm to cold: *Phos., Rumex.*
   from cold to warm: *Phos.*
becoming cold: *Ars., Hep-s., Kali-c., Nux-v.,*
   Phos., Rhus-t., Rumex., Sil.
cold air: *All-c., Caust., Nux-v., Phos., Rumex.*
   single parts of the body becoming cold:
     Hep-s., Rhus-t.
cold drinks: *Ars.*
coughing: *Ign., Sul.*
crying: *Arn.*
damp, wet weather: *Dulc., Nat-s.*
daytime: *Spo.*
deep breathing: *Bell., Bry., Con., Kali-c.*
drinking: *Dros.*
dry, cold: *Aco., Hep-s.*
eating: *Kali-b., Nux-v.*
evening: *Ars., Calc-c., Carb-v., Hep-s., Ign.,*
   Kali-c., Merc-s., Nit-ac., Puls.
evening in bed: *Calc-c., Con., Hep-s., Ign.,*
   Lach., Lyc., Merc-s., Nat-m., Sep., Sul.
evening before midnight: *Hep-s., Phos.*
excitement: *Spo.*
during fever: *Aco., Ars., Calc-c., Con., Ip.,*
   Kali-c., Nat-m., Nux-v., Phos.
fresh air: *Ars., Phos., Rumex.*
heat: *Kali-c., Kali-s., Puls.*
left side: *Rumex.*
lying on left side: *Phos.*
lying on right side: *Merc-s.*
lying down: *Ap., Ars., Caust., Con., Dros.,*
   Kali-c., Lyc., Puls., Rumex., Sep., Sul.
     must sit up: *Ars., Con., Puls., Sep.*

morning: *Calc-c., Euphr., Kali-c., Nux-v.,*
   Phos., Puls., Rumex., Sul.
    before getting up: *Nux-v.*
    after getting up: *Cina, Ferr-m., Phos.*
movement: *Ferr-m.*
physical exertion: *Puls.*
movement of chest: *Bry., Chin., Nux-v.*
moving arms: *Nat-m.*
night: *Aco., Ars., Bar-c., Bell., Calc-c.,*
   Carb-v., Cham., Kali-c., Kali-s., Lach., Lyc.,
   Merc-s., Puls., Sep., Sul.
    on going to sleep: *Lyc.*
    before midnight: *Carb-v., Hep-s.*
    after midnight: *Ars., Dros.*
playing the piano: *Calc-c.*
reading aloud: *Phos.*
right lung: *Bry.*
during sleep: *Op.*
falling sleep: *Op.*
stuffy room: *Ant-c., Cocc-c., Kali-s., Puls.*
warm room: *Kali-s.*
talking: *Dros., Kali-c., Rumex.*
teething: *Calc-p.*
touch: *Lach.*
uncovering: *Hep-s., Rhus-t., Rumex.*
   hands: *Hep-s., Rhus-t.*
   feet or head: *Sil.*
walking: *Ferr-m.*
on waking in the morning: *Kali-b., Nux-v.,*
   Op., Rumex., Sil.
warmth of bed: *Op.*
Causes:
   cold, dry wind: *Aco., Hep-s.*
   getting chilled: *Bell., Kali-c.*
   damp weather: *Dulc.*
   after measles: *Dros., Puls.*
   suppressed anger: *Stap.*
   swimming in cold water: *Rhus-t.*

Cracks at corners of mouth/around nostrils *Ant-c.*
Cramp *Calc-c., Calc-p., Caust., Coloc., Cupr., Lyc.,*
   Mag-p., Sul.
Arm: *Mag-p.*
Calf: *Calc-c., Calc-p., Cham., Coloc., Cupr., Lyc.,*
   Sul.
Foot: *Caust., Cupr.*
Fingers and hand when writing: *Mag-p.*
Hand: *Calc-c., Mag-p.*
Leg: *Coloc., Cupr., Sul.*
Soles of feet: *Calc-c., Caust., Sul.*
Thigh: *Coloc., Sul.*
Toe: *Calc-c., Caust.*
Wrist: *Mag-p.*
Better:
   heat: *Mag-p.*
Worse:
   at night: *Calc-c., Caust., Lyc., Sul.*

in bed: *Calc-c., Sul.*
childbirth: *Cupr.*
during pregnancy: *Calc-c.*
stretching leg in bed: *Calc-c.*
when walking: *Calc-p., Sul.*
Causes:
   childbirth: *Cupr.*
   prolonged use of hands: *Mag-p.*

Cravings see **Likes**
Critical *Ars., Sul.*
Croup (see **Cough** for symptoms) *Aco., Calc-s.,*
   Hep-s., Kali-b., Lach., Phos., Spo.
Only on waking: *Calc-s.*
Recurrent: *Hep-s.*
Worse:
   after sleep: *Lach.*
   on waking: *Lach.*

Cystitis *Aco., Ap., Ars., Canth., Caust., Dulc., Lyc.,*
   Merc-c., Merc-s., Nux-v., Puls., Sars., Sep.,
   Stap., Sul.
Desire to urinate:
   constant: *Ap., Canth., Merc-c., Merc-s., Sul.*
    with dragging down pain in pelvis: *Sep.*
   frequent: *Ap., Canth., Caust., Lyc., Merc-c.,*
    Merc-s., Nux-v., Puls., Stap., Sul.
   ineffectual: *Ars., Canth., Caust., Lyc.,*
    Merc-s., Nux-v., Puls., Sars.
   painful: *Merc-c.*
   urgent: *Canth., Nux-v., Puls., Sep., Sul.*
Pains:
   aching: *Lyc.*
   burning: *Ap., Ars., Canth., Caust., Merc-c.,*
    Merc-s., Nux-v., Sul.
   cutting: *Canth., Lyc., Sars.*
   pressing: *Aco., Ap., Lyc., Nux-v., Sep.*
   severe: *Merc-c.*
   spasmodic: *Puls.*
   stinging: *Ap.*
   stitching: *Lyc.*
Urination:
   burning: *Caust.*
   constant: *Ap.*
   difficult: *Caust., Merc-c.*
   dribbling: *Merc-c., Merc-s., Sars.*
   frequent: *Ap., Canth., Caust., Lyc., Merc-c.,*
    Merc-s., Nux-v., Puls., Sars., Sep., Stap.
   ineffectual: *Nux-v.*
   involuntary: *Caust., Dulc., Stap.*
   slow: *Sars.*
    can only pass urine while standing: *Sars.*
    waits long time for it to start: *Caust., Lyc.,*
     Sep.
   with unfinished feeling: *Ars., Caust.*
Urine:
   brown like beer: *Sul.*
   burning: *Nux-v., Sul.*

cloudy: *Sep.*
copious: *Puls., Sul.*
dark: *Merc-c., Merc-s.*
dark brown: *Sep.*
green: *Merc-c., Sars.*
hot: *Canth.*
pale: *Sars.*
red: *Canth., Merc-c., Sep.*
scanty: *Canth., Merc-c., Merc-s., Nux-v., Sep.,*
    Stap., Sul.
smelly: *Sep., Sul.*
with sediment: *Sars., Sep.*
with mucus: *Sars.*
Better:
    after urination: *Lyc.*
    heat: *Ars.*
    for sitting in a hot bath: *Ars.*
Worse:
    cold drinks: *Canth.*
    after getting up in the morning: *Sul.*
    after a few drops of urine have passed:
        Canth.
    after urinating: *Canth., Puls.*
    at the beginning of urinating: *Canth., Merc-s.*
    at the end of urination: *Sars.*
    before urinating: *Canth.*
    during a menstrual period: *Sars., Sep.*
    when not urinating: *Merc-s.*
    while urinating: *Canth., Caust., Merc-c.,*
        Nux-v., Sul.
    at night: *Sul.*
Causes:
    cold, wet weather: *Sars.*
    getting chilled: *Aco., Sars.*
    getting cold and wet: *Dulc., Puls.*

Dazed   (see also **Shock**; **Stupor**) *Cocc.*
Delirious   *Bell.*
Denial
Of illness: *Arn.*
Of suffering: *Arn.*
Depressed   (see also **Tearful**) *Ars., Calc-c., Carb-a.,*
    Caust., Cham., Chin., Cimi., Con., Eup-p.,
    Ferr-m., Gels., Ign., Kali-p., Lach., Lyc.,
    Merc-s., Nat-c., Nat-m., Nat-s., Nit-ac.,
    Pho-ac., Puls., Rhus-t., Sep., Sul., Zinc.
Cannot cry: *Gels., Ign., Nat-m.*
Cries on own: *Ign., Nat-m.*
Better:
    fresh air: *Puls.*
Worse:
    before menstrual period: *Nat-m., Puls.*
    stuffy room: *Puls.*
    on waking: *Lach., Lyc.*
    evening: *Puls.*
Causes:
    suppressed grief: *Ign., Nat-m., Puls.*

Desires
Company: *Arg-n., Ars., Kali-c., Lyc., Phos.*
To be alone: *Bar-c., Carb-a., Cham., Gels., Ign.,*
    Nat-m., Sep.
To be carried (infants): *Cham., Puls.*
Despair   *Ars., Calc-c., Coff.*
Of getting well: *Ars., Calc-c.*
Despondent   (see also **Depression**) *Chin.*
Diarrhoea   *Ant-c., Ap., Arg-n., Ars., Bor., Bry.,*
    Calc-c., Cham., Chin., Colch., Coloc., Dulc.,
    Ferr-m., Gels., Hep-s., Ip., Mag-c., Mag-m.,
    Merc-c., Merc-s., Nat-m., Nat-s., Nux-v.,
    Petr., Pho-ac., Phos., Podo., Puls., Rhe.,
    Rhus-t., Sil., Sul., Sul-ac., Ver-a.
Alternating with:
    constipation: *Podo.*
    constipation in elderly persons: *Ant-c.*
    headache: *Podo.*
Belly/stomach:
    bloated: *Nat-m.*
    gurgling: *Nat-s., Podo.*
    rumbling: *Nat-s., Pho-ac., Podo.*
Children: *Ip., Mag-m., Merc-s., Podo., Puls., Sul.*
Daytime only: *Nat-m., Petr.*
Drives person out of bed: *Sul.*
Elderly persons: *Ars.*
Exhausting: *Ver-a.*
Involuntary: *Ver-a.*
Morning only: *Sul.*
Pains: *Ars., Cham., Colch., Dulc., Mag-c., Merc-c.,*
    Merc-s.
    burning: *Ars., Merc-s., Sul., Ver-a.*
    colicky: *Mag-c.*
    cramping: *Mag-c., Sul.*
    cutting: *Ver-a.*
    dull/aching: *Ver-a.*
    after passing a stool: *Ars., Colch.*
    pressing: *Petr.*
    severe: *Merc-c.*
Painless: *Ap., Bor., Chin., Ferr-m., Hep-s., Nat-m.,*
    Phos., Podo., Sul.
Stools:
    blood-streaked: *Phos.*
    bloody: *Merc-c., Merc-s.*
    changeable: *Puls.*
    copious: *Ver-a.*
    frequent: *Merc-c., Phos., Podo., Ver-a.*
    frothy: *Mag-c.*
    grass green: *Ip.*
    green: *Arg-n., Cham., Coloc., Mag-c., Mag-m.,*
        Merc-c., Merc-s., Ver-a.
    greenish-yellow: *Puls.*
    gushing: *Nat-m., Podo.*
    jelly-like: *Colch.*
    hot: *Cham.*
    involuntary: *Podo.*

with mucus: *Bor.*, *Colch.*
mushy: *Rhus-t.*
painless: *Nat-m.*, *Phos.*, *Podo.*
passed with wind: *Ferr-m.*
pasty: *Coloc.*, *Rhe.*
profuse: *Pho-ac.*, *Phos.*, *Podo.*
slimy: *Mag-c.*, *Merc-c.*, *Merc-s.*, *Puls.*, *Sul.*
small, hard lumps: *Ant-c.*
smelly: *Arg-n.*, *Ars.*, *Merc-c.*, *Merc-s.*, *Nat-m.*,
  Nat-s., *Podo.*, *Sul.*
smelling of rotten eggs: *Cham.*
soft: *Sul-ac.*
sour smelling: *Calc-c.*, *Mag-c.*, *Rhe.*, *Sul.*
stringy: *Sul-ac.*
sudden: *Podo.*
thin: *Nat-s.*, *Pho-ac.*
with undigested food: *Calc-c.*, *Chin.*, *Ferr-m.*
yellow: *Dulc.*, *Merc-c.*, *Merc-s.*, *Sul-ac.*
watery: *Ant-c.*, *Arg-n.*, *Ars.*, *Calc-c.*, *Colch.*,
  Dulc., *Nat-m.*, *Nat-s.*, *Pho-ac.*, *Phos.*, *Puls.*,
  Rhus-t., *Sul.*, *Ver-a.*
white: *Pho-ac.*
Straining frequent/painful: *Merc-c.*
In teething children: *Calc-c.*, *Cham.*, *Dulc.*,
  Ferr-m., *Rhe.*, *Sil.*
Violent: *Ver-a.*
With:
  belching: *Ferr-m.*
  sour belching: *Sul-ac.*
  colic: *Coloc.*
  exhaustion: *Ars.*, *Podo.*, *Ver-a.*
  flatulence: *Arg-n.*, *Ferr-m.*, *Nat-s.*, *Sil.*, *Sul.*
  icy-cold hands and feet: *Ars.*, *Phos.*, *Ver-a.*
  indigestion: *Chin.*
  ravenous appetite: *Petr.*
  sweating: *Ars.*, *Merc-s.*, *Ver-a.*
    during/after passing stool: *Ver-a.*
    before/during/after stool: *Merc-s.*
  vomiting: *Arg-n.*, *Ver-a.*
    sour: *Sul-ac.*
  wind:
    loud: *Nat-s.*
    smelly: *Nat-s.*, *Sil.*, *Sul.*
    spluttering: *Nat-s.*
Without weakness: *Pho-ac.*
Better:
  cold food: *Phos.*
  fresh air: *Puls.*
  heat: *Sil.*
  passing wind: *Nat-s.*, *Sul.*
  warmth of bed: *Sil.*
  wrapping up warmly: *Sil.*
Worse:
  on alternate days: *Chin.*
  around 4 a.m.: *Podo.*
  5 a.m.: *Sul.*

afternoon: *Chin.*
before passing a stool (pains): *Mag-c.*,
  Merc-c.
during passing a stool: *Merc-c.*
after passing a stool: *Merc-c.*, *Merc-s.*
cold: *Ars.*, *Merc-s.*
getting chilled: *Phos.*
after drinking cold food/drinks: *Ars.*
after drinking: *Ars.*, *Arg-n.*, *Ver-a.*
after drinking water: *Ferr-m.*, *Nux-v.*, *Podo.*
immediately after drinking: *Arg-n.*, *Podo.*
after eating: *Ars.*, *Chin.*, *Coloc.*, *Podo.*, *Puls.*
while eating: *Ferr-m.*
eating cold food: *Dulc.*
eating starchy food: *Nat-m.*, *Nat-s.*, *Puls.*
evening: *Merc-s.*
after eating fruit: *Ars.*, *Coloc.*, *Nat-s.*
after getting up in the morning: *Bry.*, *Nat-s.*
hot weather: *Podo.*
during a menstrual period: *Ver-a.*
after midnight: *Ars.*
mid-morning: *Podo.*
morning: *Bry.*, *Mag-c.*, *Nat-s.*, *Phos.*, *Sul.*
movement: *Bry.*, *Ferr-m.*, *Ver-a.*
night: *Arg-n.*, *Ars.*, *Chin.*, *Dulc.*, *Ferr-m.*,
  Merc-s., *Podo.*, *Puls.*, *Sul.*
overheated: *Ant-c.*, *Puls.*
rich food: *Puls.*
solid/dry food: *Pho-ac.*
starchy food: *Nat-s.*
standing: *Sul.*
stuffy room: *Puls.*
sugar/sweets: *Arg-n.*
Causes:
  after an acute illness: *Chin.*
  alcohol: *Nux-v.*
  anger: *Coloc.*
  anticipatory anxiety: *Arg-n.*, *Gels.*
  autumn: *Colch.*
  bad or exciting news: *Gels.*
  beer: *Sul.*
  getting chilled: *Ver-a.*
  damp, cold weather: *Dulc.*
  getting cold or damp: *Dulc.*
  excitement: *Arg-n.*
  food poisoning: *Ars.*
  fright/shock: *Gels.*
  fruit: *Ars.*, *Bry.*, *Chin.*, *Coloc.*, *Nat-s.*, *Puls.*,
    Ver-a.
  hot weather: *Bry.*, *Chin.*, *Pho-ac.*
  ice-cream: *Ars.*
  milk: *Calc-c.*, *Mag-m.*
  over-eating: *Ant-c.*
  rich food: *Puls.*
  sour wine: *Ant-c.*
  sugar: *Arg-n.*

summer: *Pho-ac.*
teething: *Calc-c., Cham., Dulc., Ferr-m., Rhe., Sil.*
weaning: *Arg-n., Chin.*
getting wet: *Rhus-t.*
getting feet wet: *Rhus-t.*

Discharges
Bland (non-irritating): *Puls.*
Blood-streaked: *Calc-s., Merc-s., Phos.*
Burning: *Ars., Merc-s.*
Like ammonia: *Nit-ac.*
Like egg white: *Nat-m.*
Smelly: *Ars., Bapt., Carb-v., Merc-s., Pyr., Sul.*
Sour: *Calc-c., Mag-c., Mag-m., Nat-p., Rhe., Sul.*
Stringy/sticky: *Kali-b.*
Thick: *Calc-c., Kali-b., Kali-s., Puls.*
Watery: *Ars., Caust., Merc-s., Podo., Sul.*
White: *Kali-m.*
Yellow: *Kali-s., Lyc., Merc-s., Puls., Sep.*

Discontented   *Calc-p., Merc-s., Nat-m., Sul.*

Dislikes   (see also **Desires**)
Being alone: *Kali-c., Lyc.*
Being touched: *Ant-c., Cham., Kali-c.*
Being hugged: *Cina*
Being looked at: *Ant-c., Cham., Cina*
Being spoken to: *Cham.*
Company, see **Desires** to be alone
Consolation: *Ign., Nat-m., Sep., Sil.*
Contradiction: *Ign., Lyc., Nux-v., Petr., Sep.* (see also **Quarrelsome**)
Fresh air: *Cocc., Ign.*
Strangers: *Bar-c., Bor.*
Bread: *Chin., Nat-m., Puls.*
Coffee: *Calc-c.*
Hot drinks/food: *Phos., Puls.*
Fatty, rich food: *Chin., Petr., Puls.*
Meat: *Calc-c., Chin., Nux-v., Petr., Puls., Sep., Sil., Sul.*
Milk: *Nat-c.*

Dizzy   (see also **Faintness**) *Con.*
During pregnancy: *Nat-m.*
With:
headache: *Bell., Calc-c., Con., Nux-v., Sil.*
nausea: *Aco., Cocc., Ferr-m., Petr.*
turning sensation: *Con.*
vomiting: *Ver-a.*
Worse:
lying down: *Con.*
motion: *Bry.*
moving/turning head quickly: *Calc-c., Con.*
stooping: *Bell., Nux-v., Puls., Sul.*
stuffy room: *Nat-c.*
walking in the fresh air: *Puls., Sul.*
Causes:
downward motion (stairs, lifts etc.): *Bor.*
high places: *Calc-c., Sul.*

loss of sleep: *Cocc., Nux-v.*
mental exertion: *Nat-c., Nat-m., Nux-v.*
smoking: *Nat-m., Nux-v.*

Dreamy   (see also **Absent-minded**) *Op.*
Drowsy   (see also **Dazed**) *Bapt., Op.*
Dryness   (generally) *Ars., Bry., Nat-m.*
Dull   *Calc-s.*

Earache   *Aco., Ap., Bell., Calc-c., Calc-s., Cham., Hep-s., Kali-b., Kali-m., Kali-s., Lach., Lyc., Mag-p., Merc-s., Nit-ac., Nux-v., Puls., Sil., Sul.*
Discharge from ears:
blood-streaked: *Calc-s., Merc-s.*
smelly: *Calc-s., Hep-s., Kali-b., Merc-s., Puls.*
thick: *Calc-s., Kali-b., Puls.*
thin: *Kali-s.*
yellow-green: *Puls.*
yellow: *Kali-b., Kali-s., Puls.*
Pains
aching: *Cham., Puls., Sul.*
behind the ear: *Sil.*
boring: *Merc-s.*
burning: *Merc-s.*
lacerating: *Sul.*
outward: *Puls.*
pressing: *Cham., Merc-s., Puls.*
pressing outwards: *Puls.*
spreading down into neck: *Bell., Puls.*
shooting: *Mag-p.*
spasmodic: *Mag-p.*
splinter-like: *Nit-ac.*
stinging: *Ap.*
stitching: *Bell., Cham., Hep-s., Kali-b., Nux-v., Puls., Sul.*
tearing: *Bell., Cham., Lyc., Merc-s., Puls., Sil., Sul.*
throbbing: *Bell., Calc-c., Nit-ac., Puls.*
unbearable: *Cham.*
With:
blocked feeling in ears: *Lyc., Merc-s., Puls., Sil.*
crackling in the ears: *Nit-ac.*
when chewing: *Kali-s., Nit-ac.*
deafness: *Puls.*
deafness after a cold: *Kali-m.*
face-ache: *Bell.*
glands swollen: *Kali-m.*
itching in the ear: *Nux-v., Puls., Sil.*
has to swallow: *Nux-v.*
noises in the ear: *Bell., Calc-c., Kali-m., Lyc., Puls., Sul.*
painful: *Sul.*
redness of the external ear: *Puls.*
sensitivity to wind: *Cham., Lach.*
sore throat: *Ap., Lach., Nit-ac.*

Better:
  heat: *Mag-p.*
  firm pressure: *Mag-p.*
  wrapping up warmly: *Hep-s.*
Worse:
  bending down: *Cham.*
  cold: *Hep-s., Mag-p.*
  fresh air: *Merc-s.*
  left side: *Kali-b., Lach., Sul.*
  noise: *Sul.*
  night: *Merc-s., Puls.*
  right side: *Bell., Nit-ac.*
  swallowing: *Ap., Kali-m., Lach., Nit-ac., Nux-v.*
  turning head: *Mag-p.*
  wind: *Cham., Lach.*
  warmth of bed: *Merc-s.*
Causes:
  after a common cold: *Puls.*
  after measles: *Puls.*
  getting chilled: *Aco.*
  cold dry wind: *Aco., Mag-p.*

Exam nerves   *Arg-n., Gels., Lyc.*

Excitable   (see also **Complaints from excitement**)
  Arg-n., Bell., Cham., Coff., Lach., Nux-v., Phos., Puls.

Exhaustion   *Ant-c., Ant-t., Arg-n., Ars., Bapt., Bar-c., Bry., Calc-c., Carb-a., Carb-v., Chin., Cocc., Colch., Con., Cupr., Ferr-m., Gels., Kali-c., Kali-p., Lach., Merc-c., Merc-s., Nat-c., Nat-m., Nat-p., Nit-ac., Nux-v., Pho-ac., Phos., Puls., Rhus-t., Sep., Sil., Spo., Stap., Sul., Sul-ac., Ver-a., Zinc.*
  Extreme: *Ars., Bry.*
  In the elderly: *Bar-c.*
  Nervous: *Chin., Cocc., Kali-p., Nat-c., Nat-p., Nit-ac., Nux-v., Pho-ac., Phos., Puls., Rhus-t., Sep., Sil., Stap.*
  Paralytic: *Ars., Cocc., Gels., Pho-ac., Phos., Ver-a.*
  Sudden: *Ars., Sep., Ver-a.*
  With:
    breath cold: *Carb-v.*
    breathlessness: *Calc-c., Carb-v.*
    cold extremities: *Carb-v., Nat-c., Ver-a.*
    desire to lie down: *Ferr-m.*
    dizziness: *Calc-c., Cocc.*
    a faint feeling: *Ars.*
    fever: *Ars., Phos.*
    headache between the eyes: *Cupr.*
    heaviness: *Merc-s., Nat-c., Nat-m., Rhus-t.*
      in the limbs: *Merc-s., Nat-c.*
    nervousness: *Cocc.*
    numbness: *Cocc., Con.*
    profuse sweating: *Chin.*
    restlessness: *Ars., Rhus-t.*
    restless legs: *Zinc.*

  sleepiness: *Ant-c.*
  stiffness: *Cocc.*
  trembling: *Arg-n., Cocc., Con., Gels., Stap., Sul-ac.*
  vertigo: *Cocc.*
  weak legs: *Nat-c., Zinc.*
Better:
  being fanned: *Carb-v.*
  fresh air: *Con., Ferr-m.*
  during a menstrual period: *Sep.*
  walking in fresh air: *Rhus-t.*
  walking slowly: *Ferr-m.*
Worse:
  afternoon: *Sul.*
  after eating: *Ars., Bar-c., Pho-ac.*
  for exercise: *Ferr-m.*
  evening: *Caust., Nat-m.*
  slightest exertion: *Ars., Bry., Calc-c., Con., Lach., Nat-c., Pho-ac., Phos., Rhus-t., Spo.*
  mental exertion: *Calc-c., Cupr., Lach., Nat-c., Puls.*
  physical exertion: *Calc-c.*
  heat of sun: *Lach., Nat-c., Puls., Sul.*
  hot weather: *Ant-c.*
  after a menstrual period: *Ip.*
  during a menstrual period: *Carb-a., Sep.*
  morning: *Ars., Lach., Pho-ac., Sep.*
    in bed: *Puls.*
    after getting up: *Bry., Lach., Pho-ac., Sep.*
    on waking: *Nux-v.*
  late morning: *Ant-c.*
  mid morning: *Bry.*
  movement: *Ars., Spo.*
  sitting down: *Rhus-t.*
  after passing a stool: *Ars., Con., Merc-s., Nit-ac., Sul-ac., Ver-a.*
  stuffy room: *Puls.*
  exposure to sun: *Nat-c.*
  after sweating: *Merc-s., Sep.*
  talking: *Sul.*
  after a walk: *Ruta.*
  walking: *Ars., Bry., Calc-c., Carb-a., Con., Ferr-m., Lach., Nit-ac., Pho-ac., Phos., Rhus-t., Sep., Sul.*
    in the fresh air: *Bapt., Cocc., Rhus-t.*
    upstairs: *Calc-c.*
Causes:
  accident/injury: *Carb-v.*
  acute illness: *Carb-a., Carb-v.*
  anaemia: *Ferr-m.*
  breastfeeding: *Carb-a., Carb-v., Pho-ac.*
  carbon monoxide poisoning: *Carb-v.*
  diarrhoea: *Ars., Carb-v., Chin., Nat-s., Nit-ac., Phos., Sil., Sul., Ver-a.*
  fever: *Phos.*
  food poisoning: *Ars., Carb-v.*

flu: *Kali-p., Pho-ac., Sul.*

hunger: *Sul.*

after illness: *Carb-a., Carb-v., Chin.*

irregular sleep: *Cocc., Nit-ac., Nux-v.*

lifting: *Carb-a.*

loss of body fluids (diarrhoea, vomiting, breastfeeding etc.): *Carb-v., Chin., Pho-ac.*

loss of sleep: *Cocc., Cupr., Nit-ac.*

mental exhaustion: *Cupr., Lach.*

mental strain: *Nat-c.*

nervous exhaustion: *Cocc.*

nursing the sick: *Cocc., Nit-ac.*

over-exposure to sun: *Nat-c.*

pain: *Ars.*

surgery: *Carb-v.*

sweating: *Bry., Carb-a., Chin., Ferr-m., Merc-s., Phos., Sep.*

talking: *Sul.*

vomiting: *Carb-v.*

walking: *Sul.*

Exhilarated   (see also **Excitable**) *Coff., Lach., Op.*

Expression

Anxious: *Aco., Bor., Ver-a.*

Besotted: *Bapt.*

Confused: *Lyc.*

Fierce: *Bell.*

Frightened: *Aco.*

Haggard: *Ars., Kali-c.*

Sickly: *Ars., Cina, Lach., Lyc.*

Sleepy: *Op.*

Suffering: *Ars., Kali-c.*

Extremities cold   *Cupr.*

Eye inflammation   *Aco., All-c., Ap., Arg-n., Ars., Bell., Bry., Calc-c., Calc-s., Dulc., Euphr., Lyc., Merc-s., Nat-m., Nit-ac., Nux-v., Puls., Rhus-t., Sep., Sil., Sul., Zinc.*

Discharge:

bland (non-irritating). *All-c.*

burning: *Euphr.*

profuse: *All-c.*

purulent (mucus or pus): *Arg-n., Calc-c., Calc-s., Hep-s., Lyc., Merc-s., Puls.*

smelly: *Arg-n., Puls.*

thick: *Calc-s., Puls.*

watery: *Euphr.*

yellow: *Arg-n., Calc-s., Puls., Sil.*

In babies: *Ap., Arg-n., Ars., Calc-c., Nit-ac., Puls., Sul.*

Eyes:

aching: *Aco., Puls.*

bloodshot: *Ars., Bell., Led.*

burning: *Aco., Ap., Ars., Bell., Puls., Sep., Sul., Zinc.*

dry: *Bell., Bry.*

gritty (sandy sensation): *Ars., Calc-c., Nat-m., Sul., Zinc.*

itching: *Puls., Sul.*

red: *Aco., Ap., Arg-n.*

sensitive to light: *Aco., Arg-n., Ars., Bar-c., Bell., Calc-c., Euphr., Lyc., Merc-s., Nat-m., Nat-s., Nux-v., Op., Rhus-t., Sul.*

sore: *Ap., Bry., Rhus-t., Sil., Zinc.*

worse for moving eyes: *Bry., Rhus-t.*

stinging: *Ap.*

stitching: *Ap., Kali-c., Lyc., Rhus-t., Sul.*

watering: *All-c., Bell., Calc-c., Euphr., Lyc., Merc-s., Nat-m., Nit-ac., Puls., Rhus-t., Sul.*

Eyelids:

burning: *Ars., Euphr., Sul.*

glued together: *Arg-n., Calc-c., Lyc., Puls., Rhus-t., Sep.*

gritty: *Calc-c.*

itching: *Puls., Rhus-t., Sul.*

daytime: *Sul.*

red: *Arg-n., Euphr., Sul.*

swollen: *Ap., Euphr., Nit-ac., Rhus-t., Sep.*

With a common cold: *Aco., All-c., Bell., Calc-c., Dulc., Euphr., Merc-s., Puls.*

Better:

cold: *Arg-n., Puls.*

cold bathing: *Puls.*

cold compresses: *Arg-n.*

fresh air: *Puls.*

Worse:

cold air: *Sil.*

cold, dry wind: *Aco.*

coughing: *Euphr.*

drinking wine: *Zinc.*

evening: *Puls., Sep., Zinc.*

heat of a fire: *Merc-s.*

heat: *Ap., Bell.*

light: *Bell., Euphr.*

moving eyes: *Rhus-t.*

night: *Zinc.*

reading: *Sep.*

warm room: *Puls.*

warmth of bed: *Merc-s.*

after a walk: *Sep.*

washing eyes: *Sul.*

wind: *Euphr.*

Causes:

a foreign body in the eye: *Aco., Sil.*

getting chilled: *Aco.*

cold, wet weather: *Dulc., Rhus-t.*

Eye injuries   *Arn., Euphr., Led., Stap., Symph.*

Bruising:

to eyeball: *Arn.*

to surrounding areas: *Arn.*

and swelling: *Arn.*

and discolouration: *Led.*

Pains:

    in eyeballs: *Symph.*

    sore, bruised: *Arn., Symph.*

With eye inflammation: *Euphr.*

Wound punctured: *Stap.*

Better:

    cold compresses: *Led.*

Worse:

    touch: *Stap.*

Causes:

    a direct blow to the eyeball: *Symph.*

Eye strain *Ruta.*

Eyelids heavy *Caust., Gels.*

Eyes

Dull: *Ant-c.*

Glassy: *Op., Pho-ac.*

Shining: *Bell.*

Sunken: *Ant-c., Chin., Cina*

Face

Blue: *Carb-v., Cupr., Lach., Op., Ver-a.*

    during cough: *Dros., Ip.*

Dark red: *Bapt., Bell., Bry., Capt., Op.*

Flushes easily: *Ferr-m.*

Pale: *Ant-t., Ars., Calc-c., Calc-p., Carb-v., Cina,*
    Con., Cupr., Ferr-m., Lyc., Nat-c., Nat-p., Op.,
    Pho-ac., Tab., Ver-a., Zinc.

Pasty: *Chin., Ferr-m., Merc-s., Nat-m., Sep.*

Puffy: *Ap.*

Red: *Aco., Ap., Bell., Cham., Glon., Lach., Phos.,*
    Rhus-t., Sul.

    one-sided: *Cham., Ip.*

    from pain: *Ferr-m.*

    in spots: *Bell., Cham., Phos., Sul.*

    with toothache (teething): *Bell., Cham.*

Sallow: *Arg-n., Carb-v., Nat-m., Sul.*

Sickly: *Lyc.*

Yellow: *Sep.*

Faintness (see also **Dizzy**) *Carb-v., Op., Puls., Sep.*

Coldness after the faint: *Sep.*

After excitement: *Op.*

After fright: *Op.*

On getting up: *Carb-v.*

On waking: *Carb-v.*

Heat with the faintness: *Sep.*

In a warm room: *Puls.*

Worse:

    exercise: *Sep.*

    during a fever: *Sep.*

    during a menstrual period: *Sep.*

    stuffy room: *Sep.*

Fatigue see **Exhaustion**

Fault-finding see **Critical**

Fearful *Aco., Arg-n., Arn., Ars., Bor., Calc-c.,*
    Calc-p., Ign., Lyc., Nat-c., Phos., Puls.

Animals: *Chin.*

Being alone: *Ap., Arg-n., Ars., Kali-c., Phos.*

In a crowd: *Aco., Gels.*

Of the dark: *Phos.*

Of death: *Aco., Ap., Ars., Calc-c., Cimi., Gels.,*
    Nit-ac., Phos., Ruta.

Of dogs: *Puls., Chin.*

In the evening: *Calc-c., Caust., Puls.*

Of exams see **Exam nerves**

Of downward movement: *Bor.*

During labour: *Aco.*

Of painful death: *Coff.*

During pregnancy: *Aco.*

Of public speaking: *Arg-n., Gels., Lyc.*

Paralysing: *Gels.*

Of strangers: *Bar-c.*

Of sudden noises (sneezing, coughing etc.): *Bor.*

Of thunder: *Rhod.*

During a thunderstorm: *Phos., Rhod.*

At twilight: *Puls.*

Of being touched: *Arn.*

Fever *Aco., Ap., Bell., Bry., Cham., Cina, Eup-p.,*
    Ferr-m., Gels., Hep-s., Ign., Ip., Kali-c., Lyc.,
    Merc-s., Nat-m., Nux-v., Op., Phos., Puls.,
    Pyr., Rhus-t., Sep., Sil., Sul., Ver-a.

Heat:

    alternating with chills: *Aco., Ars., Bell., Bry.,*
        Hep-s., Merc-s., Nux-v., Rhus-t., Sul.

    burning: *Aco., Ap., Ars., Bell., Bry., Cham.,*
        Gels., Nat-m., Op., Phos., Puls., Rhus-t.

    dry: *Aco., Ap., Ars., Bell., Bry., Nux-v., Phos.,*
        Rhus-t.

    dry at night: *Aco., Ars., Bell., Phos.*

    dry in the evening: *Puls.*

    intense: *Op.*

    radiant: *Bell.*

One-sided: *Bry., Cham., Lyc., Nux-v., Phos., Puls.*

    right side: *Phos.*

    left side: *Lyc.*

Pulse:

    fast: *Aco.*

    strong: *Aco.*

Without sweating: *Bell., Bry., Gels.*

With:

    anxiety: *Aco., Ars., Ip., Sep.*

    appetite increased: *Phos.*

    backache: *Nux-v.*

    chilliness: *Ap., Nux-v., Puls., Ver-a.*

      · better for fresh air: *Ip.*

      worse for heat: *Ip.*

      extreme: *Pyr.*

      internal: *Pyr.*

    deep sleep: *Op.*

    delirium: *Ars., Bell.*

    grinding of teeth: *Bell.*

    hunger: *Cina*

    nausea: *Nat-m.*

    sensitive skin: *Ap.*

shaking: *Pyr.*

shivering: *Cham., Gels., Nux-v., Sul.*

sweating see **Sweat**

thirst see **Thirst/Thirstless**

Better:

for complete rest: *Bry.*

in bed: *Kali-c.*

drinking cold water: *Caust.*

fresh air: *Ip.*

heat: *Hep-s., Kali-c.*

hot drinks: *Rhus-t.*

for sweating: *Gels.*

for uncovering: *Aco., Ap., Ferr-m., Ign.,*
Nat-m., Op., Puls.

for urinating: *Gels.*

Worse

9 p.m.: *Bry.*

afternoon: *Ap., Bell., Gels., Ign., Phos., Puls.*

autumn: *Bry., Nat-m., Sep.*

in bed: *Merc-s., Puls.*

cold drinks: *Rhus-t.*

draughts: *Nux-v.*

after eating: *Kali-c.*

evening: *Aco., Bell., Lyc., Phos., Puls.,*
Rhus-t., Sil.

after lying down in bed: *Bry.*

fresh air: *Merc-s., Nux-v.*

front of the body: *Ign.*

for heat: *Ap., Ip., Puls.*

for light: *Bell.*

mental exertion: *Sul.*

after midnight: *Ars.*

mid morning: *Cham., Nat-m., Rhus-t.*

morning: *Ap., Ars.*

in bed: *Puls.*

movement: *Nux-v., Rhus-t., Sil.*

at night: *Aco., Ars., Bapt., Bell., Cina, Merc-s.,*
Phos., Puls., Rhus-t., Sil., Sul.

during sleep: *Op.*

slightest movement of the bedclothes:
Nux-v.

in a stuffy room: *Ap., Puls.*

for sweating: *Op., Sep., Ver-a.*

for thinking: *Sul.*

for being uncovered: *Bell., Hep-s., Nux-v.,*
Puls., Pyr., Rhus-t., Sep., Sil.

warm covers: *Ap., Ign., Puls.*

washing: *Ap., Puls.*

Causes:

anger: *Cham., Sep.*

getting chilled: *Aco.*

teething in babies: *Aco.*

Fingernails

Split: *Ant-c., Sil.*

Weak nails, split easily: *Sil.*

White spots on nails: *Sil., Zinc.*

Caused by:

injury: *Ant-c.*

Flatulence *Arg-n., Ars., Calc-c., Carb-a., Carb-v.,*
Cham., Chin., Colch., Lyc., Mag-c., Nat-s.,
Nit-ac., Podo., Puls., Sil., Sul.

Belly/stomach:

bloated: *Arg-n., Ars., Calc-c., Carb-a.,*
Carb-v., Cham., Chin., Colch., Lyc., Mag-c.,
Nux-v., Sul.

above the navel: *Chin.*

below the navel: *Carb-v., Lyc.*

gurgling: *Podo., Puls., Sul.*

before stool: *Podo.*

intolerant of tight clothing (belts etc.):
Arg-n., Calc-c., Lyc., Nux-v.

rumbling: *Carb-v., Chin., Lyc., Nat-s.,*
Nux-v., Puls., Sil., Sul.

before stool: *Mag-c.*

better for passing flatus: *Carb-v., Lyc.,*
Nat-s.

Wind:

loud: *Arg-n., Nat-s.*

during stool: *Nat-s., Podo.*

smelly: *Ars., Carb-v., Nat-s., Nit-ac., Puls.,*
Sil., Sul.

of rotten eggs: *Sul.*

obstructed (difficult to expel): *Arg-n., Chin.,*
Colch., Nit-ac., Puls., Sil.

With:

diarrhoea: *Carb-v., Nat-s.*

urging for stool but only spluttering wind is
passed: *Nat-s.*

Better:

passing wind: *Carb-v., Lyc., Nat-s., Nux-v.,*
Puls., Sul.

Worse:

after eating: *Arg-n., Lyc., Nux-v.*

after breakfast: *Nat-s.*

before/after stool: *Lyc.*

Causes:

eating fruit: *Chin.*

abdominal surgery: *Carb-a., Carb-v., Chin.*

Flu *Ars., Bapt., Bry., Dulc., Eup-p., Gels., Ip.,*
Nux-v., Pyr., Rhus-t.

Body feels bruised: *Bapt.*

Chills: *Ip.*

Eyeballs aching: *Bry., Eup-p., Gels.*

Eyelids red: *Eup-p.*

Muscles feel heavy/sore/stiff: *Bapt.*

Pains:

aching: *Ip., Pyr., Rhus-t.*

back: *Ip.*

bones: *Eup-p., Ip., Nux-v., Pyr., Rhus-t.*

bones feel broken: *Eup-p.*

joints: *Nux-v., Rhus-t.*

legs: *Ip., Pyr., Rhus-t.*

muscles: *Gels.*
shooting: *Rhus-t.*
sore, bruised: *Ip., Nux-v., Rhus-t.*
Skin sore: *Eup-p.*
With:
    chilliness, extreme, can't get warm: *Gels.,*
       Nux-v., Pyr.
    common cold: *Ars., Nux-v.*
    exhaustion: *Gels., Rhus-t.*
    fever: *Ars., Bapt., Nux-v., Pyr., Rhus-t.*
    headache: *Eup-p.*
    heaviness: *Gels.*
    nasal catarrh: *Eup-p.*
    nightmares: *Bapt.*
    numbness: *Gels.*
    restlessness: *Ars., Pyr.*
    shivering/chills in back: *Eup-p., Gels., Pyr.*
    sneezing: *Eup-p., Rhus-t.*
    extreme thirst: *Pyr.*
Better:
    warm compresses: *Nux-v.*
    for movement: *Pyr.*
    for sweating: *Eup-p., Gels.*
    for urinating: *Gels.*
    for walking: *Pyr.*
    warmth of bed: *Nux-v., Pyr.*
Worse:
    in bed: *Nux-v.*
    cold: *Nux-v.*
    during the chilly stage: *Pyr.*
    exertion: *Gels.*
    morning: *Nux-v.*
    walking: *Gels.*
    sitting: *Pyr.*
Causes:
    change of temperature: *Ars.*
    cold, damp weather: *Dulc.*

Flushed   see **Face flushed**
Food poisoning   *Ars., Carb-a., Carb-v., Lach., Lyc.,*
    Puls., Urt-u.
Causes:
    fish: *Carb-a., Carb-v., Puls.*
    meat: *Ars., Carb-v., Lach., Puls.*
    shellfish: *Lyc., Urt-u.*
    vegetables: *Carb-a.*
Forgetful   (see also **Absent-minded; Confused**)
    Arg-n., Arn., Ars., Bar-c., Caust., Cocc.,
    Colch., Con., Glon., Kali-p., Lyc., Merc-s.,
    Nat-c., Petr., Pho-ac., Sep., Stap., Ver-a.
    Following injury: *Arn.*
Fractures   see **Broken bones**
Frightened   see **Fearful**
Fussy   see **Critical; Capricious**
Gastric flu   *Ars., Bapt., Bry., Eup-p., Ip., Nux-v.*
    Pains:
       aching: *Bry.*

stomach: *Bry.*
With:
    biliousness: *Bry.*
    painless diarrhoea: *Bapt.*
    fever: *Bapt., Bry., Eup-p.*
    flu symptoms (see also **Flu**): *Ars., Bapt.,*
       Bry., Eup-p., Ip., Nux-v.
    nausea: *Eup-p.*
    retching: *Eup-p.*
    vomiting: *Eup-p.*
       bile: *Eup-p.*
       food: *Eup-p.*
Better:
    after chills: *Eup-p.*
    for belching: *Bry.*
    during fever: *Eup-p.*
Worse:
    evening: *Bry.*
    for coughing: *Bry.*
    for eating bread: *Bry.*
    for lying down in bed: *Bry.*
    for movement: *Bry.*
    for walking: *Bry.*
Gentle   *Puls.*
German measles   see **Measles**
Glands   see **Sore throat**, Tonsils swollen
    Sensitive: *Bar-c., Bell.*
    Swollen: *Bar-c., Bell., Calc-c., Merc-s., Puls.,*
       Rhus-t., Sil., Sul.
       painless: *Calc-c.*
Gloomy   (see also **Depressed; Despondent; Morose**)
    Nat-c.
Gum boils   (see also **Abscesses**) *Sil.*
Gums
    Bleeding: *Arn., Phos.*
       after tooth extraction: *Arn., Lach., Phos.*
Haemorrhoids   see **Piles**
Hair loss   *Carb-v., Lach., Lyc., Pho-ac., Phos., Sep.,*
    Sul.
    In handfuls: *Phos.*
    Causes:
       acute illness: *Carb-v., Phos.*
       childbirth: *Lyc., Sul.*
       grief: *Pho-ac.*
       menopause: *Sep.*
       pregnancy: *Lach.*
Hayfever   *All-c., Ars., Euphr., Nat-m., Nux-v., Puls.,*
    Sul.
    Eyes:
       stream: *All-c.*
       discharge:
          profuse: *All-c.*
          non-irritating: *All-c.*
          watery: *All-c.*
    Nasal catarrh:
       burning: *All-c.*

profuse: *All-c.*
watery: *All-c.*
With:
   eye inflammation: *Euphr., Sul.*
   cold sores: *Nat-m.*
   common cold symptoms: *Ars., Euphr.,*
      Nat-m., Nux-v., Puls., Sul., (see **Common**
      cold)
   cough: *Euphr.*
   sore throat: *All-c.*
   sneezing: *All-c.*
Worse:
   in the spring: *All-c.*
   in August: *All-c.*

Headache   *Aco., Agar., Ap., Arg-n., Ars., Bell., Bry.,*
   Calc-c., Calc-p., Carb-v., Chin., Cimi., Cocc.,
   Coff., Coloc., Eup-p., Ferr-m., Gels., Glon.,
   Ign., Ip., Kali-b., Kali-c., Kali-p., Kali-s., Lach.,
   Lyc., Mag-c., Mag-m., Mag-p., Merc-s., Nat-c.,
   Nat-m., Nat-p., Nat-s., Nit-ac., Nux-v., Petr.,
   Pho-ac., Phos., Puls., Rhod., Rhus-t., Ruta.,
   Sep., Sil., Stap., Sul., Zinc.
In schoolchildren: *Calc-p., Pho-ac.*
Extremities icy cold: *Sep.*
Eyes/eyelids:
   red: *Glon.*
   sensitive to light: *Nat-s.*
   smarting: *Pho-ac.*
   sore: *Nat-m.*
   twitching: *Agar.*
   watering: *Nat-m.*
Face:
   pale: *Nat-p.*
   red: *Glon.*
Head feels:
   constricted: *Nit-ac., Sul.*
   full: *Ap., Sul.*
   heavy: *Carb-v., Gels., Lach., Nat-c., Nux-v.,*
      Petr., Pho-ac.
   hot: *Ap., Lach., Sul.*
Nervous: *Chin., Coff., Kali-p., Puls., Zinc.*
Pains:
   aching: *Gels.*
   back of head: *Bell., Carb-v., Cimi., Cocc.,*
      Eup-p., Gels., Nux-v., Petr., Pho-ac.,
      Rhus-t., Sil., Stap.
   above eyes: *Kali-c.*
   behind eyeballs: *Bry.*
   in bones: *Nit-ac., Sep.*
   burning: *Aco., Ars., Calc-c., Merc-s., Phos.,*
      Sil., Sul.
   bursting: *Aco., Bell., Bry., Calc-c., Glon.,*
      Lach., Phos., Sep., Sul., Zinc.
   eyes: *Bell.*
   forehead: *Ars., Bell., Bry., Cocc., Ferr-m.,*
      Ign., Kali-c., Kali-s., Lach., Lyc., Merc-s.,

      Nat-m., Nat-p., Nux-v., Phos., Puls., Sil.,
      Stap., Sul., Zinc.
   hammering: *Bell., Ferr-m., Glon., Nat-m.,*
      Sil., Sul.
   left side of face: *Coloc.*
   maddening: *Calc-c.*
   nape of neck: *Cocc., Pho-ac.*
   one-sided: *Coff., Kali-p., Pho-ac., Puls.*
   pressing: *Carb-v., Chin., Lach., Lyc., Merc-s.,*
      Nat-c., Nat-m., Nit-ac., Nux-v., Petr.,
      Pho-ac., Phos., Puls., Sep., Sil., Stap., Sul.
   pressing out: *Cimi.*
   pressing up: *Cimi.*
   pulling: *Stap.*
   pulsating: *Bell.*
   recurring at regular intervals: *Ars., Kali-b.,*
      Mag-c., Nit-ac.
   rheumatic: *Rhus-t.*
   right side of head: *Mag-p.*
   shooting: *Kali-c., Mag-c., Mag-p., Sep.*
   sides of head: *Kali-s., Phos., Ruta., Zinc.*
   sinuses: *Kali-b., Sil.*
   sore, bruised: *Chin., Eup-p., Gels., Ip.,*
      Merc-s., Nux-v., Puls., Ruta., Sil., Stap.
   spasmodic: *Mag-c., Mag-p.*
   splitting: *Nat-m.*
   spreading to:
      back of head: *Gels., Lach.*
      forehead: *Gels.*
      top of head: *Sil.*
      to ear: *Coloc.*
      eyes: *Mag-m., Nit-ac., Sil.*
   stabbing: *Ap., Ign.*
   start and stop suddenly: *Bell.*
   stitching: *Kali-s.*
   stupefying: *Nux-v.*
   sudden: *Ap.*
   tearing: *Coloc., Kali-c., Mag-c., Nux-v., Rhod.,*
      Sep., Zinc.
   temples: *Bell., Lach., Lyc., Mag-m., Nat-m.,*
      Zinc.
   throbbing: *Aco., Ars., Bell., Chin., Eup-p.,*
      Ferr-m., Glon., Lach., Lyc., Nat-m., Phos.,
      Puls., Sep., Sil., Sul.
   top of head: *Cimi., Lach., Pho-ac., Sul.*
   violent: *Bell., Bry., Glon., Ign., Lach., Rhus-t.,*
      Sil.
   in waves: *Sep.*
   scalp feels sensitive: *Chin.*
Pupils dilated: *Gels.*
Scalp feels:
   tight: *Ap.*
   sensitive: *Chin.*
   sore: *Ap.*
Urination frequent: *Gels.*
Vision blurred: *Gels.*

With:
    belching: *Mag-m.*
    biliousness: *Nux-v.*
    cold feet: *Gels.*
    dizziness: *Nux-v.*
    eye strain: *Ruta.*
    faintness: *Glon.*
    fever: *Eup-p.*
    heaviness: *Petr.*
    hot flushes: *Glon.*
    hunger before/during headache: *Phos.*
    nausea: *Cocc., Petr., Sul.*
    sweating on the forehead: *Nat-c.*
    thirst: *Mag-m.*
    thirstlessness: *Ferr-m.*
    vomiting: *Ip.*
Better:
    for binding up the head: *Arg-n.*
    closing eyes: *Sil.*
    for cold: *Phos., Sul.*
    for cold compresses: *Bry., Glon., Phos., Sul.*
    after eating: *Lach., Sep.*
    evening in bed: *Nux-v.*
    excitement: *Nux-v., Pho-ac.*
    for fresh air: *Ars., Cimi., Kali-s., Lyc., Phos.,
        Puls., Sep., Zinc.*
    gentle walking: *Rhus-t.*
    getting up: *Nux-v., Phos., Rhod.*
        in the morning: *Nux-v.*
    heat: *Mag-p., Sil.*
    for lying down: *Calc-c., Ferr-m., Puls., Sil.*
    in a quiet, dark room: *Sil.*
    with head high: *Puls.*
    for lying in a darkened room: *Bell.*
    massage: *Phos.*
    movement: *Rhus-t.*
    for firm pressure: *Chin., Ferr-m., Mag-p.,
        Nat-m., Puls.*
    for pressure: *Bell., Bry., Glon., Mag-c.,
        Nux-v.*
    for resting head: *Bell.*
    after sleep: *Phos.*
    sunset: *Glon.*
    urinating: *Gels.*
    walking: *Mag-c., Phos., Puls., Rhod.*
        in the fresh air: *Puls., Rhod.*
    wrapping up head: *Nux-v., Rhod., Rhus-t.,
        Sil.*
Worse:
    10 a.m.–3 p.m.: *Nat-m.*
    for bending down: *Bell., Merc-s., Puls., Sep.,
        Sul.*
    blowing nose: *Puls., Sul.*
    getting chilled: *Sil.*
    for cold: *Bell., Kali-c., Mag-p., Nux-v., Phos.*
    getting head cold: *Sep., Sil.*

getting feet cold: *Sil.*
for coughing: *Bry., Lyc., Nat-m., Phos.,
    Sul.*
damp weather: *Rhod.*
daylight: *Phos., Sil.*
after drinking wine: *Zinc.*
after eating: *Nat-c., Nat-m., Nux-v., Puls.,
    Sul.*
emotions: *Nat-m.*
evening: *Kali-s.*
excitement: *Nat-m.*
moving eyes: *Nux-v.*
during a fever: *Nat-m.*
after getting up: *Bry., Sul.*
getting up from lying down: *Pho-ac., Sil.*
hot drinks: *Phos., Puls.*
jarring movement: *Glon., Nit-ac., Sil.*
for heat: *Ars., Bell., Glon., Puls.*
left side: *Kali-c., Lach.*
for light: *Bell., Calc-c.*
lying down: *Lach., Mag-c.*
during menstrual period: *Bell., Glon., Lyc.,
    Nat-m., Sep.*
mental exertion: *Glon., Nat-c., Nat-m.*
in the morning: *Agar., Sul.*
moving head: *Ferr-m., Gels.*
movement: *Gels., Nit-ac.*
at night: *Merc-s., Nit-ac.*
for noise: *Calc-c., Coff., Nit-ac.*
getting overheated: *Lyc.*
pressure: *Lach., Mag-m., Nit-ac.*
reading/writing: *Nat-m.*
on the right side of the head: *Calc-c.*
running: *Puls.*
shaking head: *Nux-v.*
smoky room: *Ign.*
warm room: *Kali-s.*
sneezing: *Sul.*
standing: *Puls.*
stuffy room: *Kali-s., Phos., Puls.*
exposure to sun: *Bell.*
summer: *Glon.*
sunrise: *Glon.*
sweating: *Eup-p.*
talking: *Nat-m.*
thinking: *Nat-c., Nat-m.*
travelling: *Sep.*
before/during a thunderstorm: *Rhod.*
touch: *Coloc., Stap.*
turning head quickly: *Nat-c.*
for tying up hair: *Bell.*
on waking: *Lach., Nat-m., Nit-ac.*
for walking: *Bell., Glon., Lach., Nit-ac., Sul.*
walking upstairs: *Sil.*
walking heavily: *Sil.*
warmth of bed: *Lyc., Sul.*

wine: *Zinc.*
wrapping up head: *Lyc., Mag-m., Phos.*
Causes:
  alcohol: *Agar., Lach., Nux-v.*
  anaemia: *Calc-p.*
  artificial light (working in): *Sep., Sil.*
  change of weather: *Bry., Rhus-t.*
  getting chilled: *Aco., Mag-p.*
  cold air: *Bell., Rhod., Rhus-t., Sil.*
  cold, damp weather: *Bry., Calc-c., Sul.*
  cold wind: *Nux-v., Rhus-t.*
  common cold: *Merc-s., Nux-v.*
  damp weather: *Nux-v., Rhus-t., Sil., Sul.*
  draughts: *Sil.*
  emotions: *Stap.*
  excitement: *Coloc., Puls., Stap.*
  excited conversation: *Sul.*
  eye strain: *Kali-c., Lyc., Pho-ac., Ruta., Sil.*
  fright: *Aco.*
  getting head wet (haircut): *Bell.*
  getting wet: *Calc-c., Rhus-t.*
  grief: *Pho-ac., Stap.*
  head injury: *Nat-s.*
  ice-cream: *Puls.*
  ironing: *Bry.*
  irregular sleep: *Cocc.*
  lifting: *Rhus-t.*
  loss of sleep: *Cocc., Nux-v.*
  menopause: *Lach.*
  mental exertion: *Calc-c., Calc-p., Kali-p., Nat-c., Nat-p., Nux-v., Pho-ac.*
  mental strain: *Chin., Lyc., Nat-c., Nux-v., Pho-ac.*
  nerves: *Agar., Chin.*
  over-eating: *Nux-v.*
  over-exposure to sun: *Bell., Bry., Glon., Lach.*
  overwork: *Calc-p., Kali-p., Sil., Zinc.*
  physical exertion: *Calc-p.*
  rheumatism: *Merc-s.*
  running: *Puls.*
  shock: *Aco.*
  summer: *Nat-c.*
  sunstroke: *Nat-c.*
  before a thunderstorm: *Phos.*
  travelling (car/coach/train etc.): *Sil.*
  vexation: *Coloc., Stap.*
  winter: *Sul.*
Head injuries see **Injuries** to head
Heartburn see **Indigestion**
Heavy feeling (see also **Sluggish**)
  Generally: *Gels., Phos., Sep.*
Herpes see **Cold sores**
Hives *Ap., Dulc., Rhus-t., Urt-u.*
  Rash:
    biting: *Urt-u.*
    burning: *Rhus-t., Urt-u.*

itching: *Rhus-t., Urt-u.*
lumpy: *Dulc.*
stinging: *Rhus-t., Urt-u.*
With:
  fever: *Ap.*
  joint pain: *Rhus-t., Urt-u.*
  sweating: *Ap.*
Better:
  rubbing: *Urt-u.*
Worse:
  cold: *Rhus-t.*
  exercise: *Urt-u.*
  heat: *Dulc., Urt-u.*
  night: *Ap., Urt-u.*
  after scratching: *Dulc., Rhus-t.*
Causes:
  getting chilled/wet: *Rhus-t.*
  getting cold: *Dulc.*
  cold air: *Rhus-t.*
  during a fever: *Rhus-t.*
  insects: *Urt-u.*
  stinging nettles: *Urt-u.*
Hoarseness *Arg-n., Bell., Calc-c., Carb-v., Caust., Phos., Rhus-t.* (see also **Voice lost**; **Sore throat**, With hoarseness)
Caused by:
  over-using voice: *Arg-n., Caust., Phos., Rhus-t.*
  voice lost: *Caust.*
Painful: *Bell., Phos.*
Painless: *Calc-c., Carb-v.*
When crying: *Bell.*
Worse:
  evening: *Carb-v., Caust., Phos.*
  morning: *Calc-c., Carb-v., Caust., Phos.*
Homesick *Ign., Pho-ac.*
Hot flushes *Cocc., Kali-c., Lach., Nat-s., Phos., Sep., Sul-ac.*
Flush moves up the body: *Sep.*
With:
  headache: *Lach.*
  palpitations: *Lach.*
  hot sweats: *Lach.*
Worse:
  during the afternoon: *Sep.*
  during the evening: *Sep.*
  after sweating: *Sep.*
Causes:
  menopause: *Lach., Sul-ac.*
Hurried *Arg-n., Hep-s., Sul-ac.*
While eating: *Hep-s., Sul-ac.*
At work: *Sul-ac.*
While speaking: *Arg-n., Hep-s.*
While waiting: *Arg-n.*
While walking: *Arg-n., Sul-ac.*
While writing: *Sul-ac.*

Idealistic *Ign.*
Impatient (see also **Irritable**) *Cham., Hep-s., Nux-v., Sul.*
Impulsive *Arg-n., Hep-s., Nux-v.*
Indecisive *Bar-c., Lyc.*
Indifferent (see also **Apathetic**) *Carb-v., Nat-m., Nat-p., Pho-ac., Rhe., Sep.*
   During a fever: *Op., Pho-ac.*
   Children: *Rhe.*
      to playing: *Rhe.*
   To everything: *Carb-v.*
   To own children: *Sep.*
   To family: *Sep.*
   To loved ones: *Sep.*
   To personal appearance (i.e., scruffy): *Sul.*
   To work: *Sep.*
Indigestion *Ant-c., Arg-n., Ars., Calc-c., Carb-v., Caust., Chin., Ign., Kali-b., Lyc., Kali-c., Kali-m., Kali-p., Mag-c., Merc-s., Nat-c., Nat-m., Nat-p., Nat-s., Nux-v., Phos., Puls., Sul.* (see **Flatulence; Taste**)
   Belches:
      acrid: *Lyc.*
      bitter: *Chin., Nat-s., Nux-v., Puls.*
      difficult: *Arg-n.*
      empty: *Ant-c., Arg-n., Carb-v., Caust., Kali-b., Lyc., Puls., Sul.*
      greasy: *Mag-c.*
      incomplete, ineffectual: *Chin., Nat-m.*
      loud: *Arg-n.*
      sour: *Calc-c., Carb-v., Chin., Ign., Kali-b., Lyc., Mag-c., Nat-c., Nat-m., Nat-p., Nat-s., Nux-v., Sul.*
      tasting of food eaten: *Ant-c., Caust., Chin., Nat-m., Puls.*
   Belly/stomach feels:
      bloated: *Ant-c., Arg-n., Calc-c., Carb-v., Chin., Kali-c., Mag-c., Nat-p., Nat-s., Nux-v., Sul.*
      empty: *Ant-c., Ign., Kali-p., Lyc., Nux-v., Puls., Sul.*
         at 11 a.m.: *Sul.*
      full: *Ant-c., Caust., Kali-c., Lyc.*
         very quickly (when eating): *Lyc.*
      hard: *Calc-c.*
      rumbling: *Mag-c.*
   Nervous: *Kali-p.*
   Pains in the stomach:
      burning: *Ars., Carb-v., Phos., Sul.*
      cramping: *Carb-v., Caust., Lyc., Nat-m., Nux-v.*
      pressing: *Calc-c., Caust., Chin., Lyc., Nat-m., Nux-v., Puls.*
      sore, bruised: *Kali-c., Nat-c., Nux-v., Phos.*
   With:
      diarrhoea: *Kali-m.*

      flatulence: *Arg-n., Calc-c., Carb-v., Sul.*
         after breakfast: *Nat-s.*
      heartburn: *Ars., Calc-c., Lyc., Mag-c., Merc-s., Nat-p., Nux-v., Puls.*
      nausea: *Arg-n., Carb-v., Mag-c., Nat-c.*
      stools pale: *Kali-m.*
      violent hiccups: *Nat-m.*
   Better:
      belching: *Arg-n., Carb-v., Ign., Kali-b., Kali-c., Lyc.*
      hot drinks: *Ars., Nux-v.*
      after passing a stool: *Nat-s.*
      passing wind: *Carb-v.*
      warmth of bed: *Nux-v.*
   Worse:
      after belching: *Chin.*
      after cabbage: *Mag-c.*
      after drinking: *Chin., Sul.*
      after eating: *Arg-n., Carb-v., Chin., Kali-b., Kali-c., Lyc., Nux-v., Phos., Puls., Sul.*
      fruit: *Chin.*
      milk: *Mag-c., Sul.*
      at night: *Puls.*
      onions: *Lyc.*
      rich/fatty food: *Carb-v., Puls.*
      starchy food: *Kali-m., Nat-m., Nat-s.*
      tight clothing: *Lyc., Nux-v.*
   Causes:
      abdominal surgery: *Chin.*
      alcohol: *Nux-v.*
      beer: *Kali-b.*
      coffee: *Nux-v.*
      grief: *Ign.*
      mental strain: *Nux-v.*
      nervous exhaustion: *Kali-p.*
      over-eating: *Nux-v.*
      overwork: *Kali-p.*
      pregnancy: *Merc-s.*
      rich/fatty food: *Nux-v., Puls.*
Injuries *Aco., Arn., Bell., Calc-s., Calen., Con., Hep-s., Hyp., Lach., Led., Phos., Ruta., Sil., Stap.* (see also **Bites/Stings; Broken bones; Bruises; Sprains; Strains**)
   Cuts/wounds:
      bleed freely: *Aco., Bell., Lach., Phos.*
      blood:
         bright red: *Phos.*
         slow to clot: *Phos.*
      crushed: *Hyp.*
      inflamed: *Hep-s., Sil.*
         with redness around: *Hep-s.*
         with dirt/splinter still inside: *Sil.*
         with pus inside: *Sil.*
         with pus oozing: *Calc-s.*
      painful: *Calen., Hep-s., Hyp., Sil., Stap.*
         shooting: *Hyp.*

sore/bruised: *Arn.*, *Hep-s.*, *Ruta.*

splinter-like: *Hep-s.*

stitching/tearing: *Stap.*

painful out of proportion to the injury: *Calen.*

suppurate: *Calc-s.*, *Calen.*, *Sil.*

with bruising: *Arn.*

To fingers/toes (crushed): *Hyp.*

Lacerated wounds (torn): *Calen.*, *Hyp.*, *Led.*

Punctured wounds (with a knife, or nail, etc.): *Hyp.*, *Led.*

Slow to heal: *Calc-s.*, *Hep-s.*, *Hyp.*, *Lach.*, *Sil.*

To glands (breasts, testicles, etc.): *Con.*

To head: *Arn.*

cold, inflamed, sensitive, stony hard lumps, swollen: *Con.*

To muscles: *Arn.*

To nerves/nerve-rich parts of the body: *Hyp.*, *Stap.*

To palm of hand or sole of foot: *Led.*

To shins: *Ruta.*

With:

shock (anxiety and fear): *Aco.*

foreign body: *Sil.*

Scars:

become lumpy: *Sil.*

become red: *Lach.*

are painful, break open and/or suppurate: *Sil.*

Better:

cold compresses: *Led.*

Worse:

heat: *Led.*

touch: *Hep-s.*, *Stap.*

Causes:

accident: *Hyp.*, *Stap.*

after dental treatment: *Arn.*, *Hyp.*, *Stap.*

childbirth: *Stap.*

episiotomy: *Hep-s.*, *Hyp.*, *Sil.*, *Stap.*

nails: *Led.*

splinter: *Hyp.*, *Led.*, *Sil.*

surgery: *Arn.*, *Hyp.*, *Sil.*, *Stap.*

Insect bites   see **Bites/Stings**

Insomnia   *Aco.*, *Ars.*, *Bell.*, *Bell-p.*, *Calc-c.*, *Calc-p.*, *Cham.*, *Cocc.*, *Coff.*, *Con.*, *Kali-c.*, *Kali-p.*, *Mag-c.*, *Mag-m.*, *Nat-c.*, *Nat-m.*, *Nit-ac.*, *Nux-v.*, *Op.*, *Pho-ac.*, *Phos.*, *Puls.*, *Rhus-t.*, *Sep.*, *Sil.*, *Sul.*

Dreams

anxious: *Aco.*, *Ars.*, *Calc-c.*, *Cocc.*, *Kali-c.*, *Nat-c.*, *Nat-m.*, *Nit-ac.*, *Phos.*, *Puls.*

nightmares: *Ars.*, *Cocc.*, *Con.*, *Kali-c.*, *Sil.*, *Sul.*

vivid: *Sil.*, *Sul.*

unpleasant: *Sul.*

vivid: *Nat-m.*

Sleep:

disturbed: *Sul.*

restless: *Aco.*, *Ars.*, *Bell.*, *Cocc.*, *Puls.*, *Rhus-t.*, *Sil.*, *Sul.*

unrefreshing: *Mag-c.*, *Mag-m.*, *Nit-ac.*, *Pho-ac.*, *Sul.*

Sleepless: *Pho-ac.*

after midnight: *Pho-ac.*, *Rhus-t.*, *Sil.*

after 2 a.m.: *Nit-ac.*

after 3 a.m.: *Bell-p.*, *Mag-c.*, *Nux-v.*

after waking: *Sil.*

before midnight: *Con.*, *Kali-c.*

Waking:

around 3 a.m.: *Nux-v.*, *Sep.*

difficult: *Calc-p.*

early: *Nat-c.*, *Nux-v.*

frequent: *Pho-ac.*, *Puls.*, *Sul.*

from cold: *Puls.*

late: *Calc-p.*, *Nux-v.*, *Sul.*

With:

empty feeling in pit of stomach: *Kali-p.*

grinding of teeth: *Bell.*

sleepiness: *Bell.*, *Cham.*, *Op.*, *Phos.*, *Puls.*, *Sep.*

Better:

short naps: *Sul.*

Worse:

around 1–2 a.m.: *Kali-c.*

after 2 a.m.: *Nit-ac.*

after 3 a.m.: *Bell-p.*, *Sep.*

after 3, 4, or 5 a.m.: *Sul.*

after midnight: *Ars.*, *Sil.*

before midnight: *Calc-c.*, *Calc-p.*, *Kali-c.*, *Puls.*

Causes:

alcohol: *Nux-v.*

anxiety: *Ars.*, *Cocc.*, *Kali-p.*

coffee: *Nux-v.*

excitement: *Kali-p.*, *Nux-v.*

grief: *Nat-m.*

mental strain: *Kali-p.*, *Nux-v.*

nervous exhaustion: *Kali-p.*

over-active mind: *Ars.*, *Calc-c.*, *Coff.*, *Nux-v.*, *Puls.*

over-excitement: *Coff.*

overwork: *Nux-v.*

repeating thoughts: *Puls.*

shock: *Ars.*

worry: *Calc-c.*

Introspective   (see also **Broody**; **Morose**; **Uncommunicative**) *Cocc.*, *Ign.*, *Nat-c.*, *Puls.*

Introverted   *Nat-m.*

Irritable   (see also **Angry**) *Ant-c.*, *Ap.*, *Ars.*, *Bry.*, *Carb-v.*, *Caust.*, *Cham.*, *Cina*, *Ferr-m.*, *Hep-s.*, *Kali-c.*, *Kali-s.*, *Lyc.*, *Mag-c.*, *Nat-c.*, *Nat-m.*, *Nit-ac.*, *Nux-v.*, *Petr.*, *Pho-ac.*, *Phos.*, *Puls.*,

Rhe., Rhus-t., Sep., Sil., Stap., Sul., Sul-ac.,
Ver-a., Zinc.
Children: Cham., Cina, Mag-c.
Before stools: Bor.
On waking: Lyc.

Jealous   Ap., Lach., Puls.

Joint pain   Ap., Arn., Bell-p., Bry., Calc-c., Calc-p.,
Caul., Caust., Cham., Colch., Dulc., Ferr-m.,
Hep-s., Kali-b., Kali-c., Kali-s., Led., Lyc.,
Merc-s., Nit-ac., Puls., Rhod., Rhus-t., Sul.
Feet cold: Kali-s.
Joints:
   icy cold: Led.
   hot: Led.
   stiff: Led.
Pains:
   aching: Rhus-t.
   acute: Colch.
   alternating with:
      indigestion: Kali-b.
      cough: Kali-b.
   arms: Ferr-m., Kali-c., Rhod.
      upper: Ferr-m.
   in back: Caust.
   bones: Nit-ac., Puls., Ruta.
   burning: Ap., Caust., Merc-s., Sul.
   cramping: Calc-c.
   drawing: Rhod.
   feet: Colch., Led., Ruta.
   fingers: Hep-s.
   fly around: Caul.
   gnawing: Caust.
   hands: Colch., Led., Ruta.
   hips: Hep-s., Kali-c., Kali-s.
      right: Led.
   irregular: Caul.
   in joints: Caust., Puls.
   legs: Kali-c., Kali-s., Nit-ac., Rhod.
   lower back: Ruta.
   in neck: Caust.
   parts lain on: Ruta.
   pressing: Caust.
   pulling: Hep-s., Puls.
   shoulders: Ferr-m., Hep-s., Kali-c., Rhod.
      left: Led.
   in small joints: Caul.
   in one spot: Kali-b.
   sore/bruised: Arn., Hep-s., Kali-b., Kali-c.,
      Puls., Rhus-t., Ruta.
   shooting: Rhus-t.
   splinter-like: Nit-ac.
   stinging: Ap.
   stitching: Bry., Caust., Ferr-m., Kali-c., Nit-ac.
   tearing: Caust., Colch., Ferr-m., Hep-s.,
      Kali-c., Lyc., Merc-s., Nit-ac., Rhod.,
      Rhus-t., Sul.

   violent: Cham.
   wandering: Kali-b., Kali-s., Puls.
With:
   heaviness: Rhus-t.
   lameness: Rhus-t., Ruta.
   numbness: Cham.
   restless legs: Kali-c.
   stiffness: Caust., Rhus-t.
   swelling: Ap., Bry., Colch.
   weakness of arms: Kali-c.
Better:
   after a common cold: Led.
   cold compresses: Led., Puls.
   cold bathing: Led.
   continued movement: Rhus-t.
   fresh air: Kali-s., Puls.
   gentle movement: Ferr-m., Puls.
   heat: Caust., Hep-s., Rhus-t.
   movement: Dulc., Kali-c., Kali-s., Lyc.,
      Rhod.
   pressure: Bry.
   complete rest: Bry.
   stretching out limb: Rhod.
   uncovering: Led.
   walking: Kali-c., Kali-s., Lyc., Puls., Rhus-t.
   warm compresses: Rhus-t.
   warmth: Caust., Colch.
   warmth of bed: Caust., Lyc., Rhus-t.
Worse:
   around 2–3 a.m.: Kali-c.
   in bed: Merc-s.
   beginning to move: Ferr-m., Lyc., Puls.,
      Rhus-t.
   bending arm backwards: Ferr-m.
   change of weather: Rhod.
   getting chilled: Rhus-t.
   cold: Bry., Calc-p., Colch., Hep-s.
   damp weather: Rhus-t.
   dry cold: Caust.
   cold, wet weather: Calc-p., Colch.
   after a common cold: Puls.
   during a fever: Lyc., Rhus-t.
   getting up from sitting: Caust.
   heat: Kali-s., Led., Puls.
   lifting arm up: Ferr-m.
   lying on the painful part: Kali-c.
   night: Dulc., Led., Merc-s., Nit-ac., Rhus-t.
   slightest movement: Bry.
   movement: Colch., Led.
   sitting down: Dulc., Lyc., Rhus-t., Rhod.
   stormy weather: Rhod.
   summer: Kali-s.
   touch: Arn.
   walking: Ruta., Sul.
   warm weather: Colch.
   warmth of bed: Led., Puls., Sul.

wet weather: *Calc-c., Merc-s., Puls., Rhod.*
wine: *Led.*
Causes:
    getting chilled after being very hot: *Bell-p.*
    getting cold: *Dulc., Hep-s.*
    damp: *Dulc.*
    wet weather: *Calc-c.*

Jumpy (see also **Anxious; Restless**) *Bar-c., Bor., Kali-c., Kali-p., Nat-c., Nat-s., Phos., Sil.*

Labour pains *Caul., Cham., Cimi., Gels., Kali-c., Puls., Sep.*
Pains:
    in back: *Gels., Kali-c., Puls.*
    distressing: *Cham., Gels., Kali-c., Sep.*
    flying around: *Cimi.*
    ineffectual: *Caul., Kali-c., Puls.*
    irregular: *Caul., Puls.*
    severe: *Cham., Sep.*
    sore, bruised: *Cimi.*
    stop: *Caul., Cimi., Kali-c., Puls.*
    unbearable: *Cham.*
    weak: *Cimi., Gels., Kali-c., Puls.*
With:
    exhaustion and trembling: *Caul.*

Lack of self-confidence (see also **Shy**) *Bar-c., Lyc., Sil.*

Laryngitis see **Sore throat**

Lazy *Sul.*

Lethargic see **Apathetic; Exhaustion; Sluggish**

Likes
boiled eggs: *Calc-c.*
bread and butter: *Merc-s.*
chocolate: *Phos., Lyc.*
cold drinks: *Aco., Bry., Cham., Chin., Cina, Eup-p., Merc-c., Merc-s., Nat-s., Phos., Ver-a.*
cold food: *Phos., Puls.*
fat/fatty foods: *Nit-ac.*
fruit: *Pho-ac., Ver-a.*
ham, salami, smoked foods: *Caust.*
hot drinks: *Ars., Bry.*
hot food: *Ars., Bry.*
ice-cream: *Phos., Ver-a.*
ice-cold drinks: *Phos., Ver-a.*
milk: *Phos., Rhus-t.*
refreshing things: *Pho-ac., Ver-a.*
salt, salty foods: *Nat-m., Phos.*
sour food: *Hep-s., Ver-a.*
spicy food: *Chin., Phos., Sul., Nux-v.*
sugar: *Arg-n.*
sweets: *Arg-n., Chin., Lyc., Sul.*
vinegar: *Sep.*

Lips
Cracked: *Ars., Nat-m., Sul.*
Blue: *Cupr., Lach.*
Dry: *Ant-c., Ars., Bry., Puls., Rhus-t., Sul.*

Licks: *Ars.*
Red: *Sul.*

Lively (see also **Excitable**) *Coff., Lach., Nat-c., Op.*

Lonely *Puls.*

Loquacious see **Talkative**

Lumbago see **Backache**

Mastitis see **Breastfeeding problems**

Measles *Aco., Ap., Bell., Bry., Euphr., Gels., Puls., Sul.*
Onset:
    slow: *Bry., Gels.*
    sudden: *Aco., Bell.*
Skin rash:
    burns: *Aco., Bell., Sul.*
    hot: *Bell.*
    itches: *Aco., Bell., Sul.*
        maddeningly: *Sul.*
    red: *Bell., Sul.*
    slow to appear: *Ap., Bry., Sul.*
With:
    common cold: *Euphr., Puls.*
    cough: *Aco., Bell., Bry., Euphr., Puls., Sul.*
    eye inflammation: *Ap., Bell., Euphr., Puls.*
    fever: *Aco., Ap., Bell., Bry., Gels., Sul.*
    headache: *Bry., Gels.*
Worse for heat: *Sul.*

Melancholic *Calc-c.*

Memory weak *Arg-n., Caust., Cocc., Colch., Con.*

Migraine see **Headache**, one-sided

Mild, gentle *Cocc., Sil.*

Moody (changeable) *Ferr-m., Ign., Lyc., Puls., Sul-ac., Zinc.*

Morose (see also **Depression; Despondent**) *Bry.*

Mouth
Burning: *Ars.*
Dark red: *Bapt.*
Dry: *Ars., Bry., Merc-s., Nat-m., Puls.*
    with thirst: *Bry., Nat-m.*
    without thirst: *Puls.*

Mouth ulcers *Lyc., Merc-s., Nit-ac.*
Ulcers:
    edges of tongue: *Nit-ac.*
    gums: *Merc-s.*
    mouth: *Merc-s.*
    painful: *Nit-ac.*
    on the tongue: *Merc-s.*
    under the tongue: *Lyc.*
Pains:
    stinging/throbbing: *Merc-s.*

Mumps *Aco., Bell., Carb-v., Jab., Lach., Lyc., Merc-s., Phyt., Puls., Rhus-t.*
Glands (parotid):
    hard: *Merc-s., Phyt.*
    swelling moves from the right side to the left: *Lyc.*

swollen/painful: *Bell., Carb-v., Jab., Lach.,
  Lyc., Merc-s., Phyt., Puls., Rhus-t., Sil.*
Onset sudden: *Aco., Bell.*
Pains spread to breasts, ovaries or testicles:
  Carb-v., Jab., Phyt., Puls.
With:
    face red: *Jab.*
    fever: *Aco., Bell., Lyc., Merc-s., Puls.,
      Rhus-t.*
    headache: *Bell.*
    copious saliva: *Jab., Merc-s., Phyt.*
    profuse sweating: *Jab., Phyt., Merc-s.*
    sore throat: *Bell., Lach., Lyc., Phyt.*
Better:
    heat: *Rhus-t., Sil.*
Worse:
    blowing nose: *Merc-s.*
    night: *Merc-s.*
    on the left: *Lach., Rhus-t.*
    on the right: *Bell., Merc-s.*
    cold: *Rhus-t., Sil.*

Nausea *Ant-c., Ant-t., Cocc., Colch., Ip., Nux-v.,
  Petr., Phos., Puls., Sep., Tab.*
Constant: *Ant-c., Ip., Nux-v.*
Deathly: *Tab.*
Intermittent: *Ant-t., Tab.*
Persistent: *Ip.*
Violent: *Ip., Tab.*
    during pregnancy: *Ant-c.*
Appetite:
    lost: *Cocc., Colch.*
Belching: *Ant-c., Cocc.*
    empty: *Ant-c., Ip.*
    sour: *Phos.*
    tasting of food eaten: *Ant-c.*
Belly/stomach feels:
    bloated: *Colch.*
    empty: *Cocc., Phos., Sep.*
Pains:
    gnawing: *Sep.*
Taste:
    metallic: *Cocc.*
With:
    dizziness: *Petr.*
    faintness: *Cocc., Colch.*
    face pallid: *Ip.*
    retching: *Ip.*
    copious saliva: *Ip.*
    vomiting: *Colch.*
Better:
    for belching: *Ant-t.*
    after eating (temporarily): *Sep.*
    fresh air: *Tab.*
    for vomiting: *Ant-t.*
Worse:
    after drinking: *Cocc., Puls.*

    after eating: *Ant-c., Cocc., Colch., Ip., Nux-v.,
      Puls., Sep.*
    afternoon: *Cocc.*
    before breakfast: *Sep.*
    coughing: *Puls.*
    eating acidic foods: *Ant-c.*
    eating bread: *Ant-c.*
    eating starchy food: *Ant-c.*
    fresh air: *Petr.*
    hot drinks: *Phos., Puls.*
    milk: *Calc-c., Nit-ac., Sep.*
    morning: *Puls., Sep.*
    morning in bed: *Nux-v.*
    movement: *Cocc., Ip.*
    pork: *Sep.*
    putting hands in warm water: *Phos.*
    sight of food: *Colch.*
    sitting up in bed: *Cocc.*
    smell of food: *Cocc., Colch., Ip.*
    stuffy room: *Tab.*
    sweating: *Nux-v.*
    tobacco: *Ip., Nux-v.*
    thought of food: *Cocc., Colch.*
    water: *Phos.*
Causes:
    ice-cream: *Puls.*
    pregnancy: *Nux-v., Sep., Tab.*
    rich food: *Puls.*
    travelling: *Nux-v., Tab.*

Nervous see **Anxious**
Nettle rash see **Hives**
Nose
    Child picks constantly: *Cina*
Nosebleeds *Arn., Carb-v., Ferr-m., Ham., Lach.,
    Phos., Sul.*
Blood:
    bright red: *Phos.*
    dark: *Carb-v., Ham., Lach.*
    persistent: *Phos.*
    thin: *Ham.*
Children: *Ferr-m.*
With:
    sweating: *Phos.*
Worse:
    before a menstrual period: *Lach.*
    blowing nose: *Phos., Sul.*
    morning: *Ham., Lach.*
    at night: *Carb-v.*
Causes:
    blowing nose: *Lach.*
    injury: *Arn.*
    menopause: *Lach.*
Obstinate see **Stubborn**
Onset of complaint
    Slow: *Bry., Gels.*
    Sudden: *Aco., Bell.*

Overconscientious: *Ign.*
Oversensitivity see **Sensitive**
Pains
    Absent: *Op.*
    Appear suddenly: *Bell.*
    Appear suddenly and disappear suddenly: *Bell.,*
        Kali-b., Nit-ac.
    Bones: *Eup-p., Merc-s., Nit-ac., Pho-ac., Ruta.*
    Burning: *Ap., Ars., Phos., Rhus-t., Sul.*
    Cramping: *Calc-c., Cupr., Mag-p., Nux-v.*
    Flying around: *Nit-ac.*
    Glands: *Arn., Bell., Lyc., Merc-s., Phos.*
    Needle-like: *Arg-n., Hep-s., Nit-ac.*
    Parts lain on: *Puls., Pyr., Ruta.*
    Pressing: *Canth., Merc-s., Rhus-t., Sep.*
    Shooting: *Bell., Hyp., Rhus-t.*
    Shoot upwards: *Phyt.*
    Sore/bruised: *Arn., Bry., Chin., Cimi., Eup-p.,*
        Ham., Pyr., Rhus-t., Ruta.
    Splinter-like see **Needle-like**
    In a spot: *Kali-b.*
    Stinging: *Ap., Sil.*
    Stitching: *Bry., Kali-c.*
    Throbbing: *Bell.*
    Unbearable: *Aco., Cham.*
    Wandering: *Kali-b., Kali-s., Led., Puls.*
    With screaming: *Aco.*
Palpitations   *Aco., Arg-n., Ars., Calc-c., Lach.*
Panic (see also **Anxious; Fearful**) *Arg-n.*
Period problems
    Belly:
        bloated: *Cocc.*
    Bleeding:
        during day time only: *Puls.*
    Blood:
        bright red: *Bell.*
        dark red: *Calc-p.*
        clotted: *Bell., Calc-p., Cham.*
    Breasts:
        lumpy before period: *Con.*
        painful before period: *Con.*
    Pains:
        aching: *Nux-v., Puls., Sep.*
        colicky: *Mag-p.*
        cramping: *Cocc., Mag-p., Nux-v.*
        cutting: *Lach.*
        dragging down: *Sep.*
        dull: *Puls., Sep.*
        gripping: *Cocc.*
        lower back: *Nux-v.*
        pressing: *Sep.*
        severe: *Cocc.*
        sore, bruised: *Sep.*
        stitching: *Con.*
        tearing: *Lach.*
        violent: *Bell.*

        wandering: *Puls.*
    Better:
        crossing legs: *Sep.*
        heat: *Mag-p.*
        once period starts: *Lach.*
        pressure: *Mag-p.*
        doubling up: *Mag-p., Nux-v., Puls.*
    Worse:
        before a menstrual period: *Bell., Con.,*
          Puls., Lach.
        during the period: *Bell., Nux-v., Puls.,*
          Sep.
        afternoon: *Sep.*
        breathing: *Cocc.*
        cold: *Mag-p.*
        morning: *Sep.*
        9 a.m.–6 p.m.: *Sep.*
        movement: *Cocc.*
        standing: *Sep.*
        walking: *Sep.*
    Causes:
        anger: *Cham.*
    With exhaustion: *Con.*
    Periods:
        heavy: *Bell., Calc-p., Nux-v.*
        late: *Aco., Puls.*
          caused by:
            fright: *Aco.*
            shock: *Aco.*
            getting chilled: *Aco.*
        painful: *Bell., Calc-p., Cham., Cocc., Con.,*
          Lach., Mag-p., Nux-v., Puls., Sep.
Perspiration   see **Sweat**
Piles   *Ham., Kali-c., Nit-ac., Nux-v.*
    Bleeding: *Ham., Nit-ac.*
    Large: *Ham., Kali-c., Nit-ac.*
    Pains:
        burning: *Nit-ac.*
        sore, bruised: *Ham.*
        splinter-like: *Nit-ac.*
    Worse:
        after a stool: *Nit-ac.*
    Causes:
        childbirth: *Ham., Kali-c.*
        pregnancy: *Ham., Nux-v.*
Pink eye   see **Eye inflammation**
Pregnancy problems   see also **Nausea, Heartburn**
    Pains:
        flying about belly: *Cimi.*
        in groin: *Bell-p.*
        while walking: *Bell-p.*
        severe: *Bell-p.*
    Worse:
        movement: *Bell-p.*
Prickly heat   *Nat-m., Sal., Sul., Urt-u.*
Pulse   rapid: *Pyr.*

Pupils

    Contracted: *Op.*

    Dilated: *Bell.*

Quarrelsome   (see also **Dislikes** contradiction; **Irritable**)

Resentful   see **Unforgiving; Complaints from** suppressed anger

Restless   *Ap., Arg-n., Ars., Bapt., Bell., Calc-p., Caust., Cimi., Cina, Coloc., Cupr., Ferr-m., Lyc., Mag-m., Merc-s., Rhus-t., Sil., Sul.*

    Evening: *Caust.*

    In bed: *Ars., Cupr., Ferr-m., Mag-m., Rhus-t.*

    Sleep: *Cina*

        body twitching/limbs jerking/grinding of teeth: *Cina*

    With anxiety: *Ars.*

Retention of urine

    In newborn babies: *Aco.*

    In children: *Ap.*

        who catch cold: *Aco.*

    Causes:

        childbirth: *Ars., Caust.*

        presence of strangers: *Nat-m.*

        shock: *Op.*

Rheumatism   see **Joint pain**

Rhinitis   see **Common cold, Hayfever**

Roseola   see **Measles**

Rushed feeling   see **Hurried**

Sad   see **Depressed; Tearful**

Saliva

    Increased: *Merc-s., Ver-a.*

        during sleep: *Merc-s.*

Scared   see **Fearful**

Scattered sensation   *Bapt.*

Sciatica   *Coloc., Ferr-m., Mag-p., Puls., Rhus-t.*

    Pains:

        tearing: *Coloc.*

    Better:

        fresh air: *Puls.*

        gentle movement: *Ferr-m.*

        heat: *Mag-p., Rhus-t.*

        movement: *Rhus-t.*

        walking: *Rhus-t.*

        walking slowly: *Ferr-m.*

    Worse:

        beginning to move: *Rhus-t.*

        cold: *Mag-p., Rhus-t.*

        cold compresses: *Rhus-t.*

        lying on painful part: *Rhus-t.*

        right side: *Coloc.*

        warm room: *Puls.*

        washing in cold water: *Rhus-t.*

        wet weather: *Rhus-t.*

Screaming   *Aco., Bell., Bor., Cham., Coff., Lyc.*

    In children: *Bor., Lyc.*

    With pain: *Aco., Bell., Cham., Coff.*

    During sleep: *Bor., Lyc.*

    On waking: *Lyc.*

Self-confidence, lack of   (see also **Shy**) *Bar-c., Lyc., Sil.*

Sense of smell

    Acute: *Colch., Nux-v., Op.*

    Lost: *Calc-c.*

Senses

    Acute   *Coff., Op.*

    Dull: *Op.*

Sensitive   *Cham., Chin., Coff., Con., Hep-s., Ign., Kali-c., Lach., Lyc., Nat-c., Nat-m., Nat-p., Nit-ac., Nux-v., Phos., Puls., Sil., Stap.*

    To light: *Bell., Nux-v., Phos.*

    To music: *Nat-c., Nux-v., Sep.*

    To noise: *Aco., Bell., Chin., Coff., Con., Kali-c., Nit-ac., Nux-v., Op., Sep., Sil., Zinc.*

    To pain: *Cham., Coff., Ign., Lach., Nit-ac., Phos., Sep., Sil., Stap.*

    To rudeness: *Hep-s., Nux-v., Stap.*

    To touch: *Lach.*

Sentimental   *Ant-c., Ign.*

Shock   *Aco., Arn., Hyp., Ign., Lach., Op., Pho-ac.*

    Causes:

        emotional trauma: *Ign., Pho-ac.*

        injuries: *Aco., Hyp., Lach., Op.*

        surgery: *Aco.*

        childbirth: *Aco.*

Shy   *Bar-c., Lyc., Nat-c., Puls., Sil.*

Sighing   *Calc-p., Cimi., Ign.*

Side   see **Symptoms**

Sinusitis   see **Common cold**

Sleepless   see **Insomnia**

Sleepy   see **Drowsy**

Slowness   *Bar-c., Calc-c., Calc-p., Con., Phos.*

    Of children: *Calc-c., Calc-p.*

        learning to walk: *Calc-c.*

        to teethe: *Calc-c., Calc-p.*

        to learn: *Bar-c., Calc-p.*

Sluggish   (see also **Apathetic; Exhaustion**) *Ant-c., Bar-c., Bry., Calc-c., Calc-p., Calc-s., Carb-v., Gels., Kali-c., Lach., Nat-c., Nat-p., Nit-ac., Sep., Sil., Sul., Zinc.*

    Children: *Bar-c., Calc-p., Sul.*

    On waking: *Lach.*

    Better for fresh air: *Lyc.*

Sore throat   *Aco., All-c., Ap., Arg-n., Ars., Bapt., Bar-c., Bell., Bry., Calc-c., Caust., Dulc., Hep-s., Ign., Kali-m., Lach., Lyc., Merc-c., Merc-s., Nat-m., Nit-ac., Nux-v., Phos., Phyt., Puls., Rhus-t., Rumex., Sil., Spo., Sul.*

    Air passages irritated: *Rumex*

    Constant: *Caust.*

    Glands:

        swollen: *Bell., Sil.*

Gums:
    bleeding: *Merc-c.*
    swollen: *Merc-c.*
Larynx:
    inflamed: *Dros.*
    irritated: *Puls.*
    tickling: *Dros., Puls., Rhus-t.*
Mouth dry: *Ap.*
Noises in ears:
    roaring: *Bar-c.*
    on swallowing: *Bar-c.*
Pains:
    burning: *Aco., Ap., Ars., Bar-c., Caust.,*
       Merc-c., Nat-m., Nit-ac., Spo., Sul.
    dry: *Caust.*
    pressing: *Nit-ac.*
    raw: *Caust., Hep-s., Lyc., Merc-c., Nit-ac.,*
       Nux-v., Phos., Puls., Sul.
    scraping: *Puls.*
    severe: *Bell.*
    sore: *Lyc., Merc-s., Phos., Rumex., Spo., Sul.*
    splinter-like: *Arg-n., Hep-s., Lach., Nit-ac.*
    spreading up to ears: *Hep-s., Lach., Merc-s.,*
       Nit-ac., Nux-v.
    spreading up to neck: *Merc-s.*
    stitching: *Aco., Bell., Bry., Ign., Merc-s.,*
       Nit-ac., Nux-v., Puls., Sil., Sul.
Throat:
    constricted: *Bell.*
    dark red: *Bapt., Phyt.*
    dry: *Calc-c., Lyc., Nat-m., Puls., Rhus-t., Sil.,*
       Spo., Sul.
    inflamed: *Bar-c.*
    irritated: *Arg-n., Bell., Rumex.*
    raw: *Arg-n., Bar-c., Bell., Rumex., Sul.*
    sore: *Rumex.*
Tonsils:
    dark red: *Bapt.*
    swollen/inflamed: *Bapt., Bar-c., Hep-s.,*
       Kali-m., Lyc., Merc-s., Nit-ac., Phos.,
       Phyt., Sil., Sul.
    ulcerated: *Merc-s., Nit-ac.*
    white: *Kali-m.*
Voice:
    lost: *Arg-n., Rumex.*
    hoarse: *Arg-n., Bry., Dros., Nat-m., Phos.,*
       Rhus-t., Spo., Sul.
With:
    choking sensation: *Caust., Ign., Lach., Sul.*
    desire to swallow: *Caust.*
    fever: *Bry.*
    hair sensation at the back of tongue: *Sil.*
    lump sensation in throat: *Ign., Lach., Lyc.,*
       Nat-m., Nux-v.
    saliva increased: *Bar-c., Merc-c.*
    ulcers in the throat: *Ars., Merc-c.*

Better:
    cold drinks: *Phyt.*
    eating: *Merc-c.*
    hot drinks: *Ars., Hep-s.*
    swallowing: *Ign.*
    swallowing liquids: *Bar-c.*
    swallowing solids: *Lach.*
    warm compresses: *Hep-s.*
    warm drinks: *Lyc.*
Worse:
    breathing in cold air: *Hep-s., Rumex.*
    breathing in: *Phos.*
    cold air: *Nux-v.*
    cold drinks: *Ars., Hep-s., Rhus-t.*
    getting cold: *Sil.*
    coughing: *Hep-s., Phos., Spo., Sul.*
    eating solid food: *Bapt.*
    evening: *Ign.*
    heat: *Lach., Puls.*
    hot drinks: *Phyt.*
    left side: *Lach.*
    morning and evening: *Phos.*
    night: *Bar-c., Lyc., Merc-s.*
    not swallowing: *Ign.*
    pressure: *Lach., Merc-c., Phos.*
    right side: *Bell., Lyc., Merc-s.*
    singing: *Spo.*
    swallowing: *Ars., Bapt., Bry., Dros., Hep-s.,*
       Merc-s., Nit-ac., Nux-v., Rhus-t., Sil., Spo.,
       Sul.
    swallowing saliva (empty swallowing):
       Bar-c., Lach.
    swallowing food: *Bar-c.*
    swallowing liquids: *Bell., Lach., Merc-c.*
    sweet drinks/food: *Spo.*
    talking: *Caust., Phos., Spo.*
    touch: *Lach., Spo.*
    turning the head: *Hep-s.*
    uncovering; *Nux-v., Rhus-t., Sil.*
    winter: *Hep-s.*
Causes:
    change of weather: *Calc-c.*
    exposure to wind: *Hep-s.*
    getting cold: *Bell., Hep-s.*
    singing: *Arg-n.*
    straining voice: *Rhus-t.*
    talking: *Arg-n.*
    getting chilled: *Aco., Bell.*

Speedy   see **Hurried**
Spiteful   *Nux-v.*
Splinters   *Sil.* see also **Injuries**
    Wound inflamed: *Sil.*
Sprains   *Arn., Calc-c., Rhus-t., Ruta.*
    Ankle: *Arn., Calc-c., Rhus-t., Ruta.*
    Foot: *Arn., Rhus-t.*
    Hand: *Calc-c.*

Wrist: *Arn., Calc-c., Rhus-t., Ruta.*
First stage: *Arn.*
Pains:
> bruised: *Ruta.*
> constant: *Ruta.*

With:
> bruising: *Arn.*
> exhaustion: *Ruta.*
> lameness: *Ruta.*
> stiffness: *Rhus-t.*
> swelling: *Arn.*
> trembling: *Rhus-t.*

Worse:
> exercise: *Ruta.*
> lifting: *Calc-c.*
> standing/walking: *Ruta.*

Causes:
> falling: *Rhus-t.*
> lifting: *Calc-c., Rhus-t.*
>> heavy weights: *Calc-c.*
> twisting: *Rhus-t.*

Stiff neck   *Calc-c., Calc-p., Rhus-t.*
In adults: *Calc-p.*
Causes:
> draughts: *Calc-p., Rhus-t.*
> getting chilled (cold): *Rhus-t.*
> lifting: *Calc-c., Rhus-t.*

Stomach-ache   see **Colic**
Strains   *Arn., Carb-a., Rhus-t., Ruta.*
Ankle: *Ruta.*
Muscles: *Carb-a.*
Periosteum: *Ruta.*
Tendons: *Carb-a., Ruta.*
Wrist: *Carb-a., Ruta.*
Pains.
> bruised: *Ruta.*
> constant: *Ruta.*
> joints: *Rhus-t.*
> sore/bruised: *Arn., Rhus-t.*

With:
> exhaustion: *Ruta.*
> lameness: *Ruta.*
> stiffness: *Rhus-t.*
> trembling: *Rhus-t.*

Better:
> continued movement: *Rhus-t.*

Worse:
> beginning to move: *Rhus-t.*
> exercise: *Ruta.*
> standing: *Ruta.*
> walking: *Ruta.*

Causes:
> childbirth: *Arn.*
> over-exertion: *Arn.*

Stubborn   *Calc-c., Cham., Nux-v.*
Stupor   (see also **Dazed**) *Bapt., Op.*

Styes   *Puls., Stap.*
Worse:
> upper eyelids: *Puls.*

Sudden onset   see **Onset**
Sulky   (see also **Moody**; **Morose**) *Ant-c.*
Sunburn   see **Burns**
Sunstroke   *Bell., Glon.*
With:
> fever: *Bell.*
> headache: *Bell., Glon.*

Sweat
Absent during fever: *Ars., Bell., Bry., Gels.*
Clammy: *Ars., Cham., Ferr-m., Lyc., Merc-s.,*
> *Pho-ac., Phos., Ver-a.*
Cold: *Ant-t., Ars., Carb-v., Chin., Cocc., Ferr-m.,*
> *Hep-s., Ip., Lyc., Merc-c., Merc-s., Sep., Ver-a.*
Exhausting: *Carb-a.*
From fright: *Nux-v.*
Head: *Calc-c.*
Hot: *Aco., Cham., Con., Ign., Ip., Nux-v., Op., Sep.*
Oily: *Mag-c.*
On covered parts of the body: *Aco., Bell., Chin.*
One-sided: *Bar-c., Nux-v., Petr., Puls.*
From pain: *Nat-s., Sep.*
Profuse: *Ant-t., Ars., Calc-c., Carb-a., Carb-v.,*
> *Chin., Ferr-m., Hep-s., Kali-c., Kali-p., Lyc.,*
> *Merc-s., Op., Pho-ac., Sep., Sil., Sul., Ver-a.*
Scanty: *Eup-p.*
Single parts of the body: *Chin., Cocc., Ign.,*
> *Kali-c., Nit-ac., Phos., Puls., Op., Sep.*
Smelly: *Carb-a., Hep-s., Lyc., Merc-s., Nit-ac.,*
> *Nux-v., Petr., Puls., Sep., Sil., Sul.*
Sour: *Ars., Calc-c., Colch., Hep-s., Lyc., Mag-c.,*
> *Merc-s., Nit-ac., Sep., Sil., Sul., Ver-a.*
With:
> diarrhoea: *Ver-a.*
> shivering: *Nux-v.*

Better:
> uncovering: *Cham., Lyc.*

Worse:
> after eating: *Kali-c.*
> at night: *Con., Puls., Sil.*
> closing eyes: *Con.*
> during sleep: *Con., Sil.*
> lying down: *Ferr-m., Rhus-t.*
> mental exertion: *Calc-c., Hep-s., Lach., Sep.,*
>> *Stap.*
> pain: *Lach., Merc-s., Nat-c., Sep.*
> slightest physical exertion: *Calc-c., Chin.,*
>> *Ferr-m., Kali-c., Kali-p., Lyc., Nat-c., Nat-s.,*
>> *Nit-ac., Phos., Rhus-t., Sep., Sul.*
> when tired: *Kali-p.*
> uncovering: *Rhus-t.*

Causes:
> fright: *Op.*

Sympathetic   *Caust., Phos.*

Symptoms

Changeable: *Puls.*

Contradictory: *Ign.*

One-sided: *Pho-ac.*

Left-sided: *Lach., Sep., Sul.*

Right-sided: *Ap., Bell., Calc-c., Lyc., Nux-v.,*
Puls.

Moving from:

left side to the right side: *Lach.*

right side to the left side: *Ap., Lyc.*

Talkative   *Lach.*

Tantrums   *Nit-ac.*

Taste   mouth tastes

Bad: *Calc-c., Merc-s., Nat-s., Nux-v., Puls., Sul.*

in the morning: *Nat-s., Nux-v., Puls.*

Bitter: *Aco., Ars., Bry., Carb-v., Chin., Merc-s.,*
Nat-m., Nat-s., Nux-v., Sul.

Metallic: *Cocc., Merc-s., Nat-c., Rhus-t.*

Salty: *Nat-m.*

Sour: *Arg-n., Calc-c., Lyc., Mag-c., Nux-v., Phos.*

Sweet: *Cupr.*

Tearful   (see also **Depression** and **Dislikes**
consolation) *Ap., Calc-c., Calc-s., Caust., Ign.,*
Lyc., Nat-m., Puls., Rhus-t., Sep., Spo., Ver-a.

During a fever: *Aco., Bell., Puls., Spo.*

Better for fresh air: *Puls.*

Difficulty crying: *Nat-m.*

Involuntary: *Ign.*

Cries on own: *Ign., Nat-m.*

Teeth

Crumbling/decaying: *Calc-f.*

Teething painful   in children (see also **Toothache**)
Aco., Bell., Calc-c., Calc-p., Cham., Mag-m.,
Mag-p., Phyt., Puls., Rhe., Sil.

Cheeks:

hot and red: *Aco., Bell., Cham.*

pale and cold: *Cham.*

red spot on one cheek: *Cham.*

swollen: *Bell.*

Slow (children late to teethe): *Calc-c., Calc-p., Sil.*

Pains:

cries out in sleep: *Cham.*

unbearable: *Cham.*

With:

colic: *Mag-m.*

diarrhoea: *Calc-c., Cham., Rhe., Sil.*

difficulty teething: *Calc-c., Calc-p., Cham.,*
Sil.

green stools: *Calc-p., Cham., Mag-m.*

restless sleep: *Aco., Bell., Cham.*

toothache: *Sil.*

Better:

biting gums together hard: *Phyt.*

cold drinks/water: *Puls.*

external heat: *Mag-p.*

walking in the fresh air: *Puls.*

Worse:

heat of bed, warm food/drinks: *Cham., Puls.*

pressure: *Cham.*

Tennis elbow   *Ruta.*

Thin   *Calc-p.*

Thirstless   *Ant-c., Ant-t., Ap., Bell., Colch., Gels.,*
Pho-ac., Puls.

Thirsty   *Aco., Ars., Bell., Bry., Eup-p., Merc-c.,*
Merc-s., Nat-m., Phos., Pyr., Sil., Sul.,
Ver-a.

Thirst with chills: *Ign.*

Thirst for:

cold drinks/hot drinks see **Likes**

large quantities: *Ars., Bry., Nat-m., Phos.,*
Sul., Ver-a.

at infrequent intervals: *Bry.*

sips: *Ars.*

small quantities often: *Ars.*

unquenchable: *Eup-p., Phos.*

water: *Phos., Sul.*

Throat   see **Sore throat**

Thrush (genital)   *Bor., Merc-s., Nat-m., Nit-ac., Sep.*

Discharge:

burning: *Bor., Merc-s., Nit-ac., Sep.*

copious: *Sep.*

like cottage cheese: *Sep.*

greenish: *Merc-s*

like egg white: *Bor., Nat-m., Sep.*

smelly: *Merc-s., Nit-ac., Sep.*

thin: *Nit-ac.*

yellow: *Sep.*

white: *Bor., Nat-m.*

With:

dryness: *Sep.*

itching: *Nit-ac., Sep.*

Worse:

before menstrual period: *Sep.*

between menstrual periods: *Bor., Sep.*

during pregnancy: *Sep.*

at night: *Merc-s.*

Thrush (oral)   in babies and children, of gums
and/or tongue: *Bor., Kali-m., Merc-s., Nat-m.,*
Sul-ac.

In breastfeeding babies: *Bor., Kali-m.*

Tongue/gums: *Sul-ac.*

coated white: *Kali-m., Nat-m.*

hot/dry/bleeds easily: *Bor.*

With:

excess saliva: *Bor., Merc-s.*

Worse:

for feeding (in babies): *Bor.*

for touch: *Bor.*

Tidy   *Ars., Nux-v.*

Time passes

quickly: *Cocc.*

slowly: *Glon.*

Timid   see **Shy**
Tired   see **Apathetic**; **Exhaustion**; **Sluggish**
Tongue

Brown-coated: *Bry.*
Cold: *Ver-a.*
Cracked: *Merc-s., Nit-ac.*
Dark red: *Bapt.*
Dirty white: *Bry.*
Fiery red: *Ap.*
Green: *Nat-s.*
Red: *Bell., Phos.*
Red-edged: *Ars., Sul.*
Red stripe down centre (white edges): *Caust.*
Red-tipped: *Arg-n., Ars., Phyt., Rhus-t., Sul.*
Strawberry: *Bell.*
White-coated: *Ant-c., Ant-t., Bell., Calc-c., Kali-b.,*
    Kali-m., Puls., Sul.
Yellow: *Kali-s., Merc-c., Merc-s., Nat-p., Puls.*
    at the back: *Nat-p.*

Toothache   (see also **Teething**) *Ant-c., Arn., Calc-c.,*
    Cham., Coff., Hep-s., Kali-c., Lach., Mag-c.,
    Mag-p., Merc-s., Nux-v., Puls., Rhod.,
    Rhus-t., Sep., Sil., Stap., Sul.

Cheeks swollen: *Lach., Merc-s.*
Children: *Cham., Coff., Stap.*
Face swollen: *Sil.*
Glands swollen: *Sil.*
Gums bleeding: *Hep-s.*
In nervous patients: *Coff.*
Pains:
    gnawing: *Ant-c., Calc-c., Puls., Stap.*
    grumbling: *Rhod.*
    in decayed teeth: *Ant-c., Stap.*
    in good teeth: *Aco.*
    pressing: *Merc-s.*
    pulling: *Puls., Sep.*
    shooting/spasmodic: *Coff.*
    spreading up to:
        ears: *Merc-s., Rhod., Sep., Stap., Sul.*
        face: *Merc-s.*
        head: *Ant-c.*
    sore, bruised: *Merc-s.*
    stitching: *Kali-c., Lach., Puls., Sep.*
    tearing: *Aco., Merc-s., Sep., Stap.*
    throbbing: *Lach., Sep., Sul.*
    unbearable: *Cham.*
Better:
    cold water: *Coff., Puls.*
    after eating: *Rhod.*
    fresh air (for walking in the fresh air): *Ant-c.,*
        Puls.
    heat: *Mag-p., Merc-s., Nux-v., Rhod., Rhus-t.*
    rubbing cheeks: *Merc-s.*
    warm compresses: *Mag-p., Merc-s., Nux-v.,*
        Rhod., Rhus-t.
    external warmth: *Nux-v.*

winter: *Nux-v.*
wrapping up head: *Nux-v., Sil.*
Worse:
    biting teeth together: *Sep.*
    brushing teeth: *Lach.*
    cold: *Mag-c.*
    cold air: *Calc-c., Merc-s., Sul.*
    cold drinks/food: *Ant-c., Hep-s., Kali-c.,*
        Lach., Rhus-t., Sep., Stap.
    drawing cold in through teeth: *Calc-c.,*
        Merc-s.
    while eating and drinking: *Kali-c., Merc-s.*
    after eating: *Ant-c., Stap.*
    fresh air: *Sul.*
    heat (compresses/hot water bottle): *Coff.,*
        Puls.
    hot drinks/food: *Calc-c., Cham., Coff., Kali-c.,*
        Lach., Puls., Sep.
    during a menstrual period: *Lach., Sep., Stap.*
    night in bed: *Ant-c., Mag-c., Merc-s., Sul.*
    during pregnancy: *Sep.*
    pressure: *Cham.*
    before a storm: *Rhod.*
    springtime: *Lach.*
    stuffy room: *Puls.*
    touch: *Sep.*
    touch of tongue: *Ant-c.*
    warmth of bed: *Cham., Merc-s., Puls.*
    washing with cold water: *Sul.*
    winter: *Hep-s., Merc-s., Nux-v., Rhus-t., Sil.*
Causes:
    abscess: *Hep-s., Merc-s., Sil.*
    anger: *Cham.*
    cold, damp weather: *Cal-c., Merc-s., Rhus-t.*
    cold, dry wind: *Aco.*
    concussion: *Arn.*
    draughts: *Calc-c., Sul.*
    after an extraction: *Nux-v.*
    after a filling: *Arn., Nux-v.*
    getting wet: *Lach.*
    pregnancy: *Mag-c., Sep.*
    teething: *Mag-p., Puls., Sil.*
    travelling: *Mag-c.*
    winter: *Sil.*

Tooth decay
Crumbling: *Calc-f.*
Decaying: *Calc-f.*

Touchy   see **Irritable**; **Sensitive**
Travel sickness   *Bor., Cocc., Nux-v., Petr., Sep.,*
    Stap., Tab.
With:
    biliousness: *Sep.*
    diarrhoea: *Cocc.*
    dizziness: *Cocc.*
    faint-like feeling: *Cocc., Nux-v.*
    headache: *Cocc., Nux-v., Petr., Sep.*

nausea: *Bor., Cocc., Nux-v., Petr., Sep., Tab.*

    deathly, intermittent, violent nausea: *Tab.*

vomiting: *Bor., Cocc., Petr., Sep., Tab.*

    food: *Sep.*

    bile: *Sep.*

Better:

    lying down: *Cocc., Nux-v.*

    fresh air: *Tab.*

Worse:

    for downward movement: *Bor.*

    after drinking: *Cocc.*

    after eating: *Cocc., Nux-v., Sep.*

    fresh air: *Cocc., Nux-v., Petr.*

    morning: *Sep.*

    movement: *Cocc., Tab.*

    sitting up: *Cocc.*

    stuffy room: *Tab.*

    tobacco: *Nux-v., Tab.*

Causes:

    pregnancy: *Sep.*

    travelling: *Petr.*

Trembling *Agar., Cimi., Cocc., Gels., Zinc.*

    From emotion: *Cocc.*

Twitchy *Agar., Zinc.*

Uncommunicative (see also **Broody; Introspective**)

    Carb-a., Cocc., Glon., Pho-ac., Phos., Ver-a., Zinc.

Unforgiving *Nit-ac.*

Urine see **Retention of urine**

Urticaria see **Hives**

Varicose veins *Ferr-m., Ham., Puls.*

    Legs and thighs: *Ham.*

    Painful:

        Pains stinging: *Puls.*

    Swollen: *Ferr-m., Ham.*

    Worse:

        during pregnancy: *Ferr-m., Ham., Puls.*

        for touch: *Ham.*

        after childbirth: *Ham.*

Voice lost *Arg-n., Carb-v., Caust., Phos.*

    In singers: *Arg-n., Caust., Phos.*

    Painless: *Phos.*

    Sudden: *Caust.*

    Worse in the evening: *Carb-v.*

Vomiting (see also **Food poisoning; Travel sickness**) *Ant-c., Ant-t., Ars., Bry., Calc-c., Cham., Chin., Colch., Ferr-m., Ip., Nux-v., Phos., Sep., Sil., Sul-ac., Tab., Ver-a.*

    Belly/stomach feel cold: *Ver-a.*

    In breastfed babies: *Ant-c., Sil.*

    Difficult: *Ant-t.*

    Easy: *Ars., Cham.*

    Exhausting: *Tab.*

    Frequent: *Ars., Chin.*

During pregnancy: *Ant-c., Nat-s., Nux-v., Sep., Tab.*

Pains in the stomach:

    burning: *Colch., Phos.*

    cramping/griping: *Ver-a.*

    sore, bruised: *Colch.*

Sudden (while eating): *Ferr-m.*

Violent: *Ars., Phos., Tab., Ver-a.*

Vomit:

    bile: *Ant-c., Ars., Cham., Ip., Nux-v., Phos., Sep., Ver-a.*

    bitter: *Bry., Nux-v., Phos.*

    curdled milk: *Ant-c., Calc-c., Sil.*

    food: *Ars., Chin., Ferr-m., Ip.*

    green: *Ip.*

    mucus: *Nux-v., Phos., Ver-a.*

    smelly: *Ars., Nux-v., Sep.*

    sour: *Ant-t., Calc-c., Chin., Nux-v., Sul-ac., Tab., Ver-a.*

    violent: *Phos., Tab.*

    watery: *Ars., Bry., Ver-a.*

    yellow: *Phos., Ver-a.*

With:

    diarrhoea: *Ars., Ver-a.*

    dizziness: *Ver-a.*

    faintness after vomiting: *Ars.*

    fever: *Ant-t.*

    headache: *Ip.*

    hiccuping after vomiting: *Ver-a.*

    retching after vomiting: *Colch.*

    sweating while vomiting: *Ars.*

Worse:

    after midnight: *Ferr-m.*

    before breakfast: *Tab.*

    bending down: *Ip.*

    coughing: *Ant-t., Bry., Ip.*

    coughing up phlegm: *Nux-v.*

    after drinking: *Ant-c., Ars., Phos., Ver-a.*

    after eating: *Ars., Chin., Ip., Phos., Sep., Sil., Ver-a.*

    a short while after eating/drinking: *Phos.*

    eggs: *Ferr-m.*

    expectorating: *Nux-v.*

    milk: *Ant-c., Sil.*

    movement: *Ars., Bry., Tab.*

    night: *Ferr-m.*

    after eating: *Ars.*

    smell of eggs: *Colch.*

Causes:

    alcohol: *Nux-v.*

    anger: *Cham., Nux-v.*

    ice-cream: *Ars.*

    measles: *Ant-c.*

    pregnancy: *Nux-v., Sep., Tab.*

    sour wine: *Ant-c.*

    travelling: *Tab.*

Warts *Thu.*
    Bleeding: *Thu.*
    Large: *Thu.*
    Stinging: *Thu.*
Weakness see **Exhaustion**
Weary *Ruta*
    Of life: *Nat-s.*
Weepy see **Tearful**
Whiny *Ap., Puls.*
Whooping cough see **Cough**
Wind see **Flatulence**
Worms *Cina*
Worry see **Anxious**
Worse see also **Complaints from**
    After midnight: *Ars., Podo.*
    Around:
        1 a.m.: *Ars.*
        3–5 p.m.: *Ap.*
        2–4 a.m.: *Kali-c.*
        10 a.m.: *Nat-m.*
        10–11 a.m.: *Sul.*
        3 p.m.: *Bell.*
        4–8 p.m.: *Lyc.*
        9 p.m.: *Bry.*
    Afternoon: *Lyc.*
    Alcohol: *Lach., Nux-v., Op., Sul-ac.*
    Autumn: *Colch., Rhus-t.*
    Bathing: *Sul.*
    Before breakfast: *Tab.*
    Beginning to move: *Ferr-m., Rhus-t.*
    Change of temperature: *Ars., Kali-s.*
    Change of weather see **Complaints from** Change
        of weather
    Cloudy weather: *Rhus-t.*
    Coffee: *Caust., Cham., Ign., Nux-v.*
    Cold: *Agar., Ars., Bar-c., Calc-c., Calc-p., Caust.,*
        Chin., Cimi., Colch., Dulc., Hep-s., Hyp.,
        Kali-b., Kali-c., Kali-p., Mag-p., Merc-s.,
        Nit-ac., Nux-v., Pho-ac., Phos., Puls., Pyr.,
        Rhod., Rhus-t., Sep., Sil.
    Cold and heat: *Merc-s.*
    Cold, dry weather: *Caust., Hep-s., Kali-c., Nux-v.*
    Cold food: *Nux-v.*
    Cold drinks/food: *Rhus-t.*
    Cold wind: *Bell., Hep-s., Nux-v., Spo.*
    Cold, wet weather: *Pyr., Rhod., Rhus-t.,* (see also
        Damp)
    Consolation see **Dislikes** consolation
    Damp (see also Cold, wet): *Ars., Calc-c., Calc-p.,*
        Colch., Dulc., Nat-s., Rhus-t., Sil.
    Draughts: *Calc-c., Calc-p., Caust., Kali-c., Rhus-t.,*
        Sil., Sul.
    After eating: *Kali-b., Nat-m., Zinc.*
    Before eating: *Nat-c., Phos.*
    Evening: *Caust., Cham., Euphr., Lyc., Mag-c.,*
        Merc-s., Nat-p., Pho-ac., Phos., Sul-ac., Zinc.

    Excitement: *Kali-p.*
    Exertion (physical): *Ars., Calc-c., Carb-v., Cocc.,*
        Kali-p., Stap., Sul.
    Exposure to sun: *Ant-c., Glon., Nat-c., Nat-m.,*
        Puls.
    Fasting: *Sep., Stap., Sul., Tab.*
    First lying down: *Con.*
    Flatulent foods (beans, etc.); *Bry., Lyc.*
    Fresh air: *Bapt., Calc-c., Calc-p., Caust., Cham.,*
        Chin., Cocc., Coff., Hep-s., Nat-c., Nit-ac.,
        Nux-v., Petr., Sil.
    Foggy weather: *Rhus-t.*
    Frosty weather: *Sep.*
    Fruit: *Ver-a.*
    Getting feet wet: *Bar-c., Puls., Sil.*
    Getting head wet: *Bell.*
    Getting wet: *Caust., Sep.*
    Getting overheated: *Ant-c., Kali-c.*
    Heat: *Ap., Arg-n., Calc-s., Glon., Kali-s., Lach.,*
        Led., Nat-m., Puls., Sul., Sul-ac.
    Heat and cold: *Merc-s.*
    Humidity: *Carb-v., Lach., Nat-s.*
    Jarring movement: *Arn., Bell., Glon., Nit-ac.*
    Light touch: *Chin., Merc-s.*
    Loss of sleep: *Cocc., Nit-ac., Nux-v.*
    Lying down: *Con., Dros., Dulc., Ferr-m., Merc-s.,*
        Nat-s., Rhus-t.
    Lying on the injured part: *Arn.*
    Lying on the painful part/side: *Hep-s., Ruta.*
    Lying on the side: *Kali-c.*
    Before a menstrual period: *Lach., Nat-m.*
    Before/during/after a menstrual period: *Sep.*
    Mental exertion: *Calc-p., Kali-p., Sep.*
    Mid-morning: *Nat-c., Nat-m., Podo., Sul-ac.*
    Midnight: *Dros.*
    Milk: *Calc-c., Calc-s., Mag-m., Sul.*
    Morning: *Lach., Nat-s., Nux-v., Petr., Pho-ac.,*
        Phos.
    Morning on waking: *Kali-b., Lach.*
    Movement: *Chin., Cocc., Colch., Led., Spo.*
    Night: *Aco., Chin., Cina, Coff., Colch., Dulc.,*
        Ferr-m., Hep-s., Ip., Kali-b., Kali-c., Mag-c.,
        Mag-m., Merc-s., Nit-ac., Sep., Zinc.
    Onions: *Lyc.*
    On one side of body: *Pho-ac.*
    Physical exertion: *Calc-s., Gels., Nat-c., Nat-m.,*
        Sep.
    Pressure: *Bar-c., Cina, Hep-s., Hyp., Lach., Lyc.,*
        Merc-c.
    Rest: *Puls., Sep.*
    Rich, fatty food: *Carb-v., Puls.*
    Sight of food: *Colch.*
    After sleep: *Lach., Spo.*
    During sleep: *Op.*
    Slightest movement: *Bry.*
    Standing: *Sul.*

Starchy food: *Nat-m., Nat-s.*
Stormy weather: *Nat-c., Rhod.*
   before a storm: *Rhod.*
   during a storm: *Nat-c.*
Stuffy rooms: *Calc-s., Lyc., Puls., Sul.*
Sugar/sweets: *Arg-n.*
Sun see **Complaints from** sunstroke
Summer: *Kali-b.*
Sweating: *Pho-ac., Sep.*
Swimming in cold water: *Ant-c., Mag-p., Rhus-t.*
Swimming in the sea: *Mag-m.*
Thinking: *Calc-c.*
Tight clothes: *Calc-c., Lach., Lyc., Nux-v., Spo.*
Tobacco: *Ign., Nux-v., Spo., Stap.*
Touch: *Aco., Ap., Arn., Bell., Cocc., Coff., Colch.,*
   Cupr., Ham., Hep-s., Kali-c., Led., Mag-p.,
   Nit-ac., Nux-v., Sep., Sil., Stap.

Travelling: *Petr.*
Twilight: *Puls.*
Uncovering: *Hep-s., Kali-c., Mag-p., Nux-v.,*
   Rhus-t., Sil.
Vomiting: *Cupr.*
On waking: *Ars., Lach., Nit-ac.*
Walking: *Nit-ac.*
   in the fresh air: *Caust., Cocc., Led., Mag-p.*
   in the wind: *Sep.*
Warmth of bed: *Dros., Op., Sul.*
Wet weather: *Ars., Calc-p., Nat-s., Puls., Sil.*
Wind: *Cham., Lyc., Nux-v., Phos., Puls., Rhod.*
Wine: *Coff., Led., Zinc.*
Winter: *Nux-v.*
Worry: *Kali-p.*
Writing: *Sep.*
Wounds See **Injuries**

PART III

PRESCRIBING GUIDELINES AND FOLLOW-THROUGH

STRESS AS A CAUSE OF DISEASE

What do we mean by 'health'? Is it simply the absence of disease? Is it more than not being ill? I believe it is a sense of well-being, of feeling good, of being in balance that is hard to dislodge. It is, above all, the ability to withstand stress.

When we are physically healthy we have strength, flexibility and a reservoir of energy on which to draw. When we are emotionally healthy we can acknowledge and express our feelings and maintain rewarding relationships. When we are mentally healthy we can think clearly, formulate ideas, solve problems and make decisions.

Disease limits our personal freedom – a broken leg, for example, limits a person's physical freedom by making it difficult to walk. Depression limits a person's emotional freedom by making it difficult to interact with others. Mental exhaustion affects a person's ability to concentrate and make decisions, therefore limiting a person's mental freedom. If you fall ill, ask yourself how that illness is limiting you.

The orthodox medical view, or germ theory of disease, is that illness is a 'bad' thing. An alternative medical view is that disease is a 'good' thing, alerting an individual to allow time off for recuperation.

Disease is neither good nor bad. That we have fallen ill simply provides us with information about how we are living and coping with stress. It alerts us to a deficiency or weakness that needs attention. An individual's susceptibility to disease determines whether or not they will fall ill (see page 13). A weakened immune system is more likely to succumb than a strong one.

We all vary enormously in our ability to adapt to and cope with stress. Understanding our own stress limits is tremendously important. I divide stress into two main categories – healthy stress and unhealthy stress.

Healthy stress might be defined as the spur that pushes you to perform better and achieve more than usual in certain circumstances: for example, to work all hours in your job during a crisis. Athletes use their naturally acquired adrenalin (stress response) to gain that little extra from their bodies in a race.

Unhealthy stress is when the stress in your life begins to limit you, bringing you too near to that 'last straw' state where your own 'coping mechanism' is overstretched, when your performance level starts to drop and you make mistakes, when you fall ill.

Under stress our bodies will let us know when the pressure is too great by producing the symptom(s) of illness. And when symptoms surface on one level then other levels will also be affected. For example, a head injury (physical) can initially cause shock (emotional) and amnesia (mental) as well as pain (physical). A difficult boss at work who is aggressive to staff can create an emotionally stressful environment for employees who may produce connected physical ailments such as headaches, indigestion, pains in the neck, etc.

At different times in our lives we may respond differently to similar stresses. Divorce of parents usually becomes less damagingly stressful as we grow older and less dependent, although a dependent older child will be as badly affected by divorce as an independent younger child. Giving birth at forty is a bigger physical stress than doing so at twenty when a woman's body is more supple and she has greater energy resources. However, an older, more mature woman may find herself less emotionally stressed by motherhood.

The body operates with the physical, emotional, mental and spiritual working together to maintain a balance. Each aspect needs nourishment, but mental and emotional nourishment is often lacking in our society. Because of the widespread rejection of religion many people do not have a time of peace or quiet in their lives to reflect or just *be*. To still the mind and let the cares of life drift away is a deeply healing process. You can do this by meditating, daydreaming, painting and writing, walking and enjoying nature or through prayer.

You also nourish yourself with food, sleep, massage, spending time with friends or family members who accept you as you are, who will listen when needed, and provide you with loving support and advice. Laughter is one of nature's great healers. Letting go of the serious business of living and having fun is essential to maintaining health.

Learn to recognise the first symptoms of being over-stressed, when the body shows early warning signs but before illness develops. Being ill can actually be a fruitful way of coping with stress, although of course, disease in itself can be stressful. Once you are stressed and weakened to the point where you become ill, the illness further stresses your body, especially if you take antibiotics or homeopathic remedies *and* carry on working as if nothing had happened. You need to stop, rest and allow time for self-healing.

The more we understand about stress the better able we are to deal with it and have some choice in how we respond to it. Observing and questioning how someone close to you has fallen ill will tell you a lot about what stresses are operating in their life, and in talking about them it is sometimes possible for that person to understand what changes are necessary to prevent a similar situation recurring.

Get to know your own stress response. What can you cope with? What are your limits? How do you recognise them? How can you stretch your limits when you have to? What nourishes you? How do you balance the stress in your life? Setting limits is an essential part of the stress-balancing mechanism.

Begin by recognising and acknowledging the forms stress takes in your life and update your stress list from time to time. Assess your reserves and strengths for dealing with stress; look at ways in which you can balance the stress(es) in your life. Avoid unnecessary stress. Learn to offload, to delegate, to say no.

Remember that you are an important person in your own life. You need to look after yourself to be a healthy mother/father/friend/employee/homeopath, etc!

As a home prescriber understanding that disease is a response to stress is important so that you can help your patient talk through the various measures they can take to make their life easier. Even children benefit from this approach. A strict teacher can affect a sensitive child who may start to have headaches. Finding out that this is the stress that is causing the headaches is the first step. Talking to your child about how to handle his or her feelings comes next. A talk with the teacher is essential so that he or she understands the effect they are having on your child. You can then prescribe if the headaches carry on or if they are specially severe.

I have only touched on stress in this chapter as there are now many good books on the subject covering every angle. The more we understand about stress the better able we are to deal with it and have some choice in how we respond to it.

DISEASES YOU CAN TREAT USING THIS BOOK

It is important to understand fully the difference between acute and chronic disease so that you know which illnesses you may safely and appropriately treat and which you need to take to a professional homeopath. For an explanation of the difference between the two, see page 14.

This section tells you whether the particular complaint you wish to treat is within your scope as a home prescriber, *before* you attempt to take the case and work out a remedy. A good general first-aid book or family medical encyclopaedia will give you more detailed information about the complaints themselves. If your complaint has an obvious cause it is important to remove the stress (for example, don't drink for a few days if your headache was caused by an excess of alcohol). Use commonsense measures and take sensible care of yourself when you are ill.

Having established that your complaint *is* within the scope of this book, turn to Chapters 4 and 5 to work out the remedy you need.

Your complaint may be treatable either by internal or external remedies, or both. You can establish this in each case by looking up your symptoms in the Repertories (pages 37 and 165–98).

I also strongly advise you to take a first-aid course with the St John Ambulance or the Red Cross to learn the mechanics of first-aid.

A criticism levelled at homeopathy is that it encourages people to take their lives in their hands by treating serious illnesses at home. *Never* treat serious injuries or complaints yourself. If in any doubt seek expert advice. Cause for concern below lists general alarm symptoms, and specific alarm symptoms to watch out for are indicated in the individual complaints that follow.

Cause for Concern

The following symptoms may indicate serious problems and so signal the need for immediate professional help. Some of them also appear in the remedy pictures, for example the laboured breathing of *Antimonium tartaricum* and the delirium of a *Belladonna* fever. If you are very worried about the general state of your patient I suggest you call for help and then give the indicated homeopathic remedy. In some instances, where the picture is very clear and/or you know from past experience that your patient is not seriously ill, you will be able to give the remedy and wait for improvement. If he or she does not show signs of improving quickly you can then call for help.

See overleaf for disease conditions *not* covered by this book.

SEEK HELP IF THERE IS:

Bleeding, unexplained, from any part of the body, including the skin

Breathing, rapid – over fifty breaths per minute at rest in children under two – over forty breaths per minute in children aged two to ten – over thirty breaths per minute in anyone over thirty

Breathing, shallow or laboured (difficult)

Chest pain, severe

Convulsions

Delirium

Fever above 105°F, 40°C

Fever, high, with a slow pulse (normal adult pulse is about 90 beats a minute and 120 in a child)

Fever, persistent – lasting for longer than 24 hours in an infant

Headache, severe – especially if accompanied by one or more of the other symptoms in this section

Mental confusion, uncharacteristic
Neck stiff
Stools, pale – grey or almost white
Urination profuse, accompanied by a great thirst
Urine dark and scanty/bloody (certain foods when eaten in quantity can change the colour of urine; beetroot for example, can turn urine red. This is nothing to worry about)
Vomiting, unexpected, repeated – comes on some time after the onset of a viral infection (i.e. a childhood illness)
Weakness, extreme
Wheezing, severe
Yellowing of the skin or whites of the eyes

IF SOMEONE SEEMS VERY ILL, EVEN IF THEY DO NOT HAVE ANY EASILY IDENTIFIABLE SYMPTOMS, ALWAYS TRUST YOUR INSTINCTS AND GET HELP.

ALWAYS SEEK PROFESSIONAL HELP IF YOUR SYMPTOMS RECUR OR DO NOT IMPROVE.

DISEASES AND CONDITIONS NOT COVERED BY THIS BOOK

With the exception of treating the acute pain of arthritis and rheumatism, this book does not cover *chronic diseases*; these are complex conditions and need careful diagnosis and treatment at all stages. The homeopathic treatment of chronic disease often requires a long-term commitment so that the homeopath can treat these underlying weaknesses in the constitution.

The following symptoms are not dealt with in this book for the reasons given in each case:

Serious degenerative diseases such as cancer, hepatitis, heart disease, AIDS, and so on, are not within the scope of the first-aid prescriber. These conditions require time and skill to treat and should not be regarded lightly.
Frequently recurring symptoms from flu, headaches, diarrhoea and coughs, to depressions, etc. Symptoms occurring as often as every week, which can be so bad that work has to be cancelled. They are *not* symptoms that occur two or three times a year and that have obvious causes, for example headaches after the stress of exams.
Skin symptoms including eczema, psoriasis, dermatitis, etc., should never be attempted by the first-aid prescriber. Read the Laws of Cure (page 15) to understand the dangers of suppressing a skin disease.

Asthma is a deep-seated chronic disease and needs careful management to cure it. The acute attacks of asthma can be alleviated, but these should always be prescribed by a homeopath who is in charge of the whole case and who is prescribing constitutional remedies between attacks so that their severity and frequency is lessened.
Hayfever for the same reasons as asthma. It is, however, possible to alleviate symptoms, and for this reason a few remedies are included in this book. However, I strongly advise that you take up constitutional treatment for the months when you are free of hayfever in order to help clear the disease from the system. It can take several years for this to happen, with the symptoms lessening in severity each year.
Persistent constipation can mask a more serious, underlying complaint that needs professional treatment, but it may simply be a result of poor diet (lots of low-fibre junk food), in which case the first step is to make the necessary dietary changes. Remedies are included for occasional constipation caused by a change in environment (although the occasional dose of a laxative will do no harm).
Persistent abdominal pain should always be checked by a professional. Never self-prescribe, except in the few instances outlined in this book. Always see your GP to make sure there is no need for urgent surgery (such as appendicitis).
Ulcers, of the skin, stomach, etc. These are evidence of a deep-seated chronic condition that needs expert attention. You may treat occasional mouth ulcers yourself. If they recur, especially frequently, then they need deeper, constitutional treatment.
Lumps and bumps – cysts, growths, warts, etc. anywhere on or in the body (except for styes, bruises and warts, as outlined in the book) must always be taken to a professional homeopath so that he or she can prescribe on the underlying weakness and prevent their recurrence.

COMPLAINTS YOU CAN TREAT

Abscesses

You can treat a simple tooth (gum) abscess yourself while waiting for your dental appointment. If the pain is greatly relieved as a result and/or the abscess discharges its pus then wait a little while before starting on antibiotics as they may not be necessary. If the pain returns, or doesn't clear completely and quickly, take the medicines prescribed by your dentist, or visit a professional homeopath who can treat these abscesses.

DO
- rest and eat well to build up your defences.
- apply hot compresses to the abscess.

Anaemia

The anaemia covered by this book is iron-deficiency anaemia, which is caused by infection, poor diet, during pregnancy when the iron count drops, and by loss of blood after an accident, tooth extraction, heavy period, nosebleed or childbirth.

Other types of anaemia need to be treated by a professional homeopath.
DO
- eat healthy, iron-rich foods such as liver, greens (not spinach as the acid in it makes the iron difficult to absorb), cabbage and dried apricots.
- rest.
- drink plenty of fluids but cut out tea (which prevents the absorption of iron).
- take a herbal iron tonic if it suits you.
DON'T
- take iron pills available from high street chemists as they often cause constipation and can make the condition worse by blocking the absorption of iron.

Arthritis see Joint pain

Athlete's foot

This is best treated with internal remedies. If it is a persistent (chronic) problem, it will require professional homeopathic treatment.
DO
- keep your feet clean and dry meticulously after bathing.
- use *Calendula* talcum powder (available from some homeopathic pharmacies) or use the cream if the skin is cracked and painful.
- go barefoot as much as possible, and wear sandals in the summer.
DON'T
- wear running shoes, which can exacerbate the problem.
- use anti-perspirants on your feet. This form of suppression can lead to more serious complaints.
SEEK HELP IF
- there is swelling or pain, especially if it spreads to the ankle.

Backache and back injuries

Homeopathic remedies will provide relief for an acute problem, but seek help from an osteopath or a physiotherapist. Chronic (long-term) back problems need long-term treatment.

There is an increased tendency to back problems in people who are overweight. The muscles in a weak back can be strengthened and further problems averted by gentle exercise.
DO
- rest as much as possible.
- use heat or cold to ease the pain.
DON'T
- further stress the back by lifting heavy bags, etc.
SEEK HELP IF
- back pain is accompanied by fever.
- the urine smells strong or is bloody (it looks pink or is flecked with red or brown).
- there is trouble with either bowels or bladder.
- it is difficult to move the legs or they feel numb.

NB NEVER ATTEMPT TO TREAT A SERIOUS BACK INJURY YOURSELF.

Bedwetting

I have included a few remedies that can help in cases of occasional bedwetting in children.
DO
- cut out all fruit juices from the diet and give water instead.
- investigate whether the bedwetting is related to emotional stress, such as problems at school or at home, and talk about it in a helpful and sympathetic way. Seek counselling help if necessary.
DON'T
- punish a child for wetting the bed.
SEEK HELP IF
- it is accompanied by an increased thirst.
- any of the symptoms below accompany the bedwetting (especially in an older child who was formerly 'dry' at night):
    pain on urinating; very copious urination; frequent urination; blood in the urine (it looks pink or reddish); pain in the abdomen; fever; pain in the kidneys (in the back just above the waist).

Bites/stings

Homeopathic remedies can be used to treat bites and stings internally and externally, and can help people who seem very susceptible to being bitten become less attractive to insects (large doses of garlic in its natural form or as pearls is also thought to be a good preventive). Some people can have severe allergic reactions to bites, with great swelling; these require urgent medical help.

DO
- use an insect repellent (homeopathic or otherwise).
- use a 'bite lotion' (see page 34) as soon as possible after being bitten.
- scrape out a bee or wasp sting with a sterilised needle-tip to prevent the poison sac from releasing more venom into the puncture. Clean the site to prevent infection, bathing it in cold water.
- be vigilant around children who are eating sweet things outdoors in the summer as wasps are attracted by the smell and sting very readily.

DON'T
- kill insects with insect sprays – these are toxic to some degree when inhaled.

SEEK HELP IF
- a bite becomes unbearably painful or itchy.
- the swelling is very severe or spreads rapidly.
- the lips, tongue or joints become swollen.
- there is difficulty breathing, or the sting is in the mouth or throat.
- the person has previously had a very severe response after being stung by the same insect.
- there is faintness or confusion.

Black eye see Eye injuries

Blisters

Blisters can result from burns (see Burns), including sunburn, friction or chemicals, and occasionally from insect bites. They can also be caused by infections such as herpes (cold sores or shingles), chicken pox or impetigo, or by chronic skin complaints like eczema; these conditions require professional treatment. Blood blisters caused by injury need to be treated like a bruise.

DO
- avoid further friction or exposure to sun.
- avoid infection by covering a blister with a sterile dressing until it has started to dry out, then expose to the air to speed healing.

DON'T
- burst the blister.

SEEK HELP IF
- blisters become infected, and the area becomes inflamed and/or swollen.
- severe pain develops.

Blood poisoning (septicaemia)

This condition, which is characterised by a high fever and a slow pulse, is always a medical emergency. It is caused by the spread of bacteria in the blood, usually through a contaminated wound or (rarely) after childbirth with some of the placenta being retained. I have

included one remedy for the treatment of this complaint in case of an emergency where you are unable to get immediate hospital help.

Boils

I have included a couple of remedies for the treatment of minor, occasional boils.

DO
- rest and eat well.
- use hot compresses to bring the boil to a 'head', and then keep covered with a dry dressing until the boil has stopped discharging, then leave open to the air to heal.

DON'T
- 'squeeze' boils until they are ready.

SEEK HELP IF
- boils are accompanied by a severe headache, high fever or a stiff neck.
- redness or swelling spreads out significantly from the site of the boil.
- there is severe pain.
- there is no improvement from self-prescribing within three days.
- the boil has opened but is still discharging pus and isn't healing after a week.
- the boil is on the face and is accompanied by swollen glands in the neck.

Breastfeeding problems

Minor complaints in the early days of breastfeeding are common. Homeopathy is wonderful at helping to deal with these without harming the baby.

DO
- use a breastfeeding counsellor for support and advice (The National Childbirth Trust and La Lèche League have a nationwide network of counsellors. Ring their London offices for your local contact.)
- rest, drink plenty of fluids and eat well and very regularly.
- wear a comfortable, supportive bra (preferably cotton).
- make sure the whole areola (especially the part *below* the nipple) is taken into the baby's mouth.
- position the baby's head properly by cradling it in your right hand when putting it to the left breast, and vice versa.
- self-prescribe for the specific problems below:

Breast abscesses (Mastitis)

Prompt treatment can clear up an acute breast infection (mastitis) and prevent a more serious abscess from developing. Breast abscesses can also occur in women who are not breastfeeding; first-aid

prescribing can help these, but a professional homeopath should always be consulted if the problem recurs.
DO
- follow the general guidelines above.
- apply hot and cold compresses alternately.
- breastfeed *more* often and in a variety of positions
  to drain all the milk from the breast.
DON'T
- stop breastfeeding.
SEEK HELP IF
- self-prescribing hasn't helped within 24–48 hours.
- there is fever.
- the glands in the armpits are swollen.

Cracked nipples
DO
- seek advice from a breastfeeding counsellor (see
  above) on how to position the baby correctly.
- keep the nipples clean and dry.
- expose the nipples to the air to promote healing.
DON'T
- use creams other than those suggested in the
  External Materia Medica.
- give up!
SEEK HELP IF
- there is bleeding or severe pain.

Engorged breasts

This common condition often occurs when the breastmilk first comes in. Homeopathic remedies can alleviate pain and discomfort and help to stabilise the milk
supply.
DO
- breastfeed frequently.
- express some milk if the baby can't 'latch on' until
  the nipple has softened – use a pump if you are
  unable to hand express.
- alternate hot and cold compresses to provide relief.

Breast lumps

These may be tender (mastitis) and can be worrying
while breastfeeding. They are harmless and respond
well to homeopathic treatment. I have included a few
remedies for breast lumps but do make sure that you
seek professional help if they don't clear within a short
time.

Broken bones

Fractures are sometimes difficult to spot, particularly
in the wrist of a child who has fallen onto an outstretched hand, or in an elderly person who has
injured a hip.
Arnica will be needed initially to reduce the swelling

and to prevent bruising around the site of the injury;
this will make the plastercast more comfortable.
Homeopathic remedies will help to alleviate the pain
and speed up the healing of a broken bone. You may
need to give the remedies for a longer period of time
than is necessary for other complaints, that is until the
bone has properly set.
DO
- take the appropriate remedy for shock.
- keep a fractured limb immobile.
- seek emergency help as soon as possible.
- apply a cold compress or ice pack (a packet of
  frozen peas is ideal) to the affected part.
- consult a good general first-aid book for how to
  deal with fractures while waiting for emergency
  help.
- take homeopathic remedies to alleviate pain and
  speed healing both before and after the bone has
  been 'set'.
DON'T
- move a fractured limb.
SEEK HELP AFTER AN INJURY IF
- there is severe pain, especially on normal
  movement.
- the injured part is swollen and the area beyond it is
  blue, cold or numb.
- the injured part cannot be used and looks an odd
  shape.
- the arm or leg is a different length.
- a joint is unnaturally loose or, conversely, it is
  impossible to straighten it.
- you have any cause to suspect a fracture.

Bruises

Treat with both the appropriate internal and external
homeopathic remedies.
DO
- have an X-ray to check for fracture following a
  severe fall (see Broken bones and Head injuries).

Burns and scalds

Burns are caused by dry heat, and scalds by moist heat
(steam or hot liquids). Minor burns and scalds produce redness and more serious burns produce blistering. Very serious burns, where the layers of skin have
burnt through, may be painless if the nerve endings
have been destroyed.
DO
- treat for shock immediately.
- plunge a minor burn into cold water immediately
  and keep it immersed until it no longer feels hot.
- cover a serious burn with a light dressing and seek
  medical help.

- learn how to deal with burns on a first-aid course or from a good book.
- soothe a burnt mouth or tongue by sucking ice cubes or an ice lolly.
- sip water frequently if you have been burned.
- take sensible safety measures to avoid burns, especially with children in the home. For example, use plug covers for empty sockets, keep matches out of reach.

DON'T
- burst blisters.
- leave children unattended near fires or cooking.
- rub butter or grease on burns.

SEEK HELP IF
- the burn is severe.
- the burn covers an area larger than the hand.
- the face or genitals are burned.
- swelling or redness develops or pus oozes from the burn.
- the burn was electrical. Don't pull someone away from the source of an electrical burn with bare hands. Use a wooden chair or broom (or anything of non-conductive material) to break the contact. Give mouth-to-mouth resuscitation if necessary.

Catarrh see Common cold, Hayfever

Chicken pox see Childhood illnesses/Fever/Cause for concern

Chilblains

DO
- keep the affected limbs warm and dry.
- take regular exercise to improve circulation.

DON'T
- subject your feet/hands to extreme changes in temperature, for example putting icy feet into hot water.
- expose the hands or feet to unnecessary cold.

SEEK HELP IF
- chilblains are severe.
- they break.
- they recur frequently throughout the winter.

Childbirth see Labour pains

Childhood illnesses

When children are subjected to new environments such as school their immune systems take time to build up strength, causing them to 'succumb' to various illnesses. This can be a trying time for parents, especially if there are several children in a family getting sick one after another. But childhood illnesses are not necessarily a 'bad' thing. They provide a child with the opportunity to develop resistance and strength. Children who have successfully come through a childhood illness without medical interference are seen to be stronger afterwards and often have a growth spurt – either physically or mentally or both.

It is important to nurse a sick child through a childhood illness. This may seem obvious, but it is becoming increasingly common to give children antibiotics and Calpol and to encourage them to carry on a normal life, including going to school. If you are a working parent you will need to prepare yourself for the fact that your children will fall ill from time to time and will need nursing, either by you or with the help of good childcare. If you are not prepared, it is easy to feel harassed and resentful whenever they do fall ill, and being sick is an event that deserves special treatment.

Encourage bedrest for a very sick child. Make up a bed in the sitting room so that he or she doesn't feel shut off from family life. Keep excitement levels down and encourage quiet activities such as reading, drawing, playing board games, watching a little television and listening to the radio. Sick children usually love being read to. Make sure they get lots of extra sleep (with early nights and naps) and encourage them to drink plenty of fluids, preferably water or diluted fruit juice (not squash or fizzy drinks). Don't feed a child who is sick and isn't hungry. In any case discourage junk food and give small, nutritious meals to a sick child who wishes to eat.

Keep a hot, feverish child cool, and a chilly feverish child warm. Don't take a child with a fever out and be careful not to overdo things in the convalescent stage of a childhood illness as relapses are common at this time.

Don't worry if sick children regress temporarily, sucking things, wetting the bed, and so on. A child who is sickening for something may regress as a first symptom that he or she is not well. In either case this behaviour will pass as they recover; it should not be punished.

Explain clearly (even to a very young child) what is wrong and say how long the illness is likely to last. Make suggestions about what the child can do to help him- or herself get better quickly.

If you are a parent nursing one child after another through a childhood illness, make sure you get out at least once a day to relieve the tedium and recharge your energy to keep you healthy and sane!

Before prescribing a homeopathic remedy, assess how well your child is coping with the disease and whether he or she *needs* a remedy.

A child who is unwell and *doesn't* recover from a childhood illness always needs constitutional treatment.

NEVER GIVE A CHILD ASPIRIN OR DISPRIN DURING OR AFTER A CHILDHOOD ILLNESS AS THIS CAN CAUSE SERIOUS COMPLICATIONS.

For general warning symptoms see Cause for Concern (page 203).

Incubation and infectious periods vary, so the information regarding them in the individual illness entries below should be used as a rough guide only.

Chicken pox

Incubation period: 7–21 days. *Infectious period:* a few days before onset, until last spot or blister has formed a scab.

Chicken pox generally occurs in a mild form in very young children and in a more severe form in older children. Adults can also suffer severe attacks – and the same virus (*Herpes zoster*) may produce shingles. Homeopathic treatment will help enormously.
DO
- take the appropriate homeopathic remedies as and when needed to speed recovery and soothe itching.
- avoid direct contact with the elderly; the chicken pox virus can occur in adults in the form of shingles, a sometimes painful and protracted disease.
DON'T
- pick the spots. This will leave scars.
SEEK HELP IF
- the spots become badly inflamed (infected).
- the spots affect the eyes (not just the eyelids).

German measles

Incubation period: 14–21 days. *Infectious period:* five days before and seven days after the rash appears.

German measles, or rubella, is generally a short-lived and very mild infection and should not need homeopathic treatment. The faint pink rash may be accompanied by watery eyes and swollen glands at the back of the neck and/or behind the ears, under the arms or in the groin. In older girls and women it may be followed by stiff joints, and homeopathic remedies are useful in treating this.
DO
- avoid anyone with German measles if you are pregnant, as the infection can damage the foetus, especially in early pregnancy; and if you have measles keep away from pregnant women during your infectious period.
- stay indoors while the rash is out.
SEEK HELP IF
- severe joint pains develop and are not alleviated by first-aid homeopathic treatment.

- pregnancy is suspected.
- there is a high fever, severe, persistent headache and marked drowsiness.

Measles

Incubation period: 8–21 days. *Infectious period:* four days before and 5–10 days after the rash appears.

You can check whether your child is in the early stages of measles by looking for small spots like grains of sand in the mouth, inside the cheeks. These spots, known as 'Koplik's spots', confirm measles before the characteristic red rash appears, usually a day or two later. Don't be tempted to suppress the fever, even if the temperature is relatively high (see Fever page 215), as it is essential that the disease burns itself out. Complications thought to be caused by suppression include ear infections, respiratory problems, pneumonia and encephalitis (inflammation of the brain), and children need careful nursing to reduce the likelihood of these.
DO
- keep a 'measly' child with sore eyes out of bright light (keep curtains partially closed and the lights dimmed, for example). Television is OK as long as your child's eyes don't hurt more from watching it.
SEEK HELP IF
- a baby under six months old contracts measles.
- there is a cough with the measles that lasts for longer than four days and doesn't respond to self-prescribing.
- the measles is accompanied by severe earache.

Mumps

Incubation period: 12–28 days. *Infectious period:* two days before and seven days after swelling appears.

Mumps usually occurs as a mild childhood infection, but it can be more severe in older children and adults. The most common symptom is the swelling of one or both of the salivary glands (in front of the ear and just above the angle of the jaw), which gives a 'hamster-cheeked' appearance. The glands under the tongue and jaw may also swell. The appropriate remedy will give relief from earache and will ease pain caused by eating, which are both common in mumps, and will speed recovery.
DO
- give soups or liquidised food if chewing is painful.
SEEK HELP IF
- there is painful swelling of the breasts or testicles.
- there is abdominal pain in girls (which might indicate swollen ovaries).
- there is difficulty hearing.

Roseola

Incubation period: 5–15 days.

Roseola is a mild, infectious illness very similar to German measles, and the two are sometimes confused. The rash will distinguish between the two: in Roseola it appears when the fever has come down and in German measles it is more likely to appear with the fever. Treat as you would German measles.

Scarlet fever

Incubation period: 2–7 days. *Infectious period:* seven days after exposure to an infected person until four weeks after the illness appears.

This highly infectious disease is rare nowadays, which is why it is not included in the Materia Medica. However, it responds extremely well to homeopathic treatment and patients usually recover without any complications. The symptoms are a sore throat, followed a day or two later by a rash of tiny spots which begins on the neck and chest and spreads over the whole body, giving the skin a texture like sandpaper; vomiting; fever and a flushed face (though the area around the mouth may be pale). The tongue may also have a red and white 'strawberry' appearance. Prescribe on the fever, sore throat and any other general and mental/emotional symptoms. The major scarlet fever remedies are *Apis, Belladonna, Lachesis, Lycopodium, Mercurius solubilis, Nitric acid* and *Rhus toxicodendron*.
SEEK HELP IF
- the joints are painful.
- there is pain in the ear.
- there is pain in the kidneys or on urination.

Whooping cough

Incubation period: 7–21 days. *Infectious period:* seven days after exposure to an infected person until four weeks after the illness appears.

The first signs of whooping cough are a slight fever, runny nose and loose cough. The mucus then thickens and great paroxysms of coughing are needed to bring it up, after which the child 'whoops' to draw air back into the lungs. Remedies can ease the coughing and speed recovery. Whooping cough can last from three weeks to four months and is a long and tiring infection for both child and parent, but complications are rare in children over a year old, so try to relax and do not be alarmed by the whooping fits.
DON'T
- smoke in the same room as a child with whooping cough.

- give proprietary cough medicines to reduce coughing – the child *needs* to cough to get the mucus up.
SEEK HELP IF
- you suspect your child under one year old has whooping cough.
- there is frequent vomiting after coughing spells.

Cold sores

Minor attacks of cold sores of the mouth respond well to the appropriate internal and external remedies. Children can have serious attacks, with numerous sores around and inside the mouth and an accompanying fever, and homeopathic remedies can help these enormously. Renewed outbreaks can be triggered by sunlight, cold or general low health so avoid over-exposure and try not to get run down.
DO
- keep the affected area clean and dry.
DON'T
- kiss (or engage in oral sex) whilst affected.
SEEK HELP IF
- cold sores recur or are especially severe.
- the area near the eyes is affected.
- there is no improvement after a week of self-prescribing.
- the sores become infected, with swelling, redness and pus.

Colic

Colic simply means sharp tummy pains or cramps. Homeopathic treatment is highly effective in the treatment of simple colic, whether in infants, children or adults. The mothers of breastfed babies with colic should experiment with their own diet, as many foods are known to affect some babies; these include dairy products, alcohol, tea, coffee, peppers, onions, garlic, cabbage (especially raw), oranges and grapes. A good breastfeeding counsellor will advise (see Breastfeeding problems). Some bottle-fed babies are allergic to cow's milk and will usually do well on soya milk although that can be too acidic for some – again, seek advice if this happens.

Colic or stomach-ache in children and adults needs careful monitoring in case it is caused by a rumbling appendix.
DO
- give small meals of bland, easily digestible foods.
- eliminate suspect foods from the diet of a baby who has just started on solids.
- try to relax when breastfeeding a colicky baby.
SEEK HELP IF
- symptoms persist (especially in young children who continue to scream inconsolably).

- severe pain is not quickly alleviated by home prescribing.
- pain is accompanied by persistent vomiting or diarrhoea.
- pain is accompanied by constipation or absence of urine.

Common cold

A cold is often the body's way of letting us know we are a little run down, and that our immune system needs recharging. If you can, take a little time off, have some early nights and deal constructively with some of the stress in your life. Neglected colds often turn into more serious chest infections, so catch them early.
DO
- get plenty of rest if you have been overdoing it.
- drink lots of fluids.
- clear the airways frequently, but gently. Teach your children to cough up phlegm and to blow their noses instead of sniffing the mucus and swallowing it. (Put your finger over one nostril and tell the child to breathe in through the mouth and breathe out hard through the nose keeping the mouth shut. Repeat with other nostril. Keep a tissue handy! You can graduate to holding a tissue over the nose once they have got the general idea. Eventually both nostrils can be blown at once!)
- use steam inhalations to dislodge stubborn mucus. Sit over a bowl of just-boiled water with a towel over the head (supervise children to avoid any possibility of an accidental burn). Or run a hot bath to get the bathroom steamed up, or use a vaporiser (filled with plain water – don't add any decongestant).
- eat plenty of fruit and vegetables and avoid dairy products, sugar, junk foods and too much bread, which all increase mucus production.
- avoid tobacco fumes.
- take some gentle exercise in the fresh air to see if this helps (and use the response as a symptom to repertorise).
DON'T
- use decongestants. These only irritate the nasal membranes and make matters worse as soon as the effect wears off.
SEEK HELP IF
- you suffer from frequent colds, as you will benefit from constitutional treatment to boost your immunity (see page 14).
- your cold seems unduly severe and you have any of the symptoms listed under Cause for Concern (page 203).

Conjunctivitis see Eye inflammation

Constipation

I have included a few remedies for use in an acute situation, but generally speaking this is not a complaint for home treatment beyond following the commonsense Dos and Don'ts listed below. A general tendency to constipation requires professional treatment. The recommendations below will help acute or long-term constipation.
DO
- make sure there is plenty of fibre in the diet by adding more fruit and vegetables.
- cut out bread and wheat products temporarily as the gluten can have a clogging effect.
- drink plenty of water.
- eat stewed prunes in the morning with a tablespoon of molasses dissolved in hot water.
- use oat bran (organically grown if possible) for occasional constipation; bran should only be taken regularly on the advice of a professional.
DON'T
- add wheat bran on a daily basis. It can irritate the bowels and interfere with the assimilation of vitamins and minerals, and your bowels can become dependent on it. Oat bran is soluble and much kinder to the bowels.
- take laxatives regularly, particularly if your diet is of mainly refined and junk foods.
SEEK HELP IF
- there has been no bowel movement for twenty-four hours and there is severe, unusual pain.
- there is difficulty in passing a stool and the stools are grey or white.
- the skin or eyes are yellow.
- there is a sudden and inexplicable change in bowel habit.
- there is alternating diarrhoea and constipation.
- the stools are extremely dark, almost black.

Convulsions

I have included some remedies for the treatment of convulsions in children as it is possible to treat this complaint as an emergency measure at the same time as calling for help. *It is essential that you get professional advice should this event occur at any time.*

Corns and bunions

DO
- use the appropriate internal and external homeopathic remedies to help alleviate the pains if they are severe.
- use a felt pad if the bunion is inflamed.
- wear sensible shoes that do not pinch or apply pressure to the corns.
- seek the advice of a good chiropodist.

Cough

Some children can cough their way through their teething years and others will suffer from repeated coughs and colds for the first year or two at school while their immune system adapts. You can use first-aid prescribing for these coughs providing you are having a good response and the moods and energy of the child remain high. If the complaints recur in spite of careful first-aid prescribing then you need to seek professional homeopathic help. Coughs and colds that recur every winter are also mostly a case for the professional homeopath. However, if you spot your own child's constitutional remedy picture from the pictures in this book then you may find that your first-aid prescribing has the side effect of preventing the recurrence of these acute episodes.

DO
- follow all the Dos for Common cold.
- rest.
- drink lots of liquids; they will help to loosen the mucus.
- cough up the phlegm as often as possible; teach young children to cough up phlegm as soon as they are able to.
- use a humidifier or vaporiser in the bedroom to fill the room with steam; this will help the chest to expel sticky phlegm. If you don't have a vaporiser, close the bathroom door and windows and leave the hot water running until you've created a humid 'fug'.
- keep the room temperature constant so that the patient isn't having to adapt to either heat or cold.

DON'T
- suppress the cough routinely with a cough medicine; this may prevent the person from coughing up mucus, and if mucus is not expelled, a more serious infection may develop.
- give cod liver oil to children, especially small children, thinking that it will boost their immunity; it may well make the cough and cold worse and make them go off their food.

SEEK HELP IF
- there is difficulty in breathing and/or wheezing and/or chest pain.
- the cough seems severe and doesn't respond to self-prescribing within forty-eight hours.
- the breathing is unduly rapid.

See also Croup and Cause for Concern.

NB PNEUMONIA (ESPECIALLY IN CHILDREN) IS NOT ALWAYS ACCOMPANIED BY A COUGH. SEEK URGENT MEDICAL HELP IF YOUR CHILD HAS A FEVER, IS BREATHING RAPIDLY AND SEEMS UNWELL (LIMP AND PALE).

Cramp

A cramp is simply a sudden muscle contraction and is often caused by a change in body temperature, a change in position or a loss of body fluids.

DO
- straighten the affected part of the body, and gently massage the affected muscle.

Croup

Croup is a frightening-sounding cough that usually occurs in children under four years old. It starts with hoarseness and fever and develops into a loud, barking, ringing, harsh cough that wakes the child at night. The breathing may also be noisy.

DO
- follow the guidelines for Common cold and Cough (see above).

SEEK HELP IF
- a steamy bathroom doesn't relieve the symptoms in half an hour.
- the cough is accompanied by a blue tinge to the lips.

Cuts/Grazes see Wounds

Cystitis

If left untreated, cystitis can develop into a serious kidney infection. I have included a few remedies for the treatment of cystitis, but symptoms should be carefully monitored and a professional consulted when symptoms give cause for concern.

DO
- drink a large amount of water to flush out the kidneys and bladder.
- keep your diet alkaline (eat lots of fruit and vegetables).
- cut out all acid foods and drinks, including tea, coffee, sugar, refined/junk food, alcohol.
- take as much rest as you can.
- keep as warm as you can (wear extra woollen clothing and carry around a hot water bottle or use a heating pad).
- be careful when wiping after urinating (women and girls): wipe from front to back so that bacteria from the anus cannot enter the urethra (this is also a general preventive measure).
- urinate frequently to keep the urethra free of bacteria.

DON'T
- use bubble baths or oils of any sort.
- wash the genitals with soap; just sponge down well with water.
- wear nylon tights or tight trousers in general.

- use vaginal deodorants or biological washing powders on underwear.
- get chilled.

SEEK HELP IF
- there are sharp pains in the area of the kidneys (in the back above the waist, on either side of the spine).
- there is blood in the urine (it looks pink, red or brown – remember that if you eat a large quantity of beetroot your urine will be red).
- the cystitis is accompanied by headache, vomiting, fever and chills.

Deafness

Deafness that occurs after a cold or ear infection is a result of catarrh in the Eustachian tubes, and this can be treated.

DON'T
- use cotton buds or other implements to remove wax from the ear as this can push it further in and make it more difficult to remove/wash out.

SEEK HELP IF
- the hearing hasn't returned more than two weeks after the original infection.
- there is a sudden loss of hearing, with or without pain.

Diarrhoea

The Dos and Don'ts listed below are written with children in mind. In general, adults with acute diarrhoea can cut out food for 24 hours and take the indicated homeopathic remedy to speed their healing.

DO
- limit the intake of food and drink.
- introduce water, freshly squeezed fruit juices, vegetable broths (simmer a selection of chopped vegetables in water for 15–20 minutes and strain), or rice water (rice cooked in double the amount of water for slightly longer than usual and strained). These can be sipped initially and gradually increased as the symptoms pass.
- introduce solid food carefully: start with white rice, toast, bananas or low-fat yogurt.
- continue to breastfeed a nursing baby.
- watch for signs of dehydration in children who refuse to drink, especially those under six months old:

    mouth and eyes are dry (no saliva/tears);
    skin tone is poor; if the skin is pressed it does not spring back;
    the eyes look sunken;
    the fontanelle (soft spot on a baby's head) is sunken;
    scanty, strong-smelling urine (fewer wet nappies in babies).

DON'T
- give rich foods that are difficult to digest.
- encourage eating if there is no appetite – a few days without food will do no harm. See also remedies for the treatment of tiredness and loss of appetite after diarrhoea.

SEEK HELP IF
- the diarrhoea persists and fluids are not being tolerated, and if there is exhaustion and loss of skin tone.
- there is acute pain in the abdomen that doesn't respond to first-aid prescribing within two to twelve hours (depending on the severity) or that is getting steadily worse.

Dizziness

Though persistent dizziness should always be investigated by a professional, you can treat minor, occasional vertigo occurring after a head injury, from overwork, travel sickness or a hangover.

DO
- rest until the dizziness has passed.
- cup your hands over your nose and mouth for a few minutes as you breathe slowly and steadily. Vertigo *can* be a result of overbreathing in which case you need to increase your levels of carbon dioxide.

DON'T
- drive

SEEK HELP IF
- there is severe vomiting alongside the dizziness.
- deafness or noises in the ear develop with the dizziness after an ear infection.

Earache

Earache often occurs during a cold and is a result of a build-up of catarrh in the Eustachian tubes. The catarrh gathers in the middle ear and presses against the eardrum itself, causing great pain. This is not necessarily a cause for concern, and the indicated homeopathic remedy will usually give speedy relief from the pain. The eardrum may perforate, which will also give instant relief from pain, and, provided the patient is in a clean environment, the drum will heal well in a couple of weeks with no troublesome consequences.

DO
- suspect earache and a possible infection in babies with a fever who cry and rub their heads.
- drink plenty of fluids.
- use a hot water bottle (or an ice pack) to relieve the pain.
- use the appropriate internal and external homeopathic remedies.

- protect a perforated eardrum from water by plugging it with cotton wool during bathing and hairwashing, and don't let the child go swimming.

DON'T

- be tempted to clean the ears – the pain is never the result of wax.
- blow the nose hard.

SEEK HELP IF

- a baby has a depressed or bulging fontanelle.
- there is swelling, redness, tenderness or pain behind the ear.
- the earache doesn't respond to first-aid prescribing within twenty-four hours.
- if pain is severe.

See also Fever (pages 215–16) and Cause for Concern (page 203).

Emotional/mental problems

The mental and emotional health of a person has a huge effect on the physical body, and keeping yourself healthy emotionally will greatly strengthen your immune system. Homeopathy is highly effective at helping with emotional stress; however, it is generally unwise to treat yourself if you are suffering from emotional problems, mainly because it is difficult to be objective about how you are behaving – you may feel depressed but are actually being irritable, for example. A trained homeopath will be able to differentiate and give you a remedy that fits your whole picture, often taking the emotional cause into account.

If you are prescribing on someone else and are very clear about what is happening emotionally you can prescribe with confidence. If the symptoms are mainly emotional and general, and if they present a very strong picture, even if the physical symptoms are not present, then the remedy required will be 'constitutional', and will help to alleviate what physical symptoms there are as well as improve the moods. It is essential that you keep detailed notes on which remedy you prescribed, why you gave it and the effect it had. If it was very effective then it may be the first remedy you think of the next time that particular person is ill.

I have included all sorts of emotional problems such as anxiety, depression, exam nerves, irritability from loss of sleep, and so on.

DO

- seek some sort of counselling help.
- seek alternative medical help in alleviating your symptoms.
- talk about your feelings to anyone who will listen.
- write about what you are going through.
- try to understand what is happening rather than fight it.

DON'T

- cut yourself off from friends and family. You need them now more than ever, even though your behaviour may be pushing them away. Tell them what you are going through and ask for their help.
- take anti-depressants, sleeping pills or other orthodox medication as these will suppress your feelings and make it more difficult for you to deal with them at a later date.

Exhaustion

I have included many remedies for tiredness in this book, for example for tiredness following a period of hard work, after an acute illness or after diarrhoea. Use commonsense measures to look after yourself and take the appropriate homeopathic remedy to hasten your recovery.

DO

- rest, and sleep – as much as you feel you need.
- eat especially well and drink plenty of fluids.
- delegate workloads for a realistic period of time while you recharge.
- take gentle exercise – this will help to create energy.
- read mindless books and magazines, the funnier the better.
- have a massage/facial/sauna, etc.
- arrange to spend time with friends doing fun things unassociated with work.

DON'T

- take remedies and carry on regardless.
- drink extra tea and coffee and carry on, as these will deplete your energy after the initial lift.

SEEK HELP IF

- the exhaustion persists in spite of following the above guidelines.

Eye inflammation

Eye infections in small babies need professional help if they don't clear quickly (within a couple of days) and easily.

DO

- bathe the eye (see page 33) and take the appropriate internal remedy if needed.
- wash your hands every time you touch the infected eye to prevent spreading the infection to the other eye or to another person.

DON'T

- rub inflamed eyes as this can make them worse.
- ever use cortisone drops in the eye unless prescribed for a specific complaint.

SEEK HELP IF

- the symptom persists, especially in a newborn baby.

- there is severe pain in the eye, especially if it is caused by bright lights.
- the sight is affected in any way.

Eye injuries

DO
- bathe the eye (see page 33); flush out immediately with lots of water if chemicals enter the eye.
- take the appropriate internal remedy if needed and apply a light bandage or scarf to a very swollen (or black) eye to rest it so that it can heal.
- remove particles of dust from the lid with a cotton bud.
DON'T
- leave eye make-up on at night as it irritates the eye.
SEEK HELP IF
- there is a foreign body that you cannot remove.
- the foreign body was made of iron – though the body itself may no longer be in your eye, it may have left rust deposits.
- the sight is affected in any way.
- there is bleeding or a clear fluid discharge from the site of the wound in the eye itself.
- chemicals get into the eye.

Eye strain

DO
- take the appropriate internal and external remedies.
- rest the eyes for as long as is needed.
- have your eyes tested fairly frequently if you suffer from recurring eye strain.
- use good light for close or fine work, or even reading in bed.

Faintness

DO
- eat if it is a long time since your last meal.
- lie down with the feet raised if exposed to strong sunshine or hot, stuffy conditions, and take in some fluids.
DON'T
- subsist on snacks if working hard.
SEEK HELP IF
- you experience your heart beating faster or slower than normal, or if the faintness is accompanied by chest pain, weakness anywhere, blurred vision, confusion or difficulty speaking.
- you feel breathless.
- your legs are swollen.

Fever

See also earache, sore throat, cough, etc., if the fever accompanies these.

In many infections fevers are an essential part of the healing process and are often underestimated partly because they evoke fear through lack of understanding of their purpose. A fever is helpful and necessary, whether associated with a cold or one of the more serious 'childhood illnesses'. Through understanding that a fever is a symptom of disease and not a disease in itself we can come to see fevers as allies and not enemies.

Some people have fevers that recur, after, say, glandular fever or malaria; these are not to be confused with the fevers we are discussing here and should always be referred to a professional homeopath.

A high temperature generally indicates that the body's defence mechanism is fighting an infection and temperature variations indicate how it is coping. During a fever the healing reactions of the body are speeded up: the heart beats faster, carrying the blood more quickly to the organs; respiration is quicker, increasing oxygen intake; and perspiration increases, helping the body to cool down naturally. Attempts to suppress or control a fever artificially with paracetamol, or even with homeopathic remedies, are likely to confuse the body's natural efforts to heal itself.

Hippocrates said, 'Give me a fever and I can cure the child.' A weak child may be endlessly 'sick', neither very ill nor very well, but with no significant rise in temperature. A more robust child whose temperature soars may look and feel very ill, therefore giving more cause for concern but is ill for a shorter time and recovers more quickly.

Each person has their own pattern of falling ill and will experience different fever symptoms; one individual may feel hot with a high fever while another may feel chilly and shiver. The latter may be irritable and intolerant of any disturbance and need to be kept warm. Another may be aching and restless, may moan and complain. Yet another may sweat profusely, be thirsty and slightly delirious. One person may want company, someone to talk to, and another will want to be alone. Each response will demand its individual, but similar, remedy.

The average normal temperature in a healthy human is said to be 98.4°F or 37°C, but it can vary quite markedly. Most people, adults and children, can run a fever of up to 104°F (40°C) for a short period – or even several days – with no danger. It is normal for healthy infants and children to throw high fevers (103°F/39.5°C and over) with an infection. A temperature of 105°F (40.5°C) is cause for concern but it is only when it passes above 106°F (41°C) that there is a risk to life.

Fevers usually peak towards night-time and drop

by the following morning, so that a temperature of 104°F/40°C registered in the evening may recur on subsequent evenings. A drop in temperature in the morning does not mean that the fever is past its peak. It can rise and fall several times over several days before finally returning to normal.

Hallucinations and tantrums in children sometimes accompany high fevers. These are distressing but not dangerous. Keep a close eye on your child and seek professional help if these symptoms don't clear up quickly with self-prescribing.

DO

- take the temperature with a thermometer for an accurate reading. A fever strip (for the forehead) is a rough guide only and a hand held on the forehead is next to useless. A temperature taken by tucking the thermometer tightly under the armpit will read a fraction lower than that taken under the tongue. The thermometer should be left under the armpit for at least five minutes rather than three minutes under the tongue.
- provide a calm environment for your feverish patient and be guided by their needs. Many children with a high fever will not wish to eat. This is a good sign: fasting encourages the body further to eliminate toxic wastes and helps it focus on recovery. Encourage a hungry patient to take light dishes such as vegetable soup, raw or stewed fruit with honey. Water, lemon and honey or diluted fresh fruit juices, warmed or cold as desired, are best to drink. Breast milk is fine for a nursing baby and is probably all that will be wanted.
- avoid tea, coffee, chocolate, alcohol and sugar as they stimulate the system when it needs to rest.
- encourage a feverish patient to drink, at least sips of water at frequent intervals. Children who are reluctant to drink will often suck on a wet sponge or flannel, especially if the water is warm. Or try an ice cube or frozen fruit juice.
- immerse a feverish but not desperately ill child in the bath from time to time to bring down the fever. Thirstless children will often drink the bathwater as an added bonus!
- sponge down if the fever goes above 103°F/104°F (40°C) and your patient feels uncomfortable (hot and sweaty). Expose and sponge one limb at a time until it feels cool to the touch. Dry and replace it under the covers before going on to the next limb. This will help the temperature to drop by one or two degrees Fahrenheit and can be repeated as often as necessary. Sponging the face and forehead alone can also give relief.
- prescribe homeopathic remedies where the fever is one of a number of symptoms, i.e. where the patient is clearly suffering from say, earache or a sore throat *and* a fever. If the first symptom to arise

is a fever then wait for other symptoms to surface before prescribing. Contain the fever, again if necessary, by sponging down (see above).

- respond to your patient's individual needs – some people feel chilly with a fever and cannot bear to be uncovered, let alone sponged down – even with a high temperature.
- make sure that your patient has a day or two on foods nutritious and easily digested once the fever has abated and the appetite returned.

DON'T

- give a homeopathic remedy, say *Aconite*, *Belladonna* or *Chamomilla*, at the first sign of a rise in temperature as this can confuse the remedy picture. Any attempt to interrupt the body's self-healing process is unwise.

SEEK HELP IF

- a baby under six months old has a fever.
- an older baby has a fever of over 103.5°F/40°C that doesn't respond to sponging and homeopathic treatment within twenty-four hours.
- a person of any age has a fever of 105°F/40.5°C or over.
- there is history of convulsions accompanying fevers.
- anyone with a fever is also refusing to drink (is thirstless) as dehydration can occur, especially if the fever continues for several days with the patient taking in or keeping down (if there is also vomiting) only small amounts of liquids.
- there is a lack of reaction (listlessness and limpness), which can imply that a serious illness such as pneumonia or meningitis has developed – see Cause for Concern page 203.

IF YOU ARE WORRIED GET IN TOUCH WITH YOUR DOCTOR AND/OR YOUR HOMEOPATH IMMEDIATELY.

Never suppress a fever in children with aspirin (or Disprin) as this has been known to lead to dangerous although rare, complications, in particular Reye's Syndrome, which affects the brain and liver. Symptoms include sudden vomiting some time after the onset of a viral infection, sleepiness, confusion, diarrhoea, and rapid, shallow breathing. Calpol (paracetamol) may be used in an emergency but the recommended dose should never be exceeded.

Flatulence

Wind is often caused by eating too much of something that is not tolerated well – meat, refined foods, alcohol (especially beer), beans or whole grains are known to cause flatulence – or by eating too hurriedly. Emotional stress, especially anxiety, and constipation can both also cause wind.

DO

- sit down and relax when eating and chew thoroughly; bolting your food on the run can stress your digestive system.
- try to reduce your intake of liquids with meals (drink more between meals).
- avoid fizzy drinks with meals.
- cook beans carefully (soak overnight, boil for twenty minutes, rinse well and then simmer till cooked).
- experiment with your diet to see if you can find the culprit if there is one and then cut it out or eat less of it.
- try a herb tea such as peppermint or fennel to aid digestion.

Flu

Look to the appropriate sections such as Sore throat, Cough and Fever, etc., depending on which particular symptoms you are suffering from. If your flu is 'gastric', i.e. accompanied by diarrhoea, colic and/or vomiting then you will need to look up these (relevant) sections also.

Use commonsense measures to look after yourself during a flu. Treat it as a bad cold and take some time off work to sleep and recharge.

DO

- go to bed.
- drink extra fluids, hot or cold as desired.

DON'T

- go to work.

Food poisoning see Vomiting and Diarrhoea

Food poisoning is caused by eating contaminated meat, fish or other foods and I have included several appropriate remedies. Certain chemicals and plants can cause vomiting and diarrhoea (including the green part of potatoes), and poisoning from these requires urgent medical help. Stomach 'bugs' which look and feel like food poisoning can be just as unpleasant and will usually be accompanied by a fever (food poisoning from contamination has no fever).

SEEK HELP IF

- there is continued abdominal pain and blood in the stools.
- there is difficulty focusing, double vision, convulsions or paralysis.

German Measles see Childhood illnesses

Gum Boil see Abscesses

Gums bleeding

I have included a few remedies that have sensitive, bleeding gums as part of their picture. However, a good diet high in fibre (fruit, vegetables, salad and wholewheat bread) and good dental hygiene are essential to maintaining healthy gums.

DO

- see your dentist for regular check-ups.
- ask your dentist or the hygienist to show you the correct way to brush your teeth.
- use dental floss and brush regularly and conscientiously.
- use a mouthwash (see page 28) and massage the gums gently after brushing.
- cut out sugar if possible for a time, at least until the gums improve.

SEEK HELP IF

- your gums still bleed in spite of taking the above measures and you also feel unwell generally (pale, exhausted, poor appetite, swollen glands).

Hair loss

I have included some remedies for the first-aid treatment of hair loss that occurs, mainly in women, after an acute illness or childbirth. If the condition persists then seek help from a professional homeopath.

Hayfever

The presence of hayfever indicates an underlying weakness that needs constitutional treatment and, though there are a few first-aid remedies here for acute hayfever, homeopaths prefer to treat a hayfever sufferer through the winter months in order to strengthen resistance to pollen and other allergens.

DO

- where possible, avoid pollen, animal hair or other substances (tobacco, dust, flowers, etc.) to which you know you are allergic, and keep dust levels low in the home. Use foam pillows and duvets filled with synthetic fibres.
- bathe the eyes if they are itchy and inflamed (see page 33).

DON'T

- take antihistamines or decongestants if you can avoid it. These suppress the body's defences and can cause a rebound effect so that the symptoms return more fiercely than ever as the effects wear off.

Headache

Occasional minor headaches that result from obvious stresses such as overwork, alcohol, loss of sleep, etc., can be treated with first-aid homeopathy. As well as finding the appropriate remedy, identify the cause of your headache and take appropriate action: remove the cause temporarily in the case of, say, alcohol, or rebalance your system with a good night's sleep if you are exhausted.

DO
- rest and relax; check your posture for tension and spend ten minutes relaxing and breathing deeply if you suspect you have a headache starting.
- get some fresh air if you've been in a stuffy room.
- have your eyes tested to make sure the cause is not poor sight.
- seek counselling or psychotherapy if you are under a lot of emotional stress.
- have a massage.
- take a long, hot bath.
- eat regular meals, and cut down (or out) on smoking, drinking tea, coffee and alcohol.
- take a nap.
- make time to see friends or pursue a hobby.

DON'T
- smoke.
- take pain relievers and carry on unless you really have to and can see a time ahead when you can rest.

SEEK HELP IF
- a headache is very severe.
- you suffer frequent or severe headaches, particularly if your eyesight is deteriorating.
- a headache is accompanied by a stiff neck.
- there is a high fever.
- there is any visual disturbance.
- there is any weakness or lack of co-ordination.
- there is any dizziness.
- a headache lasts more than three or four days.

Head injuries

Recent minor knocks and falls can be safely treated with internal and external homeopathic remedies. Give the appropriate remedies for shock and bruising but regard all head injuries as potentially serious. Keep a careful watch for any of the symptoms below, some of which may only develop hours or even days after the injury. Osteopathy can be helpful after a head injury (depending on the severity or the effect) to help any stress the spine itself may have suffered as a result of a fall. Some children continue to fall after one bad injury and are labelled 'clumsy' when their bodies have simply become misaligned. Osteopathy is therefore useful as a preventive measure.

DO
- go to hospital for an X-ray if the fall was serious (and especially if the back of the head was injured). Give *Arnica* on the way to the hospital but

if this helps do not be deceived into thinking your patient is fine and go home – by alleviating shock and pain, the seriousness of an injury can easily be masked.

DON'T
- let someone who has suffered a fall or blow go to sleep immediately afterwards; this can hide concussion and the patient may fall into a coma.

SEEK HELP IF
- there is any drowsiness or confusion.
- the person is unconscious.
- The pupils do not respond to light or are irregular in size.
- the person feels faint or is unusually thirsty.
- the person is sweaty or pale.

Heartburn see Indigestion

Hives

This 'nettle rash' may be caused by an allergic reaction to some foods – for example shellfish, eggs or strawberries – or to drugs, and it may develop at any time, when no previous reaction has been noted. Use both an internal and external remedy to reduce itching and discomfort.

SEEK HELP IF
- swelling is severe and the itching unbearable.
- the mouth or tongue is swollen.
- there is any difficulty breathing.

Hot flushes

I have included remedies to relieve the distressing hot flushes that often accompany the menopause, but it is desirable during this transition to have constitutional treatment to rebalance hormone levels and provide more long-lasting help.

DO
- talk to your friends and family and tell them what you are going through so that you are not isolated, especially if your symptoms are unpleasant.
- eat well.
- take some sort of regular exercise; a daily walk is just fine.
- be especially nice to yourself during this time.
- seek help from a counsellor or psychotherapist who is conversant with helping women through the menopause.

DON'T
- assume you can no longer fall pregnant until your menopause is complete!

Indigestion

Discomfort after eating is often caused by eating or drinking too much, so look at your diet and how you eat as well as taking the appropriate remedy. Indigestion and heartburn are also common in late pregnancy, when the foetus puts pressure on the stomach. See also Flatulence.
DO
- eat slowly and chew your food thoroughly.
- make sure you relax before meals.
DON'T
- eat too much at one sitting.
- take antacids – these only upset the balance of acidity in the stomach even further in the long run.
SEEK HELP IF
- symptoms are accompanied by a cough, loss of appetite or loss of weight.
- there is severe abdominal pain.
- pain does not respond to treatment within two or three hours.
- pain begins around the navel, then moves to the lower right abdomen (this might be appendicitis).

Injuries (cuts/wounds)

Use the appropriate external remedies to cleanse wounds, and take internal remedies to stop bleeding and promote healing when necessary.
SEEK HELP IF
- bleeding is very profuse.
- there is any numbness or tingling near the injured part (which could indicate internal damage).
- the edges of the wound cannot be held together with plasters (in which case stitches might be needed).
- the wound is on the face (these often need stitching to avoid scarring).
- the wound is not superficial and is on the palm of the hand (where it is particularly open to infection).
- there is deeply imbedded dirt or a foreign body that you cannot remove (glass is particularly tricky to remove).
- the injury is severe.
- you suspect a fracture (see Broken bones).
- the wound is near a vital organ (heart, lungs, etc.).

Insomnia

We all have very different sleep requirements. As we grow older we need less sleep and we may generally need less sleep than we think. If you are insomniac, repeat to yourself before going to sleep that you are going to sleep deeply and wake refreshed, instead of panicking about not sleeping enough and expecting to feel awful in the morning. Amazingly this really helps. If your sleep pattern has been disturbed by sick children or night work, try to have a daytime nap, or catch up by having a really early night before you fall into a pattern of sleeping badly.
DO
- take gentle exercise, such as a walk around the block or an exercise routine before bed.
- relax in a warm bath.
- read very boring books/magazines in bed.
- wear earplugs and an eye mask to cut out noise and light if necessary.
- make sure your mattress is right for you (not too hard or too soft).
- develop a regular bedtime relaxation routine, including deep breathing, and perform this twice before going to bed.
- sit up and make a list of all worries and frustrations if you can't sleep because of them.
- make sure you are warm enough (but not too hot) and that your room is well ventilated.
- take a hot, caffeine-free drink to bed: hot milk with honey, or a cup of chamomile tea if you feel tense.
- seek counselling or psychotherapy if your sleeplessness is due to emotional distress such as anxiety, depression or bereavement.
DON'T
- worry! This always makes it worse.
- read thrillers, ghost stories or material connected with your work.
- have a large meal close to bedtime.
- drink tea, hot chocolate, coffee or Coca Cola or smoke too much during the evening.
- watch too much television, work or read anything upsetting.
- get into the habit of afternoon naps or sleeping very late in the morning as this can make it more difficult to get back to normal sleeping patterns.
- take sleeping pills. These can affect your dream life so that you wake feeling unrefreshed, and many have side effects, causing drowsiness and dependence.
- drink alcohol steadily throughout the evening.

Joint pain

Although chronic rheumatism or arthritis needs professional care, I have included some remedies that will provide relief from pain as well as from those acute pains which come on after injury or after an acute illness such as German measles. See Sprains and Strains for general advice for sore joints.
DO
- keep your weight down to avoid stressing hip and leg joints.

DON'T
- over-use a painful joint more than is absolutely necessary.

Keloids

These are scars that become hard and lumpy after healing. Homeopathic self-prescribing can be effective, but do seek help as soon as possible if it has no effect after four weeks, as prompt professional treatment will be needed.

Labour pains

Homeopathic remedies do not reduce labour pains themselves but they can speed up a labour that is losing momentum and help with basic problems such as exhaustion or backache during labour. They also help a woman to cope better emotionally, and are wonderful for healing after childbirth. I have included a few basic remedies for labour and after but would advise that you seek the help of a professional homeopath while you are pregnant, who will also support you during your birth and for the time afterwards. Many homeopaths will attend a birth or be available by phone to give advice (having prepared a selection of remedies for you to have to hand).

Laryngitis see Sore throat

Lumbago

I have included a few remedies for the treatment of acute lower back pain, which is sometimes called lumbago. Follow the guidelines given under Backache.

Mastitis see Breastfeeding problems

Measles see Childhood illnesses

Mouth ulcers

You can treat occasional mouth ulcers yourself with internal and external remedies, especially if they occur after dental treatment or during temporary stress, but do seek help if they are a recurring problem.

Mumps see Childhood illnesses

Nappy rash

I have included some external remedies for this but if it is persistent a professional homeopath will be needed.

DO
- change nappies frequently.
- leave your baby with nothing on for as long as possible.
- wash and rinse thoroughly, preferably with water.
- dry the area *thoroughly*; a hairdryer on a very gentle heat is ideal for this as no further moisture will remain on the skin, but test the heat on your own skin first, and remember that a baby's skin is much more delicate than an adult's. Smear a coating of raw egg white after washing and drying as this makes an effective waterproof skin.
- cut out all fruit juice and give plain water instead.
- use almond or olive oil as a preventive, i.e. to protect the skin.
- use external ointments (see External Materia Medica) if a rash starts.

DON'T
- use zinc and castor oil cream or petroleum-based products – they are absorbed through the skin and can cause minor problems.

Nausea

See also Vomiting, Gastric flu, Travel sickness and Indigestion if appropriate. Homeopathic remedies are especially useful for nausea during pregnancy, when they are both highly effective and perfectly safe.

DO
- eat little and often.
- take frequent sips of water or a hot drink if that is better.
- get as much rest and sleep as you need.
- avoid emotional stress.

SEEK HELP IF
- nausea is severe and is accompanied by vomiting.

Nettle rash see Hives

Nosebleeds

Nosebleeds can occur for no apparent reason or can accompany a cold, violent nose-blowing or sneezing, or injury to the nose or head; they can also follow a change in pressure or occur as a result of high blood pressure.

DO
- sit with the head tilted slightly forward.
- pinch the lower, soft part of the nose between finger and thumb.
- apply a cold compress to the bridge of the nose.

SEEK HELP IF
- there is also bleeding from other parts of the body.
- the bleeding doesn't stop within a few minutes.

Pain

It is useful to remember that pain has a very positive function as a warning of disease or injury. People unable to feel pain can do themselves real harm. We all have very different pain thresholds – limits beyond which we find pain unbearable – and pain itself is experienced in many different forms. Homeopathy uses these variations to differentiate and find the appropriate remedy: *Chamomilla*, for example, is a remedy for those extremely sensitive to pain, and *Opium* for those who feel nothing when they should.

Pain acts like a red traffic light at a busy junction, warning us to stop or risk a crash. We can stop and listen to the pain and try to understand what it is telling us, what we need to do to heal. Or we can ignore the pain – at our peril – and crash!

Palpitations

The palpitations included in this book are the minor, occasional ones that result from anxiety and stress, so take care to rest and recharge (see Stress page 201).
DO
- sit quietly and practise relaxation exercises and deep breathing.
SEEK HELP IF
- the palpitations persist over several hours.
- they are accompanied by chest pain.

Period problems

In all cases of persistent period problems you will need to seek professional advice, but I have included a few remedies for occasional minor complaints.

Absence of periods (Amenorrhea)

The obvious causes of this are pregnancy and menopause, but periods can also stop as a result of shock or anxiety, a change in lifestyle (for example when teenage girls go away to college), as a consequence of anorexia, anaemia, or as a result of taking the Pill.
DO
- have a pregnancy test if you could possibly be pregnant.
- check for anaemia.
- seek counselling help if anorexia is the cause.
- stop taking the Pill if it doesn't suit you and seek advice on other forms of contraception.
SEEK HELP IF
- periods stop without any apparent explanation.
- you are over sixteen and have still not begun to menstruate.

Excessive, prolonged or irregular periods

Many women experience irregular periods or periods that vary in the amount of flow but this is rarely indicative of any major health problem. It is especially common during the menopause, but fibroids or IUDs can also cause excessive bleeding and anaemia.
SEEK HELP IF
- periods become heavier than usual and this persists for more than two periods.

Painful periods

I have included some remedies for the treatment of period pains, but you should seek professional help if these don't work.
DO
- see if using towels instead of tampons helps.
- use a hot water bottle or a heating pad to soothe the pains.
- help to prevent pain by exercising regularly, especially exercise that focuses on the pelvis/lower back.
- rest or alternatively take some vigorous exercise – this often helps.
- sex masturbation may help ease the pains when they are acute.
SEEK HELP IF
- pain is especially severe and accompanied by other symptoms, such as fainting.
- intercourse between periods is painful.
- you have any cause to suspect a pelvic infection; this is usually accompanied by a vaginal discharge (IUDs or coils increase the risk of infection).

PMT (Premenstrual tension)

Many women experience a range of symptoms such as irritability, bloating, depression, weepiness and painful breasts before a period. These can be eased by self-prescribing, but if they are severe or prolonged you should seek professional help as constitutional treatment can tackle the problem at a deeper level.
DO
- watch your diet premenstrually – cut down on salt, tea, coffee and alcohol and eat more fresh fruit and vegetables as these have a *natural* diuretic effect.
- get plenty of exercise – yoga can be particularly helpful.
- explain your problem to family (and close colleagues).
- keep a note of when your period is due and when possible avoid stressful commitments in the few days beforehand.
- try Vitamin B6 or Evening Primrose Oil for the two weeks leading up to the start of your period.

DON'T
- take diuretics – these can further upset the fluid balance and irritate the kidneys.
- overdose on 'B' vitamins.

Physical injuries – prevention

Many sports injuries can be prevented if you follow the Dos and Don'ts listed below.

DO
- train for sport/exercise under supervision (even jogging and running) to ensure you are doing things correctly and not putting yourself at risk.
- exercise regularly to strengthen muscles and tendons and protect them from sprains and strains, and to maintain suppleness.
- stop when tired. Know your limits and stay within them.
- use the right equipment and wear the right shoes – get advice from an expert.
- warm up gently before an exercise session and wind down afterwards.

DON'T
- jog on hard surfaces as the stress can damage the knee joints and, in women, the reproductive organs as well.

Piles

These are simply varicose veins of the rectum/anus. I have included both internal and external acute remedies to relieve the discomfort of piles, but they are a sign of underlying constitutional weakness, so do seek professional homeopathic help.

Pink eye see Eye inflammation

Post-operative remedies

I have included a few first-aid remedies that will help you to heal well after an operation. These include remedies for bruising, for pain, to speed the healing of scars, to help with shock, for post-operative wind (in the case of abdominal surgery), and so on.

DO
- tell your doctor/consultant that you are taking homeopathic remedies and why.
- accept all the help your hospital offers you but ask yourself whether you really need, for example, painkillers and sleeping pills as well as the other medicines you are given during your visit.

SEEK HELP IF
- you are not healing as well as is expected or have unpleasant side effects from the operation or orthodox medication.

Pregnancy problems

I have included several remedies for the treatment of minor problems in pregnancy, including anaemia, constipation, nausea, varicose veins and indigestion (see the relevant sections in this chapter).

DO
- take commonsense measures to help yourself, including resting as much as you need, sleeping more if you need it, and so on.
- eat healthily, that is, little and often.
- keep up some sort of regular exercise programme throughout your pregnancy as this has been shown to help in all ways. Walking, swimming and yoga are all good ways to exercise without overdoing it.
- seek counselling help for reassurance if you don't have family or friends that you can talk to easily and you are feeling isolated, anxious or fearful in your pregnancy.

DON'T
- 'eat for two', as this can result in an unhealthy weight gain.

SEEK HELP IF
- you are anaemic. There are safe, effective alternatives to the iron pills available from the chemist, which can cause a number of unpleasant side effects including constipation.

Prickly heat

DO
- use the appropriate internal and external remedies.
- avoid exposure to sun, especially in the middle of the day.
- wear light cotton clothing.
- bathe frequently in cool water.

DON'T
- use perfumes, scented soap, oil or bubble bath.

SEEK HELP IF
- the irritation is intolerable.
- there is accompanying weakness and lethargy.

Retention of urine

There are some acute situations where a baby or child finds it difficult to pee and I have included some of these in this book.

DO
- run a tap while trying to pee.
- try to pee in a warm bath.

SEEK HELP IF
- no urine is passed for more than fifteen hours.
- there is fever.
- there is kidney pain (which you will feel as pain in

the lower back, just above the waist on either side of the spine).
- there is nausea, vomiting or headache.

Rheumatism see Joint pain

Rhinitis see Common cold, Hayfever

Scarlet Fever see Childhood illnesses

Sciatica see Backache

Shock

The term 'shock' is used medically to refer to a serious condition in which vital functions are threatened as the result of fluid loss following an injury or during an infection or severe allergic reaction. Symptoms include: weakness; confusion or unconsciousness; shallow, irregular breathing; a weak, rapid pulse; and cold, pale skin. Get help immediately if you suspect your patient has this type of shock.

In this book, however, 'shock' refers to either the emotional response to an accident/injury or the emotional trauma that results from bad news, grief or an upsetting argument.

Sinusitis (see Common cold in Materia Medica)

Inflammation of the sinuses can accompany a common cold or hayfever and I have included several remedies for the treatment of this unpleasant and often painful condition.
DO
- use a humidifier or steam inhalation to relieve congestion.
- drink plenty of liquids.
- avoid tobacco smoke.
DON'T
- use decongestants.
- blow the nose too hard during a cold.
- expose yourself to builders' dust.
SEEK HELP IF
- there is severe pain with a high fever and a smelly discharge from the nose which does not respond to self-prescribing within forty-eight hours (or less if you are in a great deal of pain).

Sore throat

DO
- drink plenty of fluids.

- gargle with a salt or salt-and-*Hypercal* solution (see page 34).
- sip red sage tea to ease discomfort (2 teaspoons dried red sage to a pint of water); or hot lemon and honey – try adding a little grated ginger root.
- boil a kettle or use a plant mist spray to humidify a dry, centrally heated room.
SEEK HELP IF
- there is severe pain with great difficulty swallowing.
- there is excessive saliva (dribbling).
- there is difficulty breathing.

Splinters

DO
- use external remedies to cleanse the area and an internal remedy (*Silica*) to help the body to expel the splinter if necessary.
- use a sterilised needle and tweezers to remove a splinter near the surface of the skin.
- remember that glass splinters are very difficult to detect.
SEEK HELP IF
- a splinter has gone in too far to be removed at home.
- the area around a splinter becomes very red and swollen and there are red streaks going up the limb.

Stiff neck

A stiff neck can be caused by emotional stress, over-exertion or exposure to draughts, and can be helped with home-prescribing.
DO
- rest as much as possible.
- massage the neck and shoulders.
- apply heat or cold to relieve pain.
- seek the help of an osteopath, masseur or physiotherapist.
DON'T
- lift things or further stress the neck.
SEEK HELP IF
- neck pain and stiffness are accompanied by fever and any infection.

Strains/sprains

DO
- use internal and external remedies.
- use an ice pack on the injured joint (crushed ice cubes in a plastic bag wrapped in a thin towel, a hot water bottle filled with crushed ice or a packet of frozen peas).
- compress the joint by pressing the ice pack to the

injured part and wrapping it firmly (not tightly) around.
- use an elastic bandage (available from chemists) as a support to the joint while healing takes place.
- elevate the limb and rest it completely for as long as possible.
- seek the help of a trained physiotherapist, chiropractor or osteopath as soon as possible after the injury.

DON'T
- use the limb for twenty-four hours after the injury or until all the swelling has gone down.
- exercise until the joint/limb has been free of pain for ten days and then take it very gently and slowly at first.

SEEK HELP IF
- the joint seems loose or a funny shape.
- you cannot use the limb or straighten it within a day of the injury.
- a child falls onto an outstretched hand and subsequently has a sore wrist; fractures to the wrist are fairly common and difficult to spot.
- there is severe pain and/or excessive swelling.

Styes

DO
- take the appropriate internal remedy.
- apply a hot compress soaked in *Calendula* or *Hypercal*® solution for ten minutes every two or three hours to encourage the stye to come to a head.

SEEK HELP IF
- vision is affected.
- the swelling is on the inside of the eyelid.
- there is lethargy, fever or headache.
- the stye doesn't respond to treatment within forty-eight hours.

Sunburn/sunstroke

I have included internal and external remedies to treat sunburn, but the best measure is to take sensible precautions to avoid it in the first place. Sunburn can range from slight discomfort, through weakness, headache and nausea, to a very serious condition (sunstroke) which needs urgent professional attention. Keep babies and small children out of a very strong sun – they burn surprisingly easily and don't *need* a tan! If there is a strong breeze or you are in and out of a pool/the sea these precautions are doubly important as you will not *feel* yourself burning until it is too late.

PRECAUTIONS
- Use a suntan cream appropriate for your type of skin.

- Limit your exposure to the sun to thirty minutes on the first day, and increase this by thirty minutes each day until you have built up a protective tan.
- Wear a sunhat and take a shirt to cover up.
- Take care on cloudy days – you will still burn.
- Take extra care where there is reflection from snow or water.
- Don't exercise in unaccustomed heat.

If you *do* get burned, then . . .
DO
- take the appropriate remedy.
- keep the skin cool with cold compresses or cool showers.
- drink a glass of water to which half a teaspoon of salt has been added.
- keep out of the sun until healed.

SEEK HELP IF
- there is a fever of over 104°F/40°C.
- the pulse is very fast.
- the person is confused or unconscious.
- there is a headache, fever or nausea.

Teething

Some children produce teeth without any fuss or discomfort, others can be a nightmare for their entire teething period, suffering great pain and colds, diarrhoea, mood swings and sleeplessness. I have included several remedies for the treatment of these teething monsters. If they fail to have any effect, a professional homeopath can usually help.

DO
- keep teething rings in the fridge so the child has something ice cold to chew on.
- rub a little alcohol into the gums.

DON'T
- resort to giving your child Phenargan or other sedatives.
- give too much chamomile tea to your baby (several bottles every day) as it is very easy for them to prove it (see page 17). If it does help, use only while it has a soothing effect. Do not give chamomile tea if you have prescribed *Chamomilla* in potency.

Tennis elbow

This inflammation can result from any strenuous activity of the elbow, including knitting! Use external remedies to relieve soreness and the appropriate internal remedy to promote healing.

DO
- rest the joint as much as possible.
- use a support bandage.

DON'T
- use the arm until the injury has healed.

SEEK HELP IF
- the problem persists; an X-ray will be needed to check for more serious injury, or you may need physiotherapy or osteopathy.

Thrush
Oral
DO
- give live yoghurt to a child with thrush.
- sterilise dummies.

DON'T
- give sweetened drinks or fruit juice.
- use medicated mouthwash – this can destroy healthy bacteria and further upset the balance in the mouth.

SEEK HELP IF
- pus forms or the infection doesn't respond to home treatment within a few days.

Genital
I have included some remedies for the treatment of acute thrush but if this is a chronic or recurrent problem consult a professional homeopath.

DO
- wash the genitals frequently in water; don't use soap.
- add half a cup of cider vinegar to your bathwater.
- wash underwear in unscented soap or soap flakes (not detergents), and rinse well.
- apply live yoghurt to ease itching and discomfort (you can insert a tampon dipped in yoghurt. Remember to remove it after an hour or so.).
- avoid sweets, sugar and alcohol.

DON'T
- use biological soap powders for your laundry.
- use soap to wash the genital area.
- use bubble bath or oil in your bath water.
- use vaginal deodorants or talcum powder.
- wear tight jeans or nylon underwear, and wear stockings rather than tights.

SEEK HELP IF
- you have frequent attacks.
- pus forms.
- the infection doesn't respond to home treatment.

Tiredness see Exhaustion

Toothache
A few internal and external remedies for the relief of toothache are included but, as always, prevention is better than cure! Good oral hygiene with regular brushing and flossing and a healthy diet will go a long way to ensuring good teeth. Avoid giving children fruit juice (encourage them to eat fruit and drink

plenty of water), especially when given in a bottle at night.

DO
- have regular dental check-ups.
- ask your dentist for composite fillings rather than amalgam fillings, which contain mercury and can cause health problems.
- avoid refined and sweet foods.
- ask your dentist for a nightguard to wear if you grind your teeth at night (and consider whether you are failing to express your anger or confront your worries).

Travel sickness
I have included several remedies for this unpleasant complaint. Once you have found the one that works for you remember to take it before any journey.

DO
- sip a drink (especially if nausea is accompanied by vomiting).
- chew a ginger biscuit or a piece of crystallised ginger.
- sit with your head back and eyes closed and breathe deeply, or lie down if you feel very ill.
- play story tapes to distract children prone to travel sickness.

DON'T
- read on journeys if prone to queasiness.
- have a large meal or alcohol before or during a journey.
- smoke in the car.

Urticaria see Hives

Varicose veins
I have included remedies for the short-term relief of varicose veins, particularly in pregnancy. Constitutional treatment from a professional homeopath will deal with the underlying problem.

DO
- rest and elevate the limbs. Put your feet up when relaxing and raise the end of your bed with bricks to promote the flow of blood up your legs as you sleep.
- take regular exercise – good muscle tone plays a large part in moving blood along the veins. Brisk walking is ideal.
- wear support tights.
- eat a healthy diet to ensure you don't become constipated.

DON'T
- sit with your legs crossed.
- stand or sit for long periods without frequently flexing your muscles.
- become overweight.

Vertigo see Dizziness

Vomiting

DO
- rest.
- take frequent sips of cold water.
- avoid all food for several hours or until vomiting stops.
- avoid dairy produce for a further twenty-four hours *after* the vomiting has stopped.

SEEK HELP IF
- there is incessant vomiting.
- there are signs of dehydration: dry eyes and mouth, sunken eyes, and loose skin.
- the vomit is dark or bloody.
- vomiting follows an abdominal or head injury.
- a child also shows great irritability or lethargy, or screams inconsolably.
- a baby vomits a large quantity with great force (projectile vomiting).
- a baby persistently vomits moderate amounts and is not gaining weight.

Warts/verrucas

Homeopaths view warts with a certain amount of respect and have many ways of treating them with internal remedies, rather than resorting to brutal ways of removing them externally. Homeopaths have noted a connection between the suppression of warts and subsequent chronic illness (see Miasms page 14).

DO
- seek homeopathic help if self-prescribing fails to clear the warts easily.

DON'T
- burn, freeze or cut the warts out.

Weakness see Exhaustion

Whooping cough see Childhood illnesses

Wind see Flatulence

Worms

I have included a remedy (*Cina*) for the relief of complaints resulting from worms. It is essential that you seek professional help if this is a recurring problem in your household/family.

DO
- keep all pets de-wormed effectively and regularly.
- make sure children wash their hands properly after passing a stool.
- keep fingernails short and scrubbed.
- rub *Hypercal*® Ointment around the anus to soothe itching and make it harder for the worms to 'grip'.
- cut out sugar from the diet – worms thrive on sweet things.
- make sure that children wear knickers under pyjamas at night so that they can't scratch their bottoms and then put a 'contaminated' finger in their mouths.

CASE-TAKING QUESTIONNAIRE AND SYMPTOM CHECKLISTS

You can use this questionnaire as a guide or prompt when case-taking. You will need to select symptoms from each category where possible in order to construct your symptom picture.

1. **Name** _____

2. **Date** _____

3. **Date of birth** _____

4. **Complaint (its label). My . . . (headache, cough, etc.)**
   How long have you had it?
   How did it start?
   What do you think caused it?
   Have you had this before? When? How often?
   Have you taken medical advice?
   What medicines have you taken?

5. **Related symptoms. My (complaint) is . . .**
   Tell me about your (complaint).
   What affects it, makes it better or worse?
   Can you describe the pain?
   Where is it exactly?

6. **Other physical symptoms**
   HEAD: Is it sensitive to touch? Are you dizzy, worse or better for standing, walking, sitting? Hair: greasy, lifeless, dull, falling out, etc.?
   EYES: Appearance – staring, twitching, bloodshot. Pupils dilated or contracted? Sensitive to light?
   EARS: Hearing, including noises.
   NOSE: Cold sores. Cracks. Sense of smell.
   FACE: Appearance. Expression.
   MOUTH: Taste. Excess saliva/dryness. Smell of breath. Grinding of teeth. Cold sores. Teething. Ulcers. Gums.
   TONGUE: Colour/coating. Indented on edges. Cracks.
   THROAT: If throat is sore, does swallowing liquids, food, nothing, help or make worse?
   STOMACH (above navel): Appetite. Thirst. Vomiting/burping. Knot/lump felt in stomach.
   ABDOMEN (below navel): Bloated. Sensitive to touch/clothes.
   BOWELS: Constipation. Diarrhoea. Colour/consistency of stools. Piles. Wind. Worms.
   URINATION: Frequency. Difficulty. Colour, smell. Pain.
   NECK: Glands: swollen, painful. Sensitive to touch/clothes.
   BACK: Stiffness? Pain?
   LIMBS: Trembling. Twitching. Jerking. Cramps.
   SLEEP: Can you get to sleep, stay asleep, wake feeling refreshed? If not, what times do you wake? What position do you sleep in? Are you restless? Do you grind your teeth?
   DREAMS: Recurring dreams? Nightmares?

7. **General symptoms I am . . . (hot, cold, thirsty, etc.)**
   GENERALLY: Do you feel hot or cold? Does heat or cold help, either generally or when applied directly to the affected area?

Do you want fresh air? Do you feel generally better or worse for it? Is your symptom affected by it?

Are you affected by the position you are in? Are you better or worse for lying, sitting or standing?

Are you restless? Are you better or worse for moving about?

Are you better or worse at any time of day or night?

Does uncovering, touch, food, drink, sympathy, etc., affect you for better or worse?

PAINS: Do they change place? Describe them: stitching; shooting; pressing; sore, bruised; cramping; burning; throbbing, etc.

DISCHARGES: Describe them: thick; watery; sticky; ropy; burning; white; yellow; bloody, etc.

SIDE: Is your symptom one-sided? Which side? Did it start on that side?

PERSPIRATION: Smell, quantity, temperature. Is there more during the day or the night? Look for a fever without sweating.

ENERGY: At what time of day do you feel at your worst, generally?

8. Emotional/mental symptoms. I feel . . . (sad, irritable, etc.)

MOOD/BEHAVIOUR: Depressed, weepy, irritable, angry, anxious, fearful, excitable, despair, affectionate, whiny, etc.

MENTAL: Dull, confused, unable to concentrate, over-active mind. Is the memory affected?

9. Causes (or stress symptoms). It was caused by . . . (getting chilled, being very angry, unable to sleep, etc.)

What was happening in your life before you fell ill? It is important to discover what stresses pre-date the illness; these can be very useful guiding symptoms.

General symptom checklist for babies and infants

Babies cannot describe what they are feeling so you need to be specially observant to find the symptoms that will lead you to a successful prescription. Remem-ber, you are looking for any changes from their normal patterns of behaviour or health. It is a good idea to be observant of your children when they are healthy so that their changes are clear to you. You need to do lots of looking and feeling and smelling with babies as well as using your intuition in order to get a sense of how ill this baby really is. See pages 203–26 for when to seek expert advice; if you are at all unsure then do not delay in getting help and reassurance at the earliest moment. I have put together the following checklist with babies especially in mind.

Appearance: How does she look? Pale, flushed, puffy, pasty. (Skin colour, tone and texture are very important.)

Eyes: Bright and sparkly or dull? Pupils dilated or contracted.

Perspiration: Where is it? How does it feel and smell?

Sleep: What position? Restless? Crying in sleep? Nightmares?

Mood: Wanting to be carried, irritable, quiet, whiny, clingy, happy, angry on waking, fears (noise, dark or dogs, etc.)

Discharges: Catarrh. Vomit. Stools. What colour are they and if they smell can you describe it?

Energy: Any variation in energy level is an important symptom.

Side: Is the symptom one-sided? Which side? Did it stay there?

Stress: What set the complaint off? Family rows, weaning, moving house, teething, etc.

Moon: This can affect some children – some babies are sleepless at the time of the full moon.

Time of year: Winter coughs or summer colds, etc.

Fever: Temperature and reaction to it.

Heat/cold: Reaction to weather, fresh air, hot or cold baths, and so on.

At this point you can go back to the beginning of the case and see whether there is any specific information you need. You may have to check through and come back with your questions later. For example, your teenager has a sore throat that is worse for swallowing. You realise that you don't know whether she is having difficulty swallowing liquids and whether hot or cold drinks help. You may at this point ask some more specific questions. Gauge how strongly marked they are by the response you get. An unequivocal yes or no counts, a maybe or a sometimes doesn't. Finish by asking if there is anything else going on, just to check you haven't missed anything important.

Stress symptoms

All disease is caused by stress. Stress can be physical, emotional or mental. Different people are sensitive to different stresses – some to cold, some to heat, some to being told off, some to mental strain, and so on. The diseases people develop will also vary according to their own particular weaknesses. Our *patterns* of responding to stress, and of falling ill, will depend on the levels of stress and vitality, and on how weak the immune system has become as a result. Understanding and treating the cause is fundamental to homeopathic practice. It can eventually help us to identify the individual stresses that we know weaken us, so that we can avoid them or take action before we actually fall ill.

In this book I have included stresses in some of the complaints (where they are referred to as 'causes'). For example, some children (and adults) are sensitive to falls, if they bang their heads they suffer from headaches, and sometimes irritability or depression as a result. Under 'HEADACHE, Causes, head injury', you will find *Natrum sulphuricum* listed. It is vital to

build this symptom into your picture if it is strongly indicated. *Argentum nitricum* has diarrhoea caused by anticipatory anxiety. Once you know your patient you don't necessarily need to wait for symptoms to prescribe. If you have a child who is very sensitive to bangs on the head and *Natrum sulphuricum* has cured dramatically in the past then give it automatically (after *Arnica* has dealt with the bruising) to prevent the second stage of headaches developing. Give *Argentum nitricum* to a child who is studying for an important exam and who is beginning to get extremely anxious. If it has worked well in the past you don't have to wait for the sleeplessness and diarrhoea to develop.

If your prescription does not work then it is possible that you have missed the *real* cause or stress. Homeopaths are medical sleuths at heart and will delve relentlessly until they uncover what it was that actually weakened the individual, causing them to become ill.

1 REPERTORISING CHART

Name: _____ Date:

Symptoms:

Symptoms	ACO.	AGAR.	ALL-C.	ANT-C.	ANT-T.	AP.	ARG-N.	ARN.	ARS.	BAPT.	BAR-C.	BELL.	BELL-P.	BOR.	BRY.	CALC-C.	CALC-F.	CALC-P.	CALC-S.	CALEN.	CANTH.	CARB-A.	CARB-V.	CAUL.	CAUST.	CHAM.	CHIN.	CIMI.	CINA.	COCC.	COCC-C.	COFF.	COLCH.	COLOC.	CON.	CUPR.	DIOS.	DROS.	DULC.	EUP-P.	EUPHR.	FERR-M.	GELS.	GLON.	HAM.	HEP-S.	HYP.	IGN.
1.																																																
2.																																																
3.																																																
4.																																																
5.																																																
6.																																																
7.																																																
8.																																																
9.																																																
10.																																																
11.																																																
12.																																																

Symptoms	IP.	JAB.	KALI-B.	KALI-C.	KALI-M.	KALI-P.	KALI-S.	LACH.	LED.	LYC.	MAG-C.	MAG-M.	MAG-P.	MERC-C.	MERC-S.	NAT-C.	NAT-M.	NAT-P.	NAT-S.	NIT-AC.	NUX-V.	OP.	PETR.	PHO-AC.	PHOS.	PHYT.	PODO.	PULS.	PYR.	RHE.	RHOD.	RHUS-T.	RUMEX.	RUTA.	SARS.	SEP.	SIL.	SPO.	STAP.	SUL.	SUL-AC.	SYMPH.	TAB.	THU.	URT-U.	VERAT.	ZINC.
1.																																															
2.																																															
3.																																															
4.																																															
5.																																															
6.																																															
7.																																															
8.																																															
9.																																															
10.																																															
11.																																															
12.																																															

NB PHOTOCOPY THIS CHART SO THAT YOU HAVE A STOCK FOR WHENEVER YOU NEED ONE.

SAMPLE CASES

The following twelve cases will help to bring the process of first-aid prescribing to life for you. Keep in mind the five important steps you need to be familiar with in order to prescribe successfully:

1 **Check your complaint is within the scope of this book** (see pages 203–26).
2 **Take the case**, choose your symptoms and enter them on the repertorising chart (see page 230).
3 **Differentiate** between remedies, if more than one is indicated, by reading through the remedy pictures in the Materia Medica (see page 22).
4 **Prescribe** (see Chapter 5).
5 **Check the detailed list of complaints covered by this book** (pages 203–26) for additional helpful measures and advice.

Case 1
An accident/head injury

Your seven-year old daughter goes over the handlebars of her bicycle, falling on her head and grazing the side of it badly on the tarmac. She is temporarily concussed. A bottle of lemonade she was carrying has smashed and cut her hand. She comes around confused and distressed, and tries to get up and go home saying that she feels OK. She is delivered home by a kindly passer-by who tells you what has happened.

The first prescription must be for **Shock, Head injury** and **Bruising**. In the repertory you will find that *Arnica* is the only remedy that is listed for all three of these symptoms. *Arnica* is also the remedy for delayed shock, when the injured person maintains that everything is fine, when it isn't. Prescribe *Arnica* according to the urgency of the situation (see the Dosage Chart, page 27).

Next you should attend to her wounds. Check the External Repertory to see which lotion to use to bathe her cuts. It is essential to remove all the glass from her hand.

Consult the list of complaints on pages 203–26 for the other measures you need to take. You may need to visit your local hospital for a head X-ray or to have the glass removed if it is deeply embedded.

If, after the *Arnica* has helped with the shock and bruising there is severe pain in the cut hand, especially with shooting pains up the arm, then turn to the Repertory to find which remedy will help heal **Injuries** to nerves with **Pains**, shooting.

If inflammation (redness) develops around the cuts in the hand and you suspect that some bits of dirt or glass may remain then look to **Injuries**, Cuts, inflamed, and **Splinters** in the Repertory and read up the remedies listed.

Deal with one thing at a time: give one remedy at a time. You may then change to another remedy as soon as it is needed. If, for example, the bump on her head goes down after two doses of *Arnica* but the pain in her hand is very bad then prescribe for that (and the remedy you will probably need to give is *Hypericum* – see Repertory) even if it is only a few hours after her last dose of *Arnica*. Repeat this remedy until the pains abate. You may then need to go back to *Arnica* if the bruise starts to swell again. You can alternate remedies if this is called for.

Case 2
An accident/sprain

Your elderly aunt trips over uneven paving and sprains her ankle. She is helped home and prescribed bed rest by her doctor who also bandages her badly swollen ankle. By the time you see her she is taking it well and joking about her fall.

Though she doesn't appear distressed, you suspect she is suffering from delayed shock, so you note this as a potentially useful symptom. Then you turn to

Sprains, First Stage, with swelling in the Repertory and you will find *Arnica* listed. Prescribe the remedy according to the urgency of the situation (see the Dosage Chart page 27); in this case it will be every two hours, as this is a fairly serious injury. *Arnica* will bring down the swelling and will also deal with the shock.

Now turn to the External Repertory and Materia Medica to see what to put *on* the ankle, to treat the swelling and bruising. You will see that *Arnica* is indicated for bruises on unbroken skin. In fact, the doctor has bandaged the ankle firmly and ordered her not to move it, so make up a strong solution of *Arnica* tincture and soak the bandage from the outside, instructing Mary to keep it damp for at least 24 hours. This external application of *Arnica* plus the internal remedy will minimise the bruising and reduce the swelling very quickly.

You will need to continue prescribing for the sprain itself, both internally and externally, for as long as necessary, as it can take several weeks for a sprain to heal in an elderly person.

Had your aunt *fractured* her ankle, *Arnica* would still have been your first step, until the swelling had gone down. An elderly person will usually need a remedy to help to mend a fracture (these remedies are *Calcarea carbonica*, *Calcarea phosphorica* and *Silica*); they can be prescribed in low potency (6X or 6C) for up to a week at a time to assist what can be a very slow process.

Case 3
Exam nerves

Your sixteen-year-old son is taking exams in two weeks and is extremely anxious. He has been working very hard all year and is in a state of panic. He says that the more he works the less he knows. His brain won't retain information and he is exhausted. He has started having diarrhoea, due in part perhaps to all the sweets he has been eating (he has even been raiding the sugar bowl). He is also getting some indigestion after eating (he bolts his food) and this is better for burping. He paces about his room and has the windows wide open, despite the cold weather. His biggest complaint about school is the central heating: 'How am I supposed to learn anything in this heat?' he says. He feels driven but is sure he is going to fail. He was in a similar panic when he acted in the school play the year previously and had a lot of lines to learn.

You choose the following symptoms:
1 Exam nerves (Emotional/mental)
2 Anticipatory anxiety (Emotional/mental)
3 Panic (Emotional/mental)
4 Hurried (Emotional/mental)
5 Forgetful (Emotional/mental)
6 Exhaustion (Physical complaint)

7 Diarrhoea (Physical complaint)
8   caused by anxiety (Related symptom)
9 Indigestion (Physical complaint)
10   better for burping (Related symptom)
11 Likes sweet things (General)
12 Craves sugar (General)
13 Worse for heat (General)
14 Better for fresh air (General)

Argentum nitricum is listed under every symptom. There are no other remedies that have many or most of the symptoms. *Lycopodium* is the closest.

Turn to *Argentum nitricum* in the Materia Medica and read through the remedy picture. You will find that it corresponds accurately to his problems; the picture 'fits' well.

Prescribe according to the guidelines in Chapter 5.

Case 4
Cough/cold

Your three-year-old has a cough and cold. It started four days ago. The day previously, she had been caught in the rain and got drenched. Her nose started running that evening and she coughed in the night. In the morning she was very pale and pathetic and didn't want anything to eat or drink. She just wanted to sit on your lap and be cuddled. She has been like this ever since. She won't let you do anything and has regressed emotionally, wanting to be carried around. She is very weepy over little things. She isn't thirsty and is very listless. Her nose is running with lots of thick, yellow catarrh. Her cough is loose in the mornings but dry at night. It gets worse when she lies down at night and wakes her during the night, when she has to sit up to cough. The cough is worse if her room gets over-heated; she likes the window open. Oddly enough, when you had to take her out yesterday to do some shopping she was a bit better. She has no fever and isn't sweaty but she feels hot and complains of being either too hot or too cold.

You choose the following symptoms:
1 Common cold (Physical complaint)
2   with thick, yellow catarrh (Related symptom)
3 Cough (Physical complaint)
4   loose mornings (Related symptom)
5   dry at night (Related symptom)
6   worse lying down (Related symptom)
7 Whines (Emotional/mental)
8 Tearful (Emotional/mental)
9 Wants to be carried (Emotional/mental)
10 Thirstless (General)
11 Better for fresh air (General)
12 Worse for heat (General)
13 Complaints from getting wet (Stress)

1 REPERTORISING CHART

Name: __CASE 3 – EXAM NERVES (p.232)__   Date:

Symptoms:

Remedy column headers (left block): ACO. AGAR. ALL-C. ANT-C. ANT-T. AP. ARG-N. ARN. ARS. BAPT. BAR-C. BELL. BELL-P. BOR. BRY. CALC-C. CALC-F. CALC-P. CALC-S. CALEN. CANTH. CARB-A. CARB-V. CAUL. CAUST. CHAM. CHIN. CIMI. CINA. COCC. COCC-C. COFF. COLCH. COLOC. CON. CUPR. DIOS. DROS. DULC. EUP-P. EUPHR. FERR-M. GELS. GLON. HAM. HEP-S. HYP. IGN.

	1. EXAM NERVES	2. ANTICIPATORY ANXIETY	3. PANIC	4. HURRIED	5. FORGETFUL	6. EXHAUSTION	7. DIARRHOEA	8. – CAUSED BY ANXIETY	9. INDIGESTION	10. – BETTER FOR BURPING	11. LIKES SWEET THINGS	12. LIKES SUGAR	13. WORSE FOR HEAT	14. BETTER FOR FRESH AIR

Remedy column headers (right block): IP. JAB. KALI-B. KALI-C. KALI-M. KALI-P. KALI-S. LACH. LED. LYC. MAG-C. MAG-M. MAG-P. MERC-C. MERC-S. NAT-C. NAT-M. NAT-P. NAT-S. NIT-AC. NUX-V. OP. PETR. PHO-AC. PHOS. PHYT. PODO. PULS. PYR. RHE. RHOD. RHUS-T. RUMEX. RUTA. SARS. SEP. SIL. SPO. STAP. SUL. SUL-AC. SYMPH. TAB. THU. URT-U. VERAT. ZINC.

	1. EXAM NERVES	2. ANTICIPATORY ANXIETY	3. PANIC	4. HURRIED	5. FORGETFUL	6. EXHAUSTION	7. DIARRHOEA	8. – CAUSED BY ANXIETY	9. INDIGESTION	10. – BETTER FOR BURPING	11. LIKES SWEET THINGS	12. LIKES SUGAR

Name: CASE 4 – COUGH/COLD   Date:

Symptoms:

Block 1 remedies (left to right): ACO., AGAR., ALL-C., ANT-C., ANT-T., AP., ARG-N., ARN., ARS., BAPT., BAR-C., BELL., BELL-P., BOR., BRY., CALC-C., CALC-F., CALC-P., CALC-S., CALEN., CANTH., CARB-A., CARB-V., CAUL., CAUST., CHAM., CHIN., CIMI., CINA., COCC., COCC-C., COFF., COLCH., COLOC., CON., CUPR., DIOS., DROS., DULC., EUP-P., EUPHR., FERR-M., GELS., GLON., HAM., HEP-S., HYP., IGN.

Symptom	(checks)
1. COMMON COLD	ACO., ALL-C., ARS., BELL., BRY., CALC-C., CALC-F., CALC-S., CARB-V., EUPHR., HEP-S., IGN.
2. – WITH THICK (YELLOW) CATARRH	ALL-C., ANT-C., CALC-C., CALC-S., DULC., HEP-S., IGN.
3. COUGH	ACO., ANT-T., ARN., ARS., BELL., BRY., CALC-S., CHAM., CINA., CON., CUPR., DROS., DULC., EUPHR., FERR-M., HEP-S., IGN.
4. – LOOSE MORNINGS	ANT-T., ARS., CALC-C., CHAM., DROS., HEP-S.
5. – DRY AT NIGHT	AP., ARS., BELL., CAUST., CHAM., CON., DROS.
6. – WORSE LYING DOWN	AP., ARS.
7. WHINES	
8. TEARFUL	
9. WANTS TO BE CARRIED	ANT-T., CHAM.
10. THIRSTLESS	COLCH., GELS., RUMEX.
11. BETTER FOR FRESH AIR	IP.
12. WORSE FOR HEAT	CARB-V., PETR.

Block 2 remedies (left to right): IP., JAB., KALI-B., KALI-C., KALI-M., KALI-P., KALI-S., LACH., LED., LYC., MAG-C., MAG-M., MAG-P., MERC-C., MERC-S., NAT-C., NAT-M., NAT-P., NAT-S., NIT-AC., NUX-V., OP., PETR., PHO-AC., PHOS., PHYT., PODO., PULS., PYR., RHE., RHOD., RHUS-T., RUMEX., RUTA., SARS., SEP., SIL., SPO., STAP., SUL., SUL-AC., SYMPH., TAB., THU., URT-U., VERAT., ZINC.

Symptom	(checks)
1. COMMON COLD	IP., KALI-B., KALI-C., KALI-M., KALI-S., LACH., LYC., MAG-M., MERC-S., NAT-C., NAT-M., PHOS., PULS., SEP., SIL., SUL.
2. – WITH THICK (YELLOW) CATARRH	KALI-B., KALI-C., KALI-S., LACH., MERC-C., MERC-S., NAT-C., PHOS., PULS., SEP., SIL., STAP., SUL.
3. COUGH	KALI-B., KALI-C., KALI-P., LACH., PULS., SIL., SPO., STAP.
4. – LOOSE MORNINGS	PULS.
5. – DRY AT NIGHT	PULS., RHUS-T., SPO.
6. – WORSE LYING DOWN	KALI-B., PULS., RHUS-T., SPO., SUL-AC.
7. WHINES	PULS.
8. TEARFUL	PULS.
9. WANTS TO BE CARRIED	PULS.
10. THIRSTLESS	PULS.
11. BETTER FOR FRESH AIR	KALI-S., LED., PHO-AC., PULS., RHOD., SEP., THU.
12. WORSE FOR HEAT	KALI-S., LED., LYC., PULS., SEP., SUL., SUL-AC., VERAT.

On repertorising you will find that *Pulsatilla* is indicated under each symptom, and that there are no other remedies strongly indicated. You can give the indicated remedy knowing that it will help. In the unlikely event of it not working you will need to retake the case in order to check that you've taken the symptoms correctly.

Case 5a
Measles not needing treatment

After an incubation period of ten days Christopher gets mild cold symptoms, which soon develop into measles. The classic symptoms are there: he has a fever of 103°F/39.4°C in the acute phase, and an itchy rash. He is miserable but drinks a lot and sleeps most of the time. When awake he wants attention and lots of cuddles and is reasonably happy. This phase lasts for three to four days and he then convalesces with no complications.

No treatment is necessary as Christopher is coping well with the illness. He will almost certainly be stronger and healthier generally as a result of coping with the illness without interference.

Case 5b
Measles needing treatment

Christopher's friend David is also suspected of incubating measles at the same time, and he has some symptoms but not the itchy rash. A glance inside his mouth reveals Koplik's spots, a gritty rash on the inside of the cheek, which confirms that he does have measles. David, however, throws a higher fever (104°F/40°C) and is delirious with it. He feels burning hot to the touch. The rash doesn't appear and he becomes very distressed and doesn't want to eat or drink. A right-sided earache and a dry cough develop. He is very restless and irritable. Homeopathic treatment is appropriate in this case to ease the pain, to bring out the rash and to help him through the acute phase so that he won't develop complications.

You choose the following symptoms:
1 Measles (Physical complaint)
2   rash slow to come out (Related symptom)
3 Earache (Physical complaint)
4   worse right side (Related symptom)
5 Cough (Physical complaint)
6   dry (Related symptom)
7 Fever (Physical complaint)
8   burning (Related symptom)
9 Thirstless (General)
10 Delirium (Emotional/mental)
11 Restless (Emotional/mental)
12 Irritable (Emotional/mental)

This is a fairly typical case in which several remedies have many or most of the symptoms in their pictures. *Apis*, *Belladonna*, *Bryonia*, *Pulsatilla* and *Sulphur* are all partially indicated. Differentiating between these remedies is what enables you to find the correct remedy. If several remedies are strongly indicated, your symptoms are probably all too general and you need to look at the case again for less common symptoms.

In this case *Apis*, *Bryonia* and *Sulphur* all have measles with a rash that is slow to come out but only *Apis* is generally thirstless. As this is the only general symptom in this case and because of the high fever and the danger of dehydration it must be a strong guiding symptom for the remedy. We can also eliminate *Bryonia* because of the restlessness – a *Bryonia* patient lies still, like a log. We can eliminate *Bryonia* and *Sulphur* because both these patients are markedly thirsty.

Apis is restless *and* irritable – it has two of the three emotional symptoms. If you look up **Symptoms**, Right-sided, you will find *Apis* and *Pulsatilla* listed, but we can eliminate *Pulsatilla* because it doesn't have the rash that is slow to develop and our patient isn't clingy and weepy.

That leaves *Apis* and *Belladonna*. You read up both these pictures to differentiate between them and decide that *Apis* fits slightly better because David's face and eyes look puffy and he is weepy as well as irritable. You give the remedy frequently (every 2 hours) to determine whether it is correct and if there is no response after six doses change to *Belladonna*.

You may also need to change the remedy if the symptom picture changes; *Apis* or *Belladonna* are needed during the stage of the high fever with delirium and the earache, but then a *Pulsatilla* picture may emerge as the cough becomes more predominant. Remember to prescribe on the whole picture at any one time.

Case 6a
Flu not needing treatment

A thirty-five-year-old dynamic businesswoman starts to develop flu symptoms, with aching, weakness and exhaustion. She has been working extremely hard without a holiday for two years and has not been ill during this period. Her symptoms are unpleasant but not severe. She agrees (reluctantly!) to rest in bed for a few days and then to take a week's holiday to recover fully and to recharge her exhausted body. She is going to eat especially well during her convalescence, and then ease her way back into work gradually.

She does not need homeopathic treatment. It may be necessary to review the situation, however, if she gets stuck, either in the acute phase, for example with a painful, sleep-preventing cough, or in the

1 REPERTORISING CHART

Name: CASE 56 – MEASLES   Date:

Symptoms:

Remedy set A

Columns (left to right): ACO., AGAR., ALL-C., ANT-C., ANT-T., AP., ARG-N., ARN., ARS., BAPT., BAR-C., BELL., BELL-P., BOR., BRY., CALC-C., CALC-F., CALC-P., CALC-S., CALEN., CANTH., CARB-A., CARB-V., CAUL., CAUST., CHAM., CHIN., CIMI., CINA., COCC., COCC-C., COFF., COLCH., COLOC., CON., CUPR., DIOS., DROS., DULC., EUP-P., EUPHR., FERR-M., GELS., GLON., HAM., HEP-S., HYP., IGN.

#	Symptom	Remedies marked
1.	MEASLES	ACO., AP., BELL., BRY., EUPHR., GELS.
2.	– RASH SLOW TO COME OUT	ANT-T., AP., BRY.
3.	EARACHE	ACO., ALL-C., BELL., CALC-S., CHAM., HEP-S.
4.	– WORSE RIGHT SIDE	BELL.
5.	COUGH	ACO., ANT-T., BELL., BRY., CALC-C., CALC-S., CARB-V., CAUST., CHAM., CINA., COCC-C., CON., CUPR., DROS., FERR-M., HEP-S., IGN.
6.	– DRY	ACO., ANT-C., BELL., BRY., CALC-C., CHAM., CON., DROS., FERR-M., HEP-S., IGN.
7.	FEVER	ACO., ARS., BELL., BRY., CHAM., CINA., GELS., IGN.
8.	– BURNING	ACO., AP., BELL., BRY., COLCH., GELS.
9.	THIRSTLESS	ANT-C., AP., BELL., CHAM.
10.	DELERIUM	AP., ARS., BELL.
11.	RESTLESS	ARN., ARS., BAPT., BELL., CIMI., CINA., CUPR., FERR-M., HEP-S., PYR. (in set B)
12.	IRRITABLE	ANT-C., BELL.

Remedy set B

Columns (left to right): IP., JAB., KALI-B., KALI-C., KALI-M., KALI-P., KALI-S., LACH., LED., LYC., MAG-C., MAG-M., MAG-P., MERC-C., MERC-S., NAT-C., NAT-F., NAT-M., NAT-P., NAT-S., NIT-AC., NUX-V., OP., PETR., PHO-AC., PHOS., PHYT., PODO., PULS., PYR., RHE., RHOD., RHUS-T., RUMEX., RUTA., SARS., SEP., SIL., SPO., STAP., SUL., SUL-AC., TAB., THU., URT-U., VERAT., ZINC.

#	Symptom	Remedies marked
1.	MEASLES	IP., PULS., SUL.
2.	– RASH SLOW TO COME OUT	
3.	EARACHE	KALI-B., MAG-P., PULS., VERAT.
4.	– WORSE RIGHT SIDE	LYC., PHO-AC.
5.	COUGH	IP., KALI-B., KALI-M., LACH., NAT-M., OP., PHOS., PHYT., PULS., RHUS-T., SIL., STAP., SUL.
6.	– DRY	IP., KALI-M., LACH., NAT-M., OP., PHOS., PULS., RHUS-T., SIL., STAP., SUL.
7.	FEVER	KALI-C., LYC., NAT-M., OP., PHOS., PULS., SIL., SUL.
8.	– BURNING	OP., PHOS., PYR., SUL.
9.	THIRSTLESS	KALI-B., KALI-M., LYC., NIT-AC., PULS., SEP.
10.	DELERIUM	NAT-C., OP., PYR.
11.	RESTLESS	KALI-C., MERC-S., PULS., RUTA., SIL.
12.	IRRITABLE	KALI-C., LYC., MAG-M., MERC-S., NAT-M., SEP., SIL., STAP., SUL., VERAT., ZINC.

convalescent stage if her energy doesn't start to return once the acute symptoms of the flu have disappeared.

Case 6b
Flu with treatment

Your patient, a thirty-five-year-old single parent of two children, aged three and one, goes down suddenly with a severe bout of flu. She has no one to help her with the children, although a friend offers to shop for her. She feels so exhausted that she can hardly sit up. Every bone in her body aches, she has a fever and is depressed and weepy. She feels generally worse for getting cold.

Homeopathic treatment in this case is appropriate, because of the severity of the symptoms, and also because of the patient's situation. She is not able to take two weeks off.

You choose the following symptoms:
1 Flu (Physical complaint)
2   pains in bones (Related symptom)
3 Exhaustion (Physical complaint)
4   worse for exertion (Related symptom)
5 Fever (Physical complaint)
6 Depressed (Emotional/mental)
7 Tearful (Emotional/mental)
8 Worse for cold (General)

On repertorising, you find that *Rhus toxicodendron* is the only remedy that has each of the symptoms you have chosen, but when you read through the picture in the Materia Medica it doesn't quite fit. The patient isn't restless.

You go back and question her some more, and find that she is also very thirsty for cold drinks, in spite of feeling worse for getting cold. She is also lying in bed shivering and shaking and moaning with the pains.

You add the following symptoms:
9 Thirsty (General)
10 Likes cold drinks (General)
11 Flu with shivering (Physical complaint)

Eupatorium perfoliatum has a total of seven out of ten of the symptoms and on reading it through you are struck by the similarity. You ask her then if she has a headache (she has) and whether she is sweating (she isn't much) and this confirms your prescription.

Case 7
Insomnia

A friend asks for help with his insomnia. He says it hasn't been going on for very long and that he thinks it is a result of the lifestyle he has been leading, and he doesn't normally suffer from it; he's been overdoing it,

working hard, eating too much rich food, drinking coffee and alcohol in large quantities because of business lunches and dinners, and not getting enough sleep. His work commitments have been putting him under increased mental strain and he's noticed himself becoming more irritable, snapping at his secretary and even at friends. When he goes to bed he falls asleep without much difficulty, but wakes in the early hours (around 2 or 3 a.m.) feeling anxious, especially about a big contract he's working on, and he doesn't get back to sleep until shortly before the alarm goes off. He feels dreadful on waking and has to drink lots of coffee to get going.

You choose the following symptoms:
1 Insomnia (Physical complaint)
2   after 3 a.m. (Related symptom)
3   caused by mental strain (Related symptom)
4   caused by overwork (Related symptom)
5 Irritable (Emotional/mental)

In this case you have a few strong symptoms and you won't need to use the chart to repertorise; by simply looking up each symptom you will see at a glance that *Nux vomica* is listed in each symptom. On reading the picture you will recognise immediately the similarity of both the mental picture and the physical complaint. You know that he is sensitive to the cold, and that clinches it.

You give him the remedy *and* strict instructions to have a few early nights, and to stop drinking alcohol and coffee for a few days to give his liver and his nervous system a rest.

Case 8
Teething

Your baby is eight months old and is teething. A friend of yours has recommended the homeopathic 'teething granules', but you know better than to make a routine hit-or-miss prescription (!) and when you tried them once in the middle of the night in desperation they had no effect whatsoever.

He is usually a contented, easy-going baby but he has been more fractious of late and has been waking at night, when before he had been sleeping straight fhrough. Unlike his friends of the same age, he doesn't yet have any teeth. (His father was the same as a baby, with no teeth until! he was nearly a year old.) You feel desperate at the thought of endless broken nights ahead. When you go to him at night all he wants is a drink and a cuddle and he goes down quite easily. However, you notice that his head is unusually sweaty and that he smells sour.

His bowels have been upset for the past three weeks, with diarrhoea that smells sour and contains undigested food. He has also been more prone to

1 REPERTORISING CHART

Name: CASE 66 - FLU   Date:

Symptoms:

Remedy columns (left block): ACO, AGAR, ALL-C, ANT-C, ANT-T, AP, ARG-N, ARN, ARS, BAPT, BAR-C, BELL, BELL-P, BOR, BRY, CALC-C, CALC-F, CALC-P, CALC-S, CALEN, CANTH, CARB-A, CARB-V, CAUL, CAUST, CHAM, CHIN, CIMI, CINA, COCC, COCC-C, COFF, COLCH, COLOC, CON, CUPR, DIOS, DROS, DULC, EUP-P, EUPHR, FERR-M, GELS, GLON, HAM, HEP-S, HYP, IGN

Remedy columns (right block): IP, IAB, KALI-B, KALI-C, KALI-M, KALI-P, KALI-S, LACH, LED, LYC, MAG-C, MAG-M, MAG-P, MERC-C, MERC-S, NAT-C, NAT-M, NAT-P, NAT-S, NIT-AC, NUX-V, OP, PETR, PHO-AC, PHOS, PHYT, PODO, PULS, PYR, RHE, RHOD, RHUS-T, RUMEX, RUTA, SARS, SEP, SIL, SPO, STAP, SUL, SUL-AC, SYMPH, TAB, THU, URT-U, VERAT, ZINC

#	Symptom
1.	FLU
2.	- PAINS IN BONES
3.	- EXHAUSTION
4.	- WORSE FOR EXERTION
5.	FEVER
6.	DEPRESSED
7.	TEARFUL
8.	WORSE FOR COLD
9.	THIRSTY
10.	LIKES COLD DRINKS
11.	FLU - WITH SHIVERING
12.	

1 **REPERTORISING CHART** Name: CASE 7 - INSOMNIA Date:

Symptoms:

Symptoms	ACO.	AGAR.	ALL-C.	ANT-C.	ANT-T.	AP.	ARG-N.	ARN.	ARS.	BAPT.	BAR-C.	BELL.
1. INSOMNIA	✓								✓			✓
2. - AFTER 3 am.												
3. - CAUSED BY MENTAL STRAIN												
4. - " " OVERWORK												
5. IRRITABLE					✓	✓			✓			
6.												
7.												
8.												
9.												
10.												
11.												
12.												

Symptoms	BELL-P.	BOR.	BRY.	CALC-C.	CALC-F.	CALC-P.	CALC-S.	CALEN.	CANTH.	CARB-A.	CARB-V.	CAUL.
1. INSOMNIA	✓			✓		✓						
2. - AFTER 3 am.	✓											
3. - CAUSED BY MENTAL STRAIN												
4. - " " OVERWORK												
5. IRRITABLE			✓								✓	
6.												
7.												
8.												
9.												
10.												
11.												
12.												

Symptoms	CAUST.	CHAM.	CHIN.	CIMI.	CINA.	COCC.	COCC-C.	COFF.	COLCH.	COLOC.	CON.	CUPR.
1. INSOMNIA		✓				✓		✓			✓	
2. - AFTER 3 am.												
3. - CAUSED BY MENTAL STRAIN												
4. - " " OVERWORK												
5. IRRITABLE	✓	✓			✓							
6.												
7.												
8.												
9.												
10.												
11.												
12.												

Symptoms	DIOS.	DROS.	DULC.	EUP-P.	EUPHR.	FERR-M.	GELS.	GLON.	HAM.	HEP-S.	HYP.	IGN.
1. INSOMNIA												
2. - AFTER 3 am.												
3. - CAUSED BY MENTAL STRAIN												
4. - " " OVERWORK												
5. IRRITABLE						✓				✓		
6.												
7.												
8.												
9.												
10.												
11.												
12.												

Symptoms	IP.	JAB.	KALI-B.	KALI-C.	KALI-M.	KALI-P.	KALI-S.	LACH.	LED.	LYC.	MAG-C.	MAG-M.
1. INSOMNIA				✓		✓					✓	✓
2. - AFTER 3 am.											✓	
3. - CAUSED BY MENTAL STRAIN						✓						
4. - " " OVERWORK												
5. IRRITABLE				✓						✓	✓	
6.												
7.												
8.												
9.												
10.												
11.												
12.												

Symptoms	MAG-P.	MERC-C.	MERC-S.	NAT-C.	NAT-M.	NAT-P.	NAT-S.	NIT-AC.	NUX-V.	OP.	PETR.	PHO-AC.
1. INSOMNIA				✓	✓			✓	✓	✓		✓
2. - AFTER 3 am.									✓			
3. - CAUSED BY MENTAL STRAIN									✓			
4. - " " OVERWORK									✓			
5. IRRITABLE				✓	✓			✓	✓		✓	✓
6.												
7.												
8.												
9.												
10.												
11.												
12.												

Symptoms	PHOS.	PHYT.	PODO.	PULS.	PYR.	RHE.	RHOD.	RHUS-T.	RUMEX.	RUTA.	SARS.	SEP.
1. INSOMNIA	✓			✓				✓				✓
2. - AFTER 3 am.												✓
3. - CAUSED BY MENTAL STRAIN												
4. - " " OVERWORK												
5. IRRITABLE	✓			✓		✓		✓				✓
6.												
7.												
8.												
9.												
10.												
11.												
12.												

Symptoms	SIL.	SPO.	STAP.	SUL.	SUL-AC.	SYMPH.	TAB.	THU.	URT-U.	VERAT.	ZINC.	
1. INSOMNIA	✓			✓								
2. - AFTER 3 am.												
3. - CAUSED BY MENTAL STRAIN												
4. - " " OVERWORK												
5. IRRITABLE	✓		✓	✓	✓					✓	✓	
6.												
7.												
8.												
9.												
10.												
11.												
12.												

Symptoms:

Table 1

Symptom	ACO	AGAR	ALL-C	ANT-C	ANT-T	AP	ARG-N	ARN	ARS	BAPT	BAR-C	BELL	BELL-P	BOR	BRY	CALC-C	CALC-F	CALC-P	CALC-S	CALEN	CANTH	CARB-A	CARB-V	CAUL	CAUST	CHAM	CHIN	CIMI	CINA	COCC	COCC-C	COFF	COLCH	COLOC	CON	CUPR	DIOS	DROS	DULC	EUP-P	EUPHR	FERR-M	GELS	GLON	HAM	HEP-S	HYP	IGN
1. TEETHING - PAINFUL	✓											✓				✓	✓	✓								✓																						
2. " - SLOW																✓		✓																														
3. " - WITH DIARRHOEA																✓										✓																				✓		
4. SWEAT - HEAD				✓		✓	✓		✓					✓	✓	✓										✓	✓						✓	✓		✓			✓			✓	✓			✓		
5. " - SOUR									✓							✓																																
6. DIARRHOEA														✓	✓	✓										✓																✓						
7. - SOUR															✓	✓																																
8. - WITH UNDIGESTED FOOD																✓		✓																								✓				✓		
9. CATCHES COLDS EASILY																✓																														✓		
10. STUBBORN											✓	✓				✓										✓													✓							✓		
11.																																																
12.																																																

Table 2

Symptom	IP	JAB	KALI-B	KALI-C	KALI-M	KALI-P	KALI-S	LACH	LED	LYC	MAG-C	MAG-M	MAG-P	MERC-C	MERC-S	NAT-C	NAT-M	NAT-P	NAT-S	NIT-AC	NUX-V	OP	PETR	PHO-AC	PHOS	PHYT	PODO	PULS	PYR	RHE	RHOD	RHUS-T	RUMEX	RUTA	SARS	SEP	SIL	SPO	STAP	SUL	SUL-AC	SYMPH	TAB	THU	URT-U	VERAT	ZINC
1. TEETHING - PAINFUL	✓												✓													✓											✓										
2. " - SLOW																																					✓										
3. " - WITH DIARRHOEA																														✓							✓										
4. SWEAT - HEAD			✓								✓	✓					✓			✓			✓	✓	✓			✓				✓					✓				✓					✓	
5. " - SOUR																	✓													✓							✓			✓							
6. DIARRHOEA	✓									✓	✓	✓		✓	✓					✓								✓								✓	✓			✓						✓	
7. - SOUR																																															
8. - WITH UNDIGESTED FOOD											✓		✓																								✓										
9. CATCHES COLDS EASILY											✓	✓			✓					✓	✓															✓	✓										
10. STUBBORN	✓			✓								✓			✓		✓			✓	✓																			✓							
11.																																															
12.																																															

catching colds over the past few months and they seem to be running into each other so that he has a constantly runny nose.

Finding a mental/emotional symptom is more difficult. Recently he has been more stubborn about what he wants, although in the past he was a very placid baby.

You choose the following symptoms:
1 Teething painful (Physical complaint)
2 Teething slow (Physical complaint)
3   with diarrhoea (Related symptom)
4 Sweat – head (General)
5 Sweat – sour (General)
6 Diarrhoea (Physical complaint)
7   sour (Related symptom)
8   with undigested food (Related symptom)
9 Catches colds easily (General)
10 Stubborn (Mental/emotional)

Calcarea carbonica has each of these symptoms in its picture. You read through the picture in the Materia Medica and in spite of the fact that you have only one emotional/mental symptom you recognise your son in the description.

This remedy will not only help him through the pains of the teething and clear up his diarrhoea and nasal catarrh, but will actually speed up the process of producing teeth.

Case 9
Food poisoning

You took your mother out to dinner last night and she has been up since midnight with the most terrible vomiting and diarrhoea. She ate pâté and steak, so it looks as if the meat was off. She is in a sorry state and asks for help. The diarrhoea is very painful and utterly exhausting. She feels faint after vomiting, and can only take small sips of water, otherwise she vomits up all she has drunk. She is extremely anxious and doesn't want to be left alone.

You list her symptoms as follows:
1 Food poisoning (Physical complaint)
2   caused by meat (Related symptom)
3 Diarrhoea (Physical complaint)
4   painful (Related symptom)
5 Vomiting (Physical complaint)
      feels faint after (Related symptom)
6 Thirsty for sips (General)
7 Exhaustion from diarrhoea (Physical complaint)
8 Anxious (Emotional/mental)
9 Anxious – worse when alone (Emotional/mental)

Arsenicum is strongly indicated, and you remember that you needed it a year ago for a similar attack. You

don't even need to read through the picture. You are sure that it is right and you give it every half hour until she starts to improve.

Case 10
Sore throat

Your eleven-year-old son has a bad sore throat. He complains of constant pain and says that it feels as if there is a lump in his throat. The only relief from the pain is when he is eating or drinking. He is off school and moping around, spending most of the time on his own in his room. He is morose and withdrawn and looks as if he might have been crying but denies that anything is wrong when you ask him.

His adored pet rabbit died last week and he has been increasingly quiet since then. You remember he had a similar sore throat last year when his best friend moved to another part of the country. Antibiotics did not help and it took him weeks to recover. He only talked about his feelings about his friend leaving once and did seem incredibly sad.

You talk to him about how he feels and he admits to being grief-stricken about his rabbit, to the extent of crying himself to sleep every night. When you sympathise with him he gets cross and changes the subject.

You choose the following symptoms based on what you know generally about him – that he is a private, introspective child – as well as on what is actually happening.

1 Sore throat (Physical complaint)
2   with lump sensation (Related symptom)
3   better for swallowing (Related symptom)
4   worse when not swallowing (Related symptom)
5 Symptoms – contradictory (General)
6 Introspective (Emotional/mental)
7 Tearful – cries on own (Emotional/mental)
8 Dislikes consolation (Emotional/mental)
9 Complaints from grief (Emotional/mental)

After repertorising it is clear that the emotional and the physical symptoms are present in the *Ignatia* picture. You remember that *Natrum muriaticum* has a similar picture and read it through just to make sure that it is *Ignatia* he needs. The contradictory nature of the symptoms (the sore throat is worse when not swallowing) convinces you that *Ignatia* is the correct remedy. You prescribe according to the urgency – one tablet every two hours in this case – and not only avoid the antibiotics but also help him to recover emotionally. You realise how sensitive he is and suggest that you have a proper burial complete with service in the garden to give him a chance to grieve properly instead of hiding away with his pain.

1 **REPERTORISING CHART** Name: CASE 9 - FOOD POISONING Date:

Symptoms:

		ACO.	AGAR.	ALL-C.	ANT-C.	ANT-T.	AP.	ARG-N.	ARN.	ARS.	BAPT.	BAR-C.	BELL.	BELL-P.	BOR.	BRY.	CALC-C.	CALC-F.	CALC-P.	CALC-S.	CALEN.	CANTH.	CARB-A.	CARB-V.	CAUL.
1.	FOOD POISONING									✓													✓	✓	
2.	- CAUSED BY MEAT									✓														✓	
3.	DIARRHOEA				✓		✓	✓		✓					✓	✓	✓								
4.	" - PAINFUL									✓															
5.	VOMITING				✓	✓				✓						✓	✓								
6.	" - FEELS FAINT AFTER									✓															
7.	THIRSTY FOR SIPS									✓															
8.	EXHAUSTION - FROM DIARRHOEA									✓														✓	
9.	ANXIOUS	✓						✓		✓			✓			✓	✓		✓	✓				✓	
10.	" - WORSE WHEN ALONE									✓															
11.																									
12.																									

		CAUST.	CHAM.	CHIN.	CIMI.	CINA.	COCC.	COCC-C.	COFF.	COLCH.	COLOC.	CON.	CUPR.	DIOS.	DROS.	DULC.	EUP-P.	EUPHR.	FERR-M.	GELS.	GLON.	HAM.	HEP-S.	HYP.	IGN.
1.	FOOD POISONING																								
2.	- CAUSED BY MEAT																								
3.	DIARRHOEA		✓	✓						✓	✓					✓			✓	✓			✓		
4.	" - PAINFUL		✓							✓						✓									
5.	VOMITING		✓	✓						✓									✓						
6.	" - FEELS FAINT AFTER																								
7.	THIRSTY FOR SIPS																								
8.	EXHAUSTION - FROM DIARRHOEA			✓																					
9.	ANXIOUS	✓		✓			✓				✓														
10.	" - WORSE WHEN ALONE																								
11.																									
12.																									

		IP.	JAB.	KALI-B.	KALI-C.	KALI-M.	KALI-P.	KALI-S.	LACH.	LED.	LYC.	MAG-C.	MAG-M.	MAG-P.	MERC-C.	MERC-S.	NAT-C.	NAT-M.	NAT-P.	NAT-S.	NIT-AC.	NUX-V.	OP.	PETR.	PHO-AC.
1.	FOOD POISONING								✓		✓														
2.	-CAUSED BY MEAT								✓																
3.	DIARRHOEA	✓										✓	✓		✓	✓		✓		✓		✓		✓	✓
4.	-PAINFUL											✓			✓	✓									
5.	VOMITING	✓																				✓			
6.	-FEELS FAINT AFTER																								
7.	THIRSTY FOR SIPS																								
8.	EXHAUSTION-FROM DIARRHOEA																			✓	✓				
9.	ANXIOUS				✓		✓	✓			✓		✓				✓				✓				
10.	-WORSE WHEN ALONE																								
11.																									
12.																									

		PHOS.	PHYT.	PODO.	PULS.	PYR.	RHE.	RHOD.	RHUS-T.	RUMEX.	RUTA.	SARS.	SEP.	SIL.	SPO.	STAP.	SUL.	SUL-AC.	SYMPH.	TAB.	THU.	URT-U.	VERAT.	ZINC.
1.	FOOD POISONING				✓																	✓		
2.	-CAUSED BY MEAT				✓																			
3.	DIARRHOEA	✓		✓	✓		✓		✓					✓			✓	✓					✓	
4.	-PAINFUL																							
5.	VOMITING	✓											✓	✓				✓		✓			✓	
6.	-FEELS FAINT AFTER																							
7.	THIRSTY FOR SIPS																							
8.	EXHAUSTION-FROM DIARRHOEA	✓												✓			✓						✓	
9.	ANXIOUS	✓			✓				✓				✓		✓		✓							
10.	-WORSE WHEN ALONE	✓																						
11.																								
12.																								

1 REPERTORISING CHART

Name: CASE 10 – SORE THROAT (p. 241)   Date:

Symptoms:

Block 1 — Remedies: ACO, AGAR, ALL-C, ANT-C, ANT-T, AP, ARG-N, ARN, ARS, BAPT, BAR-C, BELL, BELL-P, BOR, BRY, CALC-C, CALC-F, CALC-P, CALC-S, CALEN, CANTH, CARB-A, CARB-V, CAUL, CAUST, CHAM, CHIN, CIMI, CINA, COCC, COCC-C, COFF, COLCH, COLOC, CON, CUPR, DIOS, DROS, DULC, EUP-P, EUPHR, FERR-M, GELS, GLON, HAM, HEP-S, HYP, IGN

Symptom	Remedies marked (✓)
1. SORE THROAT	ACO, ALL-C, ANT-T, AP, ARG-N, BAR-C, BELL, BRY, CALC-C, CAUST, DULC, IGN
2. –WITH LUMP SENSATION	HEP-S, IGN
3. –BETTER SWALLOWING	IGN
4. –WORSE NOT SWALLOWING	IGN
5. SYMPTOMS CONTRADICTORY	CAUST, COCC, IGN
6. INTROSPECTIVE	IGN
7. TEARFUL – CRIES ON OWN	COCC, IGN
8. DISLIKES CONSOLATION	IGN
9. COMPLAINTS FROM GRIEF	
10.	
11.	
12.	

Block 2 — Remedies: IP, IAB, KALI-B, KALI-C, KALI-M, KALI-P, KALI-S, LACH, LED, LYC, MAG-C, MAG-M, MAG-P, MERC-C, MERC-S, NAT-C, NAT-M, NAT-P, NAT-S, NIT-AC, NUX-V, OP, PETR, PHO-AC, PHOS, PHYT, PODO, PULS, PYR, RHE, RHOD, RHUS-T, RUMEX, RUTA, SARS, SEP, SIL, SPO, STAP, SUL, SUL-AC, SYMPH, TAB, THU, URT-U, VERAT, ZINC

Symptom	Remedies marked (✓)
1. SORE THROAT	IP, KALI-M, LACH, LYC, MERC-C, MERC-S, NAT-C, NAT-M, NIT-AC, NUX-V, PHOS, PHYT, PULS, RHUS-T, RUMEX, SPO, SUL
2. –WITH LUMP SENS.	LYC, NAT-M, NUX-V
3. –BETTER SWALLOWING	
4. –WORSE NOT SWALLOWING	
5. SYMPTOMS CONTRADICTORY	
6. INTROSPECTIVE	PULS
7. TEARFUL – CRIES ON OWN	NAT-C, NAT-M, SEP, SIL
8. DISLIKES CONSOLATION	LACH, NAT-M, PULS, SEP, SIL
9. COMPLAINTS FROM GRIEF	NAT-M, PHO-AC, PULS, SPO
10.	
11.	
12.	

PART IV
THE APPENDICES

LIST OF REMEDIES

External Materia Medica

Aesculus and Hamamelis, 32
Arnica, 32
Calendula, 32
Euphrasia, 33
Hamamelis, 33

Hypercal®, 33
Hypericum, 34
Ledum, 34
Phytolacca, 34
Plantago, 34

Pyrethrum, 35
Rescue Remedy, 35
Rhus toxicodendron, 35
Ruta graveolens, 35
Symphytum, 35

Tamus, 36
Thiosinaminum, 36
Thuja, 36
Urtica urens, 36
Verbascum oil, 36

Internal materia Medica

Aconitum napellus, 38
Agaricus muscarius, 40
Allium cepa, 41
Antimonium crudum, 42
Antimonium tartaricum, 43
Apis mellifica, 44
Argentum nitricum, 46
Arnica montana, 47
Arsenicum album, 49
Baptisia tinctoria, 51
Baryta carbonica, 53
Belladonna, 53
Bellis perennis, 56
Borax veneta, 57
Bryonia alba, 58
Calcarea carbonica, 60
Calcarea fluorica, 62
Calcarea phosphorica, 63
Calcarea sulphurica, 64
Calendula officinalis, 65
Cantharis vesicatoria, 66
Carbo animalis, 67
Carbo vegetabilis, 67
Caulophyllum, 69

Causticum, 70
Chamomilla, 71
China officinalis, 73
Cimicifuga, 75
Cina, 76
Cocculus indicus, 77
Coccus cacti, 78
Coffea cruda, 79
Colchicum autumnale, 80
Colocynthis, 81
Conium maculatum, 82
Cuprum metallicum, 83
Dioscorea, 84
Drosera rotundifolia, 85
Dulcamara, 86
Eupatorium perfoliatum, 87
Euphrasia, 88
Ferrum metallicum, 89
Gelsemium sempervirens, 91
Glonoine, 92
Hamamelis virginica, 93
Hepar sulphuris calcareum, 94
Hypericum perfoliatum, 95
Ignatia amara, 96

Ipecacuanha, 98
Jaborandi, 99
Kali bichromicum, 100
Kali carbonicum, 101
Kali muriaticum, 102
Kali phosphoricum, 103
Kali sulphuricum, 104
Lachesis, 105
Ledum palustre, 107
Lycopodium, 108
Magnesia carbonica, 110
Magnesia muriaticum, 111
Magnesia phosphorica,112
Mercurius corrosivus, 113
Mercurius solubilis, 114
Natrum carbonicum, 116
Natrum muriaticum, 117
Natrum phosphoricum, 120
Natrum sulphuricum, 120
Nitric acidum,122
Nux vomica, 123
Opium, 126
Petroleum, 128
Phosphoric acid, 129

Phosphorus, 130
Phytolacca decandra, 132
Podophyllum, 133
Pulsatilla, 134
Pyrogen, 138
Rheum, 139
Rhododendron, 140
Rhus toxicodendron, 141
Rumex crispus, 144
Ruta graveolens, 144
Sarsaparilla, 146
Sepia, 146
Silica, 149
Spongia tosta, 152
Staphysagria, 153
Sulphur, 155
Sulphuric acid, 158
Symphytum, 159
Tabacum, 159
Thuja occidentalis, 160
Urtica urens, 161
Veratrum album, 162
Zincum metallicum, 163

GLOSSARY

Acute illness An illness that is generally short lived. It has three stages, the *incubation period* when there may be no symptoms, the *acute stage* when the disease itself surfaces, and the *convalescent* stage when a person usually improves (see page 14).

Aggravation A temporary worsening of symptoms during the process of cure. It is a common occurrence in the constitutional treatment of chronic disease, but relatively rare in the treatment of acute disease.

Allopathy From the Greek root *allo* meaning 'other' or 'opposite', and *pathos* meaning 'suffering'. A term coined by Hahnemann to describe orthodox medicine and to distinguish it from homeopathy.

Antidote Anything that counteracts the effect of a homeopathic remedy, which may hamper or prevent the remedy working (see page 27).

Case taking The interview in which information is gathered from the patient. Homeopathic casetaking is very thorough, as the specific and detailed symptoms experienced by the patient are important in leading to the prescription of the correct homeopathic remedy.

Centesimal The scale of dilution of substances based on diluting one part in a hundred (see page 13).

Chronic illness Chronic disease develops slowly and does not usually resolve itself without some sort of healing intervention. It is usually accompanied by a general deterioration in health. See page 14.

Common symptoms Symptoms that are commonly found in a particular disease, for example spots in measles or swollen glands in mumps.

Constitution A person's overall state of health. This includes inherited tendencies, personal history, lifestyle, environmental factors and past medical treatment.

Constitutional treatment aims to treat the whole person, rather than the symptoms alone. In so doing, it also enhances the general level of health rather than just getting rid of the symptoms.

Cure The homeopath defines cure as more than the disappearance of the pain or disease itself. It implies a sense of well being on all levels, including the mental and emotional, as well as a lasting physical improvement.

Defence mechanism see Immunity.

Differentiate The art of distinguishing between remedies where more than one is indicated, to find the 'similimum' or the remedy whose picture best fits that of the sick person.

Disease 'Dis-ease' – a departure from our normal, healthy self that limits our physical, mental or emotional expression (see page 15).

Emotional symptoms Feelings or moods.

General symptoms Symptoms that may be present in any disease, regardless of what it is; for example, *Aconite* is indicated generally for *any* complaint that comes on suddenly and is caused by getting chilled.

Healing crisis see Aggravation.

Immunity is simply our resistance to disease. It is partly innate (inherited) and partly shaped by the lives we lead. Our ability to ward off disease is determined by the strength of our immune system.

Infinitesimal dose see Minimum dose.

Laws of Cure are the principles that govern the healing process. They are mostly appropriate to constitutional treatment and are described on page 15.

Materia Medica A collection of homeopathic remedy pictures, giving detailed indications for their uses (see page 12).

Mental symptoms Thinking processes, memory, concentration, etc.

Miasm A block to health, usually left by a disease. This can be inherited or acquired and is an obstacle to cure (see pages 14–15).

Minimum dose   The potentised substance, which stimulates healing without side effects.

Mother tincture   see Tincture

Orthodox medicine   see Allopathy

Particular symptoms   Symptoms related to parts of the body, for example a pain in the knee or a headache.

Placebo   An unmedicated pill that has no active effect (see page 18).

Polycrest   A remedy which has produced a wide range of symptoms in the provings and can therefore treat a wide range of problems.

Potency   denotes the strength of the remedy according to the number of times it has been diluted and succussed (see pages 12–13).

Potentisation   The process whereby substances are prepared homeopathically by repeated dilution and succussion (see page 13).

Proving   The testing of a substance on healthy volunteers to discover the symptoms it is capable of producing (and therefore able to cure).

Remedy   The term for a homeopathic medicine.

Remedy picture   The jigsaw of symptoms that a remedy is known to produce, including mental and emotional, general and physical symptoms. It is this totality of symptoms that is called the remedy picture.

Repertorise   To look up symptoms in the Repertory to find which remedy (or remedies) is common to the presenting symptoms.

Repertory   An index of symptoms (based on the Materia Medica) with a list of remedies indicated for each particular symptom.

Sac lac   Saccharin lactose, the sugar and milk base of homeopathic tablets (see page 25).

Similimum   The similimum is the remedy that matches the symptom picture of the patient most closely. Based on the law *Similia similibus curentur* ('Let like be cured with like'), the principle states that a substance is capable of curing a sick person of the same symptoms it is capable of producing in a healthy person.

Specific remedies   Remedies that are given for a particular symptom or disease *without* taking the whole person into account, for example *Arnica* for bruises and *Hypericum* for crushed fingers.

Stress   Anything that produces mental, emotional or physical strain or tension. Stress itself may be mental, emotional or physical (see page 201).

Succussion   The process of vigorous shaking that accompanies dilution during the preparation of a homeopathic remedy.

Suppression   The driving inward of disease(s), so that a person experiences more serious symptoms than those originally presented, and there is a general deterioration in health.

Susceptibility   Vulnerability to disease (see also Immunity).

Symptom picture   The whole range (or totality) of symptoms experienced by a person that emerges during the casetaking. The symptom picture is matched to a remedy picture with the same or similar symptoms.

Symptom   Any change in the body's functioning on a mental, emotional or physical level. Usually associated either with a particular disease or a specific stress.

Tincture   A solution of a substance in alcohol; it is not succussed but is used as the starting material for all homeopathically prepared remedies. Some pharmacies call these mother tinctures.

Trituration   The process of grinding an insoluble substance with 'sac lac' in order to render it soluble.

Uncommon symptoms   Symptoms which seem odd or unusual, and, because of this, point clearly to a particular remedy. For example, lack of pain where it is expected would point to *Opium*. A high fever without sweating may point to *Belladonna*.

Vital force   A term used by Hahnemann to describe the energy that animates all living beings. It is the vital force that is stimulated by the potentised remedy to enable the sick person to cure him or herself (see page 14).

FIRST-AID KITS, PHARMACIES AND COURSES

You can make up your own first-aid kit, in which case I suggest that you make a rough list of the complaints you wish to be able to treat at home/self-prescribe on and make up your kit accordingly. For example, if you are a single person who travels frequently to exotic places then remedies for accidents and injuries as well as stomach upsets will be priorities. You may also need travel sickness remedies if you are a sufferer, and so on. If, however, you are a mother of small children then in addition to accidents and injuries you may also choose remedies for burns, teething, coughs and colds.

If you can't afford an extensive kit at the beginning, then build it up slowly; as far as we know, homeopathic remedies have an indefinite shelf life, providing they are properly stored.

Miranda Castro's First Aid Kits

The following first aid kits are available from Helios in soft tablets. They make good basic kits on which to build. Each kit comes with its own instruction booklet giving guidelines on prescribing.

Accidents and Injuries

This kit contains ten remedies for common accidents and injuries including shock, cuts, falls, bruises, bites and stings, burns, sprains and strains. I keep one in the car as well as one at home.

1	*Aconite* 30	6	*Hepar-sul* 12
2	*Apis* 12	7	*Hypericum* 30
3	*Arnica* 12	8	*Ledum* 30
4	*Calendula* 6	9	*Rhus-tox* 12
5	*Cantharis* 30	10	*Ruta* 12

Everyday Complaints

This kit contains ten remedies for everyday complaints including general 'inflammations' such as coughs, colds, flu's, fevers, earaches, sore throats, and for minor digestive upsets.

1	*Arsenicum* 12	6	*Mag phos* 12X
2	*Belladonna* 12	7	*Merc sol* 12
3	*Bryonia* 12	8	*Nux vomica* 12
4	*Carbo veg* 12	9	*Pulsatilla* 12
5	*Chamomilla* 12	10	*Sulphur* 12

Ointments and Lotions

This kit contains seven external remedies for common complaints – in their most needed form.

1	Bruises ointment	5	Eye drops
2	Burns ointment	6	Sprains ointment
3	Cuts cream	7	Rescue Remedy drops
4	Earache oil		

The homeopathic pharmacies listed below all stock first-aid boxes in varying shapes and sizes. It is wise to decide which kit you are going to build on from which pharmacy so that your additional remedies will slot in easily each time and you do not end up with six different shapes of bottle. Don't forget to specify what types of pills you require – soft or hard tablets, small globules (see page 25).

Caution: If you are a traveller, do not put your homeopathic remedies through an airport X-ray machine as this has been known to antidote them; carry them in your pocket as the metal detector you walk through will not affect them.

Ainsworths Homeopathic Pharmacy
38 New Cavendish Street
London W1M 7LH
Tel: 01-935 5330 (daytime number and shop)
01-487 5253 (24-hour answering machine service)
Ainsworths produce many different types of first-aid kit. Their smallest, a plastic wallet holding twenty-four small vials of cane-sugar or hard tablet-form remedies, will fit in a pocket and is ideal for travellers.

Helios Homeopathic Pharmacy
97 Camden Road
Tunbridge Wells
Kent TN1 2QP
*Tel: 0892 36393 (daytime number and answering machine
which will take orders outside shop opening hours)*
Helios makes most of its fine remedies by hand (as
opposed to by machine). It produces several types of
first-aid kit. Details available on request. Remedies are
available in all forms (hard and soft tablets, etc.).

A. Nelson and Co. Ltd
Customer Services
5 Endeavour Way
London SW19 9UH
Tel: 01-946 8527
Nelsons produce remedies to a high standard and a
selection of these are available in many chemists and
whole food shops in this country. They also make up
first-aid kits that include ointments and tinctures.
Contact the address above for further details of all
their mail order services or visit their shop at 73 Duke
Street, London W1M 6BY (01-629 3118) if you wish to
buy direct.

Weleda
Heanor Road
Ilkeston
Derbyshire DE7 8DR
Tel: 0602 303151
Weleda grow many of the plants organically for their
homeopathic remedies, which are made in their own
laboratories to a high standard. They use hard tablets
and are useful for those who wish to build up a kit of
larger bottles. The remedies are also freely available
in many chemists and whole food shops. Remedies
can be ordered by phone and will be sent out with an
invoice. They do not (at time of going to press) have a
special kit or box.

Rescue Remedy

Rescue Remedy is a combination of five of Edward
Bach's Flower Remedies and is not, strictly speaking,
homeopathic. Bach was a homeopath who devoted his

energies to finding healing plants which would act on
negative emotions alone, and by so doing restore
peace of mind which would lead to physical health.

There are few complaints that are not helped, even
temporarily, by Rescue Remedy, including shock
(after an accident, bad news, the dentist, etc.); panic:
emotional upset or distress of any sort; sunburn; travel
sickness; fear (stage fright, exam nerves, sleeplessness
through anxiety or fear, fainting from fright); childbirth (before, during and after); headaches from emotional stress, and so on.

Take a few drops on the tongue and repeat this as
often as needed – once for a minor injury and every
few minutes for a serious situation. The drops can also
be added to water and sipped frequently, or applied
neat externally (there is also ready-made cream) for
headaches, rashes, bruises, etc., as often as needed.
Or if you are under a lot of emotional stress add seven
drops to a bath and soak well.

First-aid courses

It is valuable to take a basic first-aid course so that you
can deal with accidents and emergency situations
effectively and confidently. Both the British Red Cross
and St John Ambulance run excellent training courses
for the interested lay person. Contact your local
branch for details. The addresses of their head offices
are:

British Red Cross Society
9 Grosvenor Crescent
London SW1X 7EJ
Tel: 01-235 5454

St John Ambulance
1 Grosvenor Crescent
London SW1X 7EF
Tel 01-235 5231
The authorised manual of St John Ambulance, St
Andrew's Ambulance Association and The British Red
Cross Society (published by Dorling Kindersley) is a
comprehensive, clear and informative guide for treat-
ing casualties of all ages in any emergency or first-aid
situation.

HOMEOPATHS AND HOMEOPATHIC ORGANISATIONS

Homeopathic practitioners in the UK are either professional homeopaths who study medical sciences as part of their homeopathic training or doctors who have completed an additional training in homeopathy. It is important to ask for credentials as there are some practising homeopaths in this country who are not medically qualified, many of whom have completed only short postal courses in homeopathy. The best referral to a professional homeopath is by personal recommendation. Failing that, consult the Society of Homœopath's register (see below) to locate a fully trained homeopath in your area.

Professional homeopaths

Professional homeopaths work independently and are not connected with the National Health Service. Their fees vary from about £20 to £40 for a first consultation, which lasts from one to two hours, with follow-up consultations costing from £10 to £30 depending on the time taken. Most homeopaths see their patients about once a month although this varies. Many homeopaths offer concessions to children, the unwaged and to pensioners, etc. There is a growing number of homeopathic clinics offering low-cost treatment to those who need it.

Professional homeopaths are examined and represented by the Society of Homœopaths, a member of the Council for Complementary and Alternative Medicine, the umbrella organisation fighting to establish a high standard of alternative medical practice in this country. Professional homeopaths may use the initials RS Hom. or FS Hom. (Fellow) after their names.

The Society of Homœopaths publishes a register of homeopaths, information sheets, details of courses for training in homeopathy and contact names and addresses for local groups, etc. The general public may take associate membership and/or become Friends of the Society; members receive a quarterly journal, newsletter, and discounts at seminars and conferences. For further details/application form send an SAE (24 × 16cm) to:

The Society of Homœopaths
2 Artizan Road
Northampton NN1 4HU
Tel: 0604 21400

Doctor homeopaths

Doctors practising homeopathy are entitled to use the initials MFHom. on passing the London Faculty of Homœopathy examination after a relatively short training. Most doctors are in private practice, although some work under the NHS (with difficulty as their time is severely limited). There are homeopathic hospitals in London, Glasgow, Bristol, Tunbridge Wells, Liverpool and Birmingham.

The British Homœopathic Association is a charitable association open to membership by the general public. Members receive a bi-monthly magazine and are entitled to use the extensive library. As well as publishing some homeopathic books, they produce a booklist (for mail order), various lists including doctor homeopaths – distinguishing between private and NHS practice – and vets and dentists who practise homeopathy. They do not take telephone orders. For further information send an SAE (24 × 16cm) to:

The British Homœopathic Association
27a Devonshire Street
London W1
Tel: 01-935 2163

USEFUL READING AND BOOKSHOPS

Homeopathy

Blackie, Margery, *The Challenge of Homœopathy* (Unwin Hyman, 1981).
Interesting anecdotes from the doctor who was the Queen's homeopathic physician for many years.

Campbell, Anthony, *The Two Faces of Homœopathy* (Jill Norman/Robert Hale, London 1984).
A fascinating look at the relationship between homeopathy and orthodox medicine outlining the conflicts that have traditionally existed between the two disciplines.

Coulter, Harris L., *Homœopathic Science and Modern Medicine: The Physics of Healing with Microdoses* (North Atlantic Books, 1987).
A brief but interesting defence of homeopathy with accounts of trials that have proved the efficacy of homeopathy.

Shepherd, Dorothy: *Magic of the Minumum Dose* (Health Science Press, 1964). *More Magic of the Minimum Dose* (Health Science Press, 1974). *A Physician's Posy* (Health Science Press, 1969). *Homœopathy in Epidemic Diseases* (Health Science Press, 1967).
Dorothy Shepherd writes in an accessible, anecdotal style which is both fascinating and informative. All these books are worth a read. *Homœopathy in Epidemic Diseases* is especially useful for those with children as it draws on her experience of disease while running a homeopathic GP practice, dealing successfully with diseases from Measles to Typhoid.

Tyler, Margaret, *Homœopathic Drug Pictures* (Health Science Press, 1970).
A full description of 125 remedy pictures compiled from a lifetime's experience and the work of many other great homeopaths of repute.

Vithoulkas, George, *Homœopathy: Medicine of the New Man* (Thorsons, 1985).
An exciting introduction to homeopathic thinking.

He is also the author of *The Science of Homœopathy* (Thorsons, 1986). A thorough textbook for those who wish to go deeper into homeopathic philosophy and prescribing.

General

Kapit, Wynn and Elson, Lawrence M., *The Anatomy Colouring Book* (Harper & Row, 1977)
Become familiar with the ins and outs of your body. A book that all the family will enjoy.

Parish, Peter, *Medicines: A Guide for Everybody* (Penguin, 1976).
An indispensable drug reference book written for the lay person.

Ornstein, Robert and Sobel, David, *The Healing Brain* (Macmillan, 1988).
A beautifully written book on the dynamics of health and healing from an orthodox (very unorthodox) medical perspective. A real treat.

First Aid Manual
The Authorised Manual of St John Ambulance, St Andrew's Ambulance Association and The British Red Cross Society (Dorling Kindersley).
A comprehensive first-aid guide.

Reader's Digest Family Medical Adviser (Reader's Digest Association, London, 1983).
A comprehensive and easy-to-read A–Z guide to everyday ailments, their causes and symptoms. Includes first-aid section.

Bookshops

Ainsworths (see below) and the British Homœopathic Association (see page 251) have booklists of homeopathic books, and they both operate a mail order service. All high street bookshops will order books (including most of the homeopathic ones listed above) for you on request if they are not in stock, and many take credit card orders over the phone.

Ainsworths Pharmacy
38 New Cavendish Street
London W1M 7LH
Tel: 01-935 5330
 08834 0332 (book department)
Homeopathic books only. Ring for a comprehensive booklist. Books can be purchased either over the counter or by phone. Access and Visa accepted.

Changes Bookshop
242 Belsize Road
London NW6 4BT
Tel: 01-328 5161
Books related to personal development and alternative health care. Ring for their comprehensive booklist. Access, American Express and Visa accepted for telephone orders.

Watkins Books
19 Cecil Court
Charing Cross Road
London WC2N 4EZ
Tel: 01-836 2182
Large range of books on all matters concerned with 'body, mind and spirit'. General catalogue available. Access and Visa accepted for telephone orders.

INDEX

to Parts I, III and IV

abdominal pain, 204
abscesses: breast, 206–7; tooth, 204–5
accidental provings, 11–12
accidents, 24, 231–2
Aconite, 24, 249
acute illness, 14, 24, 27, 203
aggravation of symptoms, 27–8, 247
AIDS, 204
alchemy, 3, 6
alcohol: antidotes, 27; bases, 25
allopathy, 5, 247
amenorrhea, 221
American Medical Association, 8, 9
anaemia, 205
animals, 18, 26
antibiotics, 10, 26
antibodies, 18
antidotes, 4, 24, 28, 247
Antimonium tartaricum, 203
anxiety, 16
Apis, 235, 249
Arab states, 10
Argentina, 9
Argentum nitricum, 229
Arnica, 24, 207, 229, 231, 232, 249
Arsenicum, 241, 249
arthritis, 14, 219–20
Asia, 9
aspirin, 216
asthma, 15, 204
Athens, 10
athlete's foot, 205
Australia, 9

babies, 18, 24; nappy rash, 220; symptom checklist, 228; taking

remedies, 25, 26; teething, 224, 237–41
back injuries, 205
backache, 205
Bangladesh, 9
bedwetting, 205
bee stings, 205
Belladonna, 12, 203, 235, 249
Birmingham, 252
bites, 205–6
bleeding, 203
blisters, 206
blocks, miasmic, 6, 15, 247
blood blisters, 206
blood-letting, 8
blood poisoning, 206
Board of Health (Britain), 8
boils, 206
bones, broken, 207, 232
Brazil, 9
breastfeeding problems, 206–7; abscesses, 206–7; cracked nipples, 207; engorged, 207; lumps, 207
breath, smells, 21
breathing: laboured, 203; rapid, 203
Bristol, 10, 252
Britain, 8–9, 10
British Homœopathic Association, 247
British Homœopathic Society, 8
broken bones, 207, 232
bruises, 207, 231
Bryonia, 22, 23, 235, 249
Bryonia alba, 6
bunions, 211–12
burns, 207–8
bushmaster snake, 7

Calcarea carbonica, 232
Calcarea phosphorica, 232
Calendula, 28, 224, 249
Calomel, 8
Camphor, 6, 8, 28
cancer, 14, 15, 204
cannabis, 28
Cantharis, 249
case-taking, 21–2, 227–9, 247
catarrh, 213
centesimal scale, diluting substances, 13, 247
Chamomilla, 17, 18, 25, 221, 249
chest pain, 203
chicken pox, 14, 206, 209
chilblains, 208
children, 24; bedwetting, 205; illnesses, 14, 208–10; safety, 25; symptom checklist, 228; taking remedies, 25; teething, 224, 237–41
cholera, 6, 8
Chronic Diseases and Their Homœopathic Cure (Hahnemann), 6
chronic illness, 14–15, 20, 203, 226, 247
Cinchona, 4, 5
cloves, oil of, 28
coffee, 28
cold sores, 23, 206, 210
colds, 14, 27, 211, 232–5
colic, 17, 210–11
combination remedies, 9, 12
common symptoms, 247
confusion, mental, 204
Conium, 12
conjunctivitis, 20
constipation, 204, 211

constitution, 13–14, 247
contraception, 16
convalescence, 14
convulsions, 203, 211, 216
corns, 211–12
coughs, 14, 20, 21, 212, 232–5
Coulter, Harris, 19
Council for Complementary and
    Alternative Medicine, 252
cow's milk, 24–5
cracked nipples, 207
cramp, 212
Crimean War, 8
croup, 212
Cullen, Dr William, 4
Cuprum metallicum, 6
cure, definition, 247
Cure, Laws of, 7, 15, 247
cured symptoms, 12
curries, 28
cuts, 219, 231
cystitis, 20, 212–13
cysts, 204

Darwinism, 8
deadly nightshade, 11–12
deafness, 213
decimal scales, diluting
    substances, 13
defence mechanisms, 14
degenerative diseases, 204
dehydration, 216
delirium, 203
Denmark, 9
dentists, 28
dermatitis, 204
diarrhoea, 27, 213, 217, 241
differentiation, 22, 247
dilution of remedies, 5, 12–13
disease, definition, 247
dizziness, 213
doctor homeopaths, 247
Doctrine of Signatures, 4
doses: how many and how often,
    26, 27; minimum, 5, 12–13, 248;
    shaking, 5; size of, 25–6; *see
    also* remedies
drugs, 9, 28
Dudgeon, Robert, 8

earache, 26, 27, 213–14
Eastern Europe, 9
eczema, 15, 20, 204, 206
elbow, tennis, 224–5
electromagnetism, 13
emergencies, 24

emotional health, 15–16
emotional problems, 214, 247
energy, 14, 15, 18
engorged breasts, 207
Enlightenment, 4
environmental pollution, 14
epidemics, 6, 8, 13
Ernst, Duke of Saxe-Coburg, 9
eucalyptus, 28
Eupatorium perfoliatum, 249
Europe, 9
exam nerves, 232
exhaustion, 214
eyes: eye strain, 215;
    inflammation, 214–15; injuries,
    215; styes, 224

Faculty of Homeopathy, 8
faintness, 215
fasting, 216
feet: athlete's foot, 205; bunions,
    211–12; chilblains, 208; corns,
    211–12
fever, 203, 215–16
first-aid kits, 25, 249
first-aid prescribing, 13, 20, 26
flatulence, 216–17
flu, 14, 23, 26, 28, 216, 235–7
flushes, hot, 218
folk-medicine, 3, 6
food poisoning, 14, 217, 241
fractures, 207, 232
France, 9
Frederick Augustus I, King of
    Saxony, 7

Gelsemium, 28, 249
general symptoms, 247
genetics, 13
genital thrush, 225
germ theory of disease, 3, 6, 9,
    13, 16, 201
German measles, 209
Germany, 3–4, 9
glandular fever, 215
Glasgow, 10, 252
globules, 25
gonorrhoea, 15
Greece, 10
gums: abscesses, 205; bleeding,
    217

Hahnemann, Marie Melanie d',
    6
Hahnemann, Samuel, 3–7, 8–9,
    10, 11, 14–15

Hahnemann Medical College,
    Philadelphia, 7
hair loss, 217
hallucinations, 216
hayfever, 204, 217
head injuries, 26, 27, 218, 231
headaches, 21, 203, 217
'healing crisis', 27
health, 15–16
heart disease, 14, 15, 204
heartburn, 218, 219
hemlock, 11–12
Hepar sulphuricum, 249
hepatitis, 204
herbalism, 18
Hering, Constantine, 7, 8, 12, 15
herpes, 206
high-potency prescribing, 7, 8, 9,
    13, 28
Hippocrates, 3, 5, 215
history, 3–9
hives, 218
homeopaths, professional, 252
homeostasis, 14
hospitals, homeopathic, 10, 252
hot flushes, 218
House of Lords, 8
Hughes, Richard, 8–9
Hungary, 6
hygiene, 6
Hypercal®, 224
Hypericum, 24, 231, 249

Iceland, 9
Ignatia, 241
immune system, 14, 18, 208, 211,
    214
immunity, 247
impetigo, 206
incubation period, 14
India, 9
indigestion, 219
inherited tendencies to disease,
    6, 13–14
injuries, 219, 222, 231
insect bites and stings, 205–6
insomnia, 219, 237
iron-deficiency anaemia, 205
isopathy, 7
Israel, 10

joints: pain, 219–20; strains,
    223–4

keloids, 220
Kent, James Tyler, 7, 8, 10, 17

Kentians, 7
Kothen, 6

labour pains, 220
Lachesis, 7, 12, 22
laughter, 202
Law of Similars, 11
Laws of Cure, 7, 15, 247
Ledum, 249
Leipzig, 5, 8
Leipzig Homeopathic Hospital, 6
Leipzig University, 4, 5, 7
leprosy, 15
'like cures like', 4–5, 11, 248
liquid remedies, 25
listening, 21–2
Lister, Joseph, 6
Liverpool, 10, 252
London, 8, 10, 252
London Faculty of Homeopathy,
    252
London Homeopathic Hospital,
    8
low-potency prescribing, 8, 9, 13,
    26, 28
lumbago, 220
lumps, 204, 207

Magnesia phosphorica, 249
malaria, 4, 215
Materia Medica, 11–12, 247
Materia Medica (Kent), 7
Materia Medica Pura
    (Hahnemann), 6
measles, 209, 235
Meissen, 3
meningitis, 216
menopause, 218
menstruation, 221
mental health, 15–16
mental problems, 14, 204, 214,
    247
menthol, 28
Mercurius chloride, 8
Mercurius solubilis, 249
mercury poisoning, 8
metals, 13
Mexico, 9
miasms, 6, 7, 14–15, 247
milk sugar, 24–5
minimum dose, 5, 12–13, 248
mint, 28
Montmartre, 6
mother tinctures, 11, 13
mouth: mouthwashes, 28;
    thrush, 225, ulcers, 204, 219

mumps, 209
muscles, cramp, 212

Napoleonic Laws, 9
Napoleonic Wars, 3, 5
nappy rash, 220
National Health Service, 10, 252
Natrum muriaticum, 23, 241, 249
Natrum sulphuricum, 229
nausea, 220
neck, stiff, 204, 223
Nelson's, 25
Nepal, 9
nervousness, 232
nettle rash, 218
New Era Tissue Salts, 25
New Zealand, 9
Nightingale, Florence, 8
nightshade, deadly, 11–12
nipples, cracked, 207
nosebleeds, 220
note-taking, 21–2, 227–9, 247
nursing, children, 208–9
Nux vomica, 17, 249

Opium, 221
The Organon (Hahnemann), 5, 6,
    7, 11

pain, 221
Pakistan, 9
palpitations, 221
Paracelsus, 3
Paris, 6, 8
particular symptoms, 248
Pasteur, Louis, 6
penicillin, 9
peppermint, 28
Père Lachaise cemetery, 6
period problems, 221–2
perspiration, 21
Peruvian bark, 4
pharmaceutical industry, 9
Philadelphia, 7
Philosophy (Kent), 7
physical injuries, 222
piles, 222
placebos, 18–19, 248
plants, herbalism, 18
pneumonia, 216
poisons, 11–12
Poland, 9
pollution, 14
polycrest, 248
post-operative remedies, 222
potencies, 5, 7, 13, 26, 248

potentisation, 5, 248
powders, 25, 26
pregnancy, 220, 222
premenstrual tension, 221–2
prescribing: self-prescribing, 17,
    18, 20, 24; when to prescribe,
    24; whom to prescribe for, 24
prickly heat, 222
Provers' Union, 7
proving, 11–12, 17, 248
Psora, 15
psoriasis, 204
Pulsatilla, 235, 249

questionnaire, symptoms, 227–9
Quin, Frederick Hervey Foster, 8
quinine, 4

Raab, 6
rashes, nappy, 220
recreational drugs, 28
remedies: assessing response to,
    26–7; classifying symptoms,
    22–3; combined, 9, 12;
    confusion of symptom
    picture, 17–18; forms
    available, 24–5; how many
    doses and how often, 26, 27;
    list of, 246; Materia Medica,
    12; minimum dose, 5, 12–13,
    248; potency, 13, 26, 248; remedy
    picture, 248; self-prescribing,
    17, 18, 20, 24; shaking, 5; single,
    12; size of doses, 25–6; specific,
    248; storing, 25; taking, 25–6;
    treating the whole person, 13;
    unintentional provings, 17;
    when to prescribe, 24; whom
    to prescribe for, 24; *see also*
    doses
repertorising, 22, 248
Repertory, 12, 248
Repertory (Kent), 7
retention of urine, 222–3
Reye's Syndrome, 216
rheumatism, 18, 219–20
Rhus toxicodendron, 6, 18, 249
roseola, 210
rubella, 209
Ruta, 249

saccharin lactose (*sac lac*), 25, 248
safety, 25
St Helena, 8
sample cases, 231–41
Saxony, 3, 9

scalds, 207–8
scarlet fever, 210
scars, keloids, 220
self-prescribing, 17, 18, 20, 24
septicaemia, 206
shingles, 206, 209
shock, 223, 231
Signatures, Doctrine of, 4
Silica, 223, 232, 249
similars, curing with, 3, 4, 5, 11, 248
similia similibus curentur, 11
similimum, 248
single remedies, 12
sinusitis, 223
skin: blisters, 206; burns, 207–8; diseases, 15, 204; eruptions, 18, 20; feel of, 21; hives, 218; injuries, 219; keloid scars, 220; scalds, 207–8; ulcers, 204; yellowing, 204
sleeping difficulties, 219, 237
smell, 21
snake venom, 11–12
Society of Homœopaths, 10, 252
Socrates, 12
soft tablets, 25
sore throat, 223, 241
South Africa, 10
South America, 7, 9
Spain, 9
specific remedies, 248
splinters, 223
sports injuries, 222
sprains, 223–4, 231–2
Sri Lanka, 9
Staphysagria, 249
stiff neck, 223
stings, 205–6
stomach disease, 15; ulcers, 204
stools, pale, 204
storing remedies, 25
strains, 223–4

stress, 11, 13, 14, 15–16, 28, 201–2, 214, 228–9
styes, 224
succussion, 5, 12–13, 248
sucrose, 25
Sulphur, 7, 13, 23, 235, 249
sunburn, 224
sunstroke, 224
suppression, 18, 248
surgery, post-operative remedies, 222
susceptibility, 13–14, 248
Swedenborg, Emanuel, 8
Sycosis, 15
symptoms, 11; aggravation, 27–8, 247; case-taking, 21–2, 227–9, 247; cause for concern, 203–4; classifying, 22–3; common, 247; confusion of symptom picture, 17–18; definition, 248; emotional, 247; general, 247; homeostasis, 14; Laws of Cure, 7, 15, 247; Materia Medica, 12; mental, 247; particular, 248; provings, 11–12; questionnaire, 227–9; Repertory, 12, 248; symptom picture, 20–2, 202; uncommon, 248; unintentional provings, 17
syphilis, 8, 15

tablets, 24–6
talking, 21–2
tantrums, 216
teeth: abscesses, 204; bleeding gums, 217; teething, 18, 224, 237–41; toothache, 225
temperature, 215–16
tennis elbow, 224–5
Thackeray, William Makepeace, 8
throat, sore, 223, 241
thrush, 17, 225
tinctures, 13, 248

tiredness, 214
toothache, 225
toothpaste, 28
travel sickness, 225
trituration, 13, 248
tuberculosis, 7
Tunbridge Wells, 10, 252

ulcers, 204; mouth, 220
uncommon symptoms, 248
United States of America, 7, 8, 9, 10, 11
urine: profuse urination, 204; retention of, 222–3; unusual, 204
USSR, 9

vaccination, 18
varicose veins, 224
Veratrum album, 6
verrucas, 226
vertigo, 213
vital force, 14, 18, 248
Vithoulkas, George, 10, 13
vomiting, 204, 217, 226, 241

wafers, 25
warts, 204, 226
wasp stings, 206
weakness, 204
Weleda, 25
West Germany, 9
wheezing, 204
'whole person', 13
whooping cough, 210
William IV, King of England, 9
wind, 216–17
worms, 226
wounds, 219, 231

X-rays, 28

yellowing of skin, 204

LAST WORD

I do not pretend to have written a definitive homeopathic first-aid book, however I have attempted to produce a more thorough and detailed one than those currently available. Although there has been much diligent checking and re-checking it is entirely possible (probable even!) that some errors (including omissions) have slipped through the net. Please feel free to send them to me so that I can correct these for future reprints. Thank you.

Miranda Castro
c/o Macmillan London Limited
4 Little Essex Street
London WC2R 3LF